PRINCIPLES OF
NEURAL DEVELOPMENT

PRINCIPLES OF NEURAL DEVELOPMENT

Dale Purves and Jeff W. Lichtman
WASHINGTON UNIVERSITY SCHOOL OF MEDICINE   ST. LOUIS

SINAUER ASSOCIATES INC. PUBLISHERS SUNDERLAND MASSACHUSETTS

THE COVER: Halo response of an embryonic chick
ganglion after incubation with nerve growth factor;
see Chapter 7. (Courtesy of R. Levi-Montalcini.)

PRINCIPLES OF NEURAL DEVELOPMENT

Copyright © 1985 by Sinauer Associates, Inc.

Library of Congress Cataloging in Publication Data
Purves, Dale.
Principles of neural development.
Bibliography: p.
Includes index.
1. Developmental neurology.   I.   Lichtman,
Jeff W., 1951–   . II. Title.
QP363.5.P87   1984   591.3′33   84-10566
ISBN 0-87893-744-7

Printed in U.S.A.

5 4 3 2 1

Contents

3   PATTERN AND POSITIONAL INFORMATION   53

4   MOVEMENT AND MIGRATION OF NEURONS   81

PRINCIPLES OF
NEURAL DEVELOPMENT

Early Events in Neural Development

INTRODUCTION

The development of the nervous system is difficult to separate, as a topic, from the development of the rest of the animal. The nervous system is ultimately the collection of cells that organizes an animal's behavior. But embryos do not behave, at least in the beginning, and there is really no reason to imagine that neural development is fundamentally different from the generation of other organ systems. Moreover, the nervous system does not, of course, develop in isolation: it both is influenced by and influences the motor and sensory organs that allow an animal to act and to react. Finally, the development of the nervous system depends on a metabolic and hormonal context. Thus, it is no more sensible to talk about neural development without reference to the general course of embryogenesis than it is to discuss the performance of a conductor without reference to the orchestra; it is often done, but not very usefully.

Throughout this account, then, we have tried to relate the development of the nervous system to development generally, and the views of neurobiologists to the ideas of experimental embryologists.

THE RISE OF EXPERIMENTAL EMBRYOLOGY

Although many historical controversies seem outdated in retrospect, surprisingly few fundamental issues in development have really been settled; they have simply taken on different guises as technical and intellectual styles have changed. "It is easy to sneer at our ancestors," wrote T. H. Huxley, ". . . but it is much more profitable to try to discover why they, who were not really one whit less sensible persons than our excellent selves, should have been led to entertain views which strike us as absurd" (Meyer, 1939).

Perhaps it was Aristotle who began what must surely be one of the most protracted debates in the history of science: Is the development of animals based on preformation, or is it the result of an initial plan operating in conjunction with "external" factors? The idea that the zygote is simply a miniature individual that grows seemed so cogent that many philosophers took this notion of development for granted.

3

"In the seed," the Roman philosopher Seneca declared about 2000 years ago, "are enclosed all the parts of the body of the man that shall be formed. The infant that is borne in his mother's wombe hath the rootes of the beard and hair that he shall weare one day. In this little masse likewise are all the lineaments of the bodie and all that which Posterity shall discover in him" (quoted from Needham, 1959). Even with the advent of the microscope, the appeal of preformation was so strong that biologists claimed to see a homunculus in the head of a human sperm and a microscopic horse in equine semen. There were, of course, arguments against preformation (Meyer, 1939; Needham, 1959; Oppenheimer, 1967). For example, this view logically requires the inclusion of all humanity in a single ancestral homunculus. In spite of such counter arguments, the thrust of developmental inquiry well into the nineteenth century was not so much to question preformation but to decide whether the key element in this scheme was the egg or the sperm.

By the middle of the nineteenth century, the idea of preformation was in decline, largely as a result of the observations and arguments of C. F. Wolff and K. E. von Baer. In particular, von Baer's *Entwicklungsgeschichte der Thiere* (roughly *Developmental History of the Animals*), published in 1828, convinced many people that embryos simply did not look like miniature replicas of the adults they would become. In fact, embryos, regardless of species, resembled the embryos of other animals much more than they resembled the adults of their own kind (Figure 1). As concern shifted from homunculi to heritability, debates about development took on a decidedly more modern ring; it seemed that gametes might contain information needed to *create* an organism rather than animal rudiments in miniature form (Wilson, 1911; Jacob, 1982). A major proponent of this new view was W. Roux, who is generally credited with founding the discipline of experimental embryology and, indirectly, the more specialized field of neuroembryology (Hamburger, 1981).

Roux, who lived from 1850 to 1924, was the son of the fencing master at the University of Jena, where he became a student of the biologist and philosopher E. Haeckel. Haeckel was the foremost exponent of the biological approach to embryonic development in the late nineteenth century: the key to ontogeny, he argued, lay in phylogeny (see Box A). Haeckel's teachings apparently impressed Roux in two ways. On the one hand, Roux found Haeckel's emphasis on phylogeny unsatisfactory and metaphysical; on the other hand, he was intrigued by Haeckel's interest in the physicochemical basis of development (Gould, 1977). Roux did not accept Haeckel's verdict that phylogeny is a sufficient cause for ontogeny; he realized that proximate causes had to be analyzed. In consequence, he emphasized the importance of discovering a causal scheme of embryogenesis; he called this scheme "Developmental Mechanics" (in an analogy to Newton's laws of mechanics).

A central question that absorbed Roux's interest was the cause of embryonic differentiation: How do cells that develop from a single fertilized egg become so different in form and function? To attack this

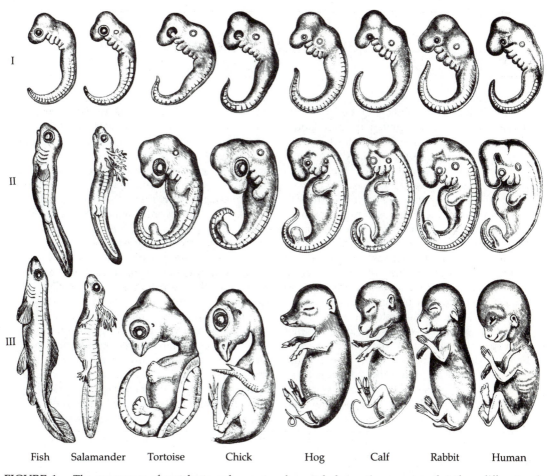

| Fish | Salamander | Tortoise | Chick | Hog | Calf | Rabbit | Human |

FIGURE 1.   *The appearance of vertebrate embryos at various stages of development. The similarity of different embryos during early development is striking; this fundamental observation suggests that these different animals share both a common ancestor and the same basic mechanisms of development. (From Romanes, 1901.)*

problem Roux took up an experiment initially performed by Haeckel in 1869. Haeckel had tried to kill one of the first two cells produced by the cleavage of a fertilized frog egg, but he met with little success. Roux realized that the embryo arising from the remaining cell should indicate whether each cell generates a unique part or whether individual cells have a broader potential. In 1888 Roux published the results of experiments in which he succeeded in killing one blastomere at the 2-cell stage (Roux, 1888). The structures that grew from the residual cell appeared to constitute half an embryo, and Roux therefore concluded that each blastomere develops independently. On the basis of this result he proposed a mosaic theory of development that held that the fate of cells is preordained: each cell was regarded as having only the information necessary to create a particular part of the embryo.

Three years later, in 1891, H. Driesch tested Roux's conclusion more

Ontogeny and Phylogeny

An important controversy that bears on the modern view of development is the relationship of embryogenesis to the obvious hierarchy of animal species (Gould, 1977). Although the argument can be traced earlier, the modern portion of the story begins with K. E. von Baer (1792–1876). A popular idea in the eighteenth century was that the embryos of higher animals recapitulate the *adult* features of lower forms. Von Baer (who figured in the discovery of the mammalian ovum, put forward the germ-layer theory and discovered the notochord in chick embryos, among other accomplishments) vigorously attacked this notion of recapitulation (von Baer, 1828). He suggested instead that the more general features of animals appear earlier than special features and that developing embryos of different species simply depart more and more from an early form common to all (see Figure 1). This sensible argument was temporarily eclipsed by E. Haeckel's assertion that the normal events of early development are a recapitulation of biological history (Haeckel, by the way, coined the terms *ontogeny* and *phylogeny*). For Haeckel, development was simply an accelerated version of evolution. However, Haeckel's idea that development proceeds through a series of adult stages of lower forms (a human embryo is first a fish) simply did not fit the facts. Embryonic men are not really like fish at some point; rather, human embryos and fish embryos are at early times very similar.

The similarity of early embryos is relevant to theories of evolution because it implies that more complex forms arose from a common ancestor—evidently the strategy of early development is highly conserved. In accord with this idea is the fact that the genes of closely related species (man and monkey, for instance) differ very little. This presumably means that the profound differences between the two species do not arise from major differences in genetic programs. One view of speciation is that many differences between animals arise from

carefully with sea urchin eggs at the Zoological Station in Naples (Figure 2). Instead of killing one of the first two blastomeres, Driesch separated them so that each cell could develop independently. In this circumstance Driesch found that the isolated blastomeres developed into fully formed, if smaller, larvae (Driesch, 1892). Subsequently, H. Spemann and others confirmed Driesch's work in vertebrates, thus invalidating Roux's major experimental contribution. The reason for Roux's misinterpretation was probably that the damaged cell, which remained in contact with the other blastomere, caused development to proceed abnormally.

In the end, however, it was Driesch who gave up science after a few years to become a professor of philosophy; in this post he argued that the "harmonious equipotential system" that the embryo represents is beyond analysis. He felt that no system of mechanics could explain how a part could be transformed into a whole. Roux, on the other hand, became a leader of German science, lectured widely, and continued to promote experimental embryology. Not the least of his achievements was founding the *Archiv für Entwicklungsmechanik* (Archives of Developmental Mechanics) in 1894 (now *Wilhelm Roux's Archives*). Influenced

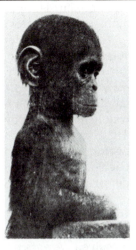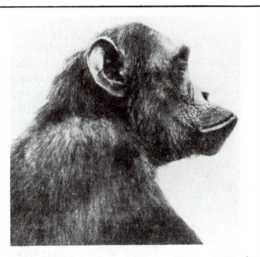

A juvenile and an adult chimpanzee. The resemblance of the juvenile chimp to adult man suggests that differences in the duration of development pro-

duce major differences in form. (From A. Naef, 1926.)

modulations of the regulatory systems that govern quite general aspects of development, such as rate. S. J. Gould and others have argued that humans and primates may differ because of the more protracted development of humans (Gould, 1977). For instance, by the criterion of ossification, a newborn infant (40 weeks) is comparable to an 18-week monkey fetus (macaque), and the bones of a macaque at birth (24 weeks) are similar in their development to a child of several years! Indeed, the physiognomy of an adult human bears a much greater resemblance to a baby chimp than to a full-grown ape (see figure).

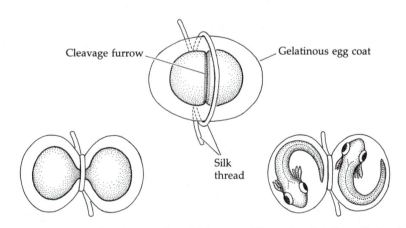

FIGURE 2. *Induced twinning of amphibian eggs. The notion that the earliest embryonic cells in every animal are preordained to give rise to only a part of the embryo had to be discarded when the German zoologist and philosopher H. Driesch showed that each of the first two blastomeres of the sea urchin egg could give rise to a complete larva. This point was confirmed in an experiment carried out by H. Spemann in which a salamander egg was constricted by a fine thread in the plane of the first cleavage furrow, as illustrated here. (After Hamburger, 1963.)*

by Roux's approach, T. H. Morgan, E. G. Conklin, H. Spemann, E. B. Wilson, F. R. Lillie, R. G. Harrison, and others rapidly provided a body of classic experiments in this field (Wilson, 1911; Morgan, 1927; Detwiler, 1936; Waddington, 1936). Before Roux, embryology as a discipline was either a philosophical or an entirely descriptive pursuit; Roux made it an experimental and analytical science. "In zoology," Spemann wrote in 1938, ". . . the speculations on evolution have, partly, perhaps for accidental . . . reasons, outweighed and overpowered every other interest for a number of decades. Here, the initiative of an original thinker was necessary to remind investigators of the fundamental principle [of strict causation]. We owe this achievement to Wilhelm Roux. He will always be honored as the founder of a new discipline in animal embryology" (Spemann, 1938).

In fact, the controversy about whether the fate of early embryonic cells is preordained or determined by interactions with other cells and the environment has never been fully resolved. A variety of observations and experiments indicate that both preordination and flexibility are important in different aspects of development (Chapter 2).

SOME MAJOR EVENTS IN EARLY EMBRYONIC DEVELOPMENT

Respective roles of nucleus and cytoplasm in the earliest stages of development

Development begins with the activation of the egg, usually stimulated by the penetration of a sperm. At the turn of the nineteenth century, the relative importance of the egg nucleus and cytoplasm in development was unclear. In the 1890s, T. Boveri, who later showed that chromosomes are qualitatively different from one another, found that fragments of sea urchin egg that contained only cytoplasm and the genetic material contributed by a sperm developed into an embryo, all parts of which were characteristic of the paternal species (Wilson, 1911). This observation suggested what is now taken for granted: the nuclear material rather than the cytoplasm carries the genetic information. These experiments were extended by I. J. Lorch and J. F. Danielli, who were able to remove (and subsequently reimplant) nuclei from amoebae (Lorch and Danielli, 1950). The enucleated cells failed to survive; they could, however, be rescued by subsequent nuclear implantation.

Other experiments, however, showed that the cytoplasm of the egg also plays a critical role in development. The egg cytoplasm has an uneven distribution of cytoplasmic inclusions such as lipid droplets and yolk granules; such asymmetries are the basis for describing eggs as having an animal pole and a vegetal pole (Figure 3). Different parts of the egg cytoplasm have special functions in development. A striking example is the egg of *Styela* (a sea squirt). Before fertilization the egg has three distinct regions: a peripheral layer that is yellow, a central mass of gray yolk, and a clear germinal vesicle. E. G. Conklin was one of the first embryologists to note that the egg cytoplasm is rearranged within a few minutes of fertilization (Conklin, 1905, 1932). The yellow

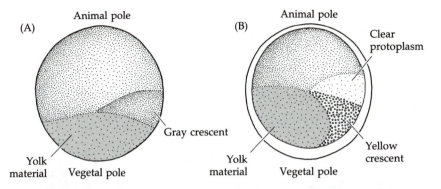

FIGURE 3. *Fertilized eggs of some animals have asymmetrical features before cell division begins. The distribution of yolk and pigment in a frog egg (A) and a* Styela *(sea squirt) egg (B) permits the definition of the animal and the vegetal poles, as well as dorsal and ventral sides. The preexisting features in these eggs, which bear a constant relationship to the initial cleavage planes, indicate that significant organization is already present at the outset of development. (A after Hamburger, 1963; B after Conklin, 1905.)*

material segregates largely into two blastomeres which give rise to muscle cells; the gray yolk gives rise to endoderm, and the clear material gives rise to the ectoderm (see later). Thus, *Styela* eggs are already organized in developmentally significant ways before cell division, a fact that Conklin confirmed by centrifugation. When the different regions of egg cytoplasm were rearranged by centrifugal force, the resulting structures and organs followed suit (Conklin, 1931). Although other eggs, particularly mammalian eggs, are not so obviously heterogeneous, the importance of egg cytoplasm for subsequent events demonstrates that, from the earliest stages, development involves local interpretation of genetic instructions.

In general, some eggs (those of ascidians and mollusks, for example) are mosaic in the sense that the progeny of the earliest cell divisions are already different from one another and generate different parts of the adult animal. On the other hand, the cells of early mammalian embryos are more nearly equipotential (Chapter 2). Because sooner or later all cells generate only a restricted range of progeny, the underlying issue is simply how and when this restriction occurs. From this vantage, both the preformationist and interactivist (epigenetic) arguments have some merit.

Cell cleavage and formation of the blastula

The first step in the course of early development is the division of the fertilized egg into a number of cells called blastomeres, which arrange themselves around a central cavity called the blastocoel. This hollow sphere of cells is called the blastula and is recognized as the first major developmental stage (Figure 4). The formation of the blastula—and other early steps in development—are common to most metazoans, although the shape of the blastula can differ; for example, in birds and

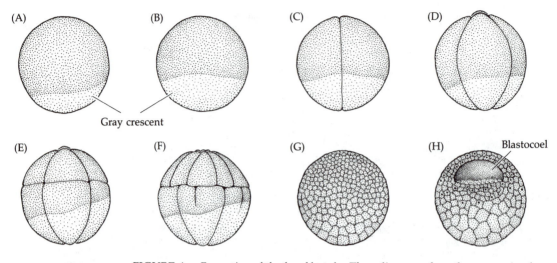

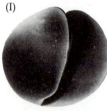

FIGURE 4. *Formation of the frog blastula. These diagrams show the progression from the uncleaved zygote (A,B), through the first cleavage (C) to the early blastula stage (H) (one side in H is cut away). In frog eggs, the initial cleavage planes bear a consistent relationship to preexisting features, such as the gray crescent (the orientation of the egg is somewhat different than Figure 3A). (I,J) Scanning electron micrographs of the earliest stages of egg division (I; comparable to C) and of an 8-cell frog (J; comparable to E). (A–H after Saunders, 1970; I,J from Beams and Kessel, 1976.)*

mammals the blastula extends as a sheet over the yolk rather than forming a sphere.

The division of the fertilized egg into blastomeres occurs with little or no increase in the size of the embryo and is thus really a form of partitioning. The particular style of division varies greatly from one species to another. In eggs that have a large amount of yolk, this nutritive material remains external to the developing embryo itself; therefore, cleavage occurs only in the appropriate part of the egg (the animal pole). Such partial (meroblastic) cleavage is characteristic of some fishes, birds, and reptiles. Complete (holoblastic) cleavage occurs in eggs that have relatively little yolk such as those of annelids, mollusks, amphibians, and mammals. In amphibians, which have more yolk than most other holoblastic embryos, cleavage of the vegetal part of the embryo is somewhat retarded, giving rise to fewer (and larger) cells in the vegetal half than in the animal half. A special sort of cleavage takes place in insects; here the nuclei divide many times without any partitioning of the cytoplasm. Eventually the nuclei move to the periphery of the egg and establish discrete cells by rapidly acquiring cell membranes.

As diverse as these events may seem in different animals, the common denominator is clear enough: with little or no growth, the egg is transformed from a single cell into many hundreds of cells that eventually form the wall of a blastula.

Formation of the gastrula

The next developmental step, also common to most animals, is called gastrulation (Figure 5). In this process, an indentation forms at a particular point on the surface of the blastula (the blastopore), and a portion of the cellular sphere begins to invaginate. The cellular movements of

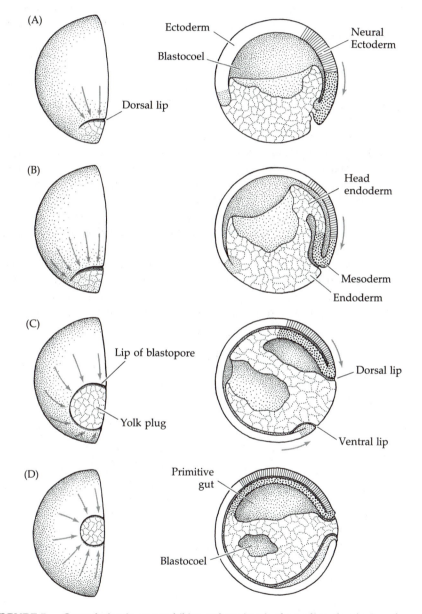

FIGURE 5. *Gastrulation in an amphibian embryo (cut in the median plane). A surface view of successive stages (A–D) is shown on the left, and a corresponding view of the cut surface is shown on the right. Invagination of cells at the blastula stage (A) ultimately results in a three-layered embryo (D). (After Saunders, 1970.)*

gastrulation ultimately give rise to three different tissue layers. The details of this phenomenon have been studied in a number of animals, perhaps most thoroughly in amphibians. The invaginating cells, which form an internal layer or endoderm, send out processes that attach to the outer layer (ectoderm), thus pulling the external and internal layers of the inverted ball together. In this way the blastocoel is gradually obliterated as the primitive gut forms (Figure 5). Some cells from the inner and/or outer layer detach to form an intermediate layer called the mesoderm (Figure 6).

Because of the accessibility of embryos developing in ovo, gastrulation has also been studied intensively in chicks and other avians. Indeed, studies of avian embryos provide the basis of much of the experimental neuroembryology discussed in later chapters (Hamburger and Hamilton, 1951; Waddington, 1952). In birds, the invagination of the cells of the blastula occurs along the primitive streak, a groove on the surface of the blastula (Figure 6). The structure that corresponds to the amphibian blastopore is called Hensen's node and is a deeper pit found at the anterior end of the primitive streak. Gastrulation in mammals is generally similar to that in birds.

Although styles differ, the result of gastrulation in different animals is a three-layered structure surrounding the primitive gut, which is open to the outside through the blastopore. Thus, by the late gastrula stage, embryos have an outside layer (the ectoderm), a middle layer (the mesoderm), and an inner layer (the endoderm); the embryo also has a front and a back and bilateral symmetry (the posterior end is identified by the position of the blastopore in amphibians or of Hensen's

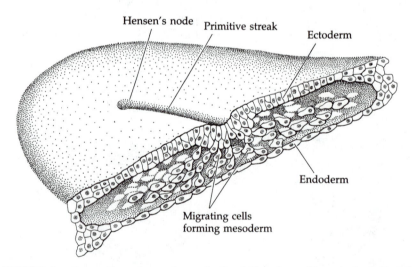

FIGURE 6. *Segregation of germ layers in the chick embryo. The anterior half of the embryo is cut transversely to show the cellular movements equivalent to gastrulation in amphibians (Figure 5; see Figures 7 and 8). As in amphibians, the mesoderm is formed by invagination of a well-defined region of the embryonic surface (the primitive streak). (After Balinsky, 1975.)*

node in birds and mammals). The three layers of the gastrula are called the germ layers. The endoderm gives rise to the gut and many of the major organs associated with the gut; the mesoderm forms muscle, skeleton, connective tissue, and the cardiovascular and urogenital systems; and the ectoderm forms the skin and the nervous system. It is at this stage that the formation of the nervous system proper begins.

INITIAL FORMATION OF NEURAL STRUCTURES IN VERTEBRATES

Neurulation

Because of the conspicuous appearance of the primitive nervous system, the embryo is called the neurula during the next stage of development. In vertebrates, the earliest specialization recognized as a neural antecedent is an anterior–posterior groove in the ectoderm. The formation of this groove proceeds cranially from the blastopore or its equivalent in birds and mammals (Hensen's node). As the neural groove widens, the ectoderm lateral to it thickens to form a flattened structure called the neural plate on the dorsal surface of the embryo (Figure 7). The

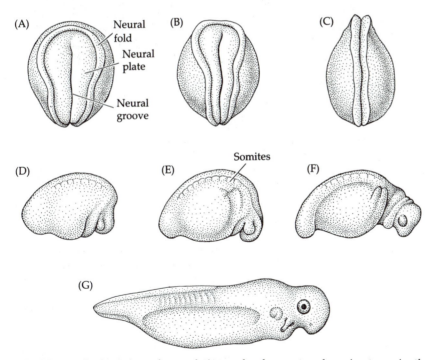

FIGURE 7. *Surface view of neurulation and subsequent embryonic stages in the amphibian (Ambystoma). (A–C) Views showing formation of the neural plate and neural folds; the neural folds eventually fuse in the midline. (D–G) Further developmental stages viewed from the right side. (After Hamburger, 1947.)*

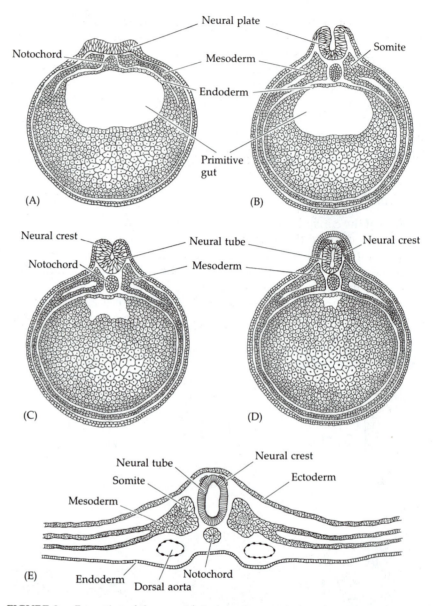

FIGURE 8. *Formation of the neural tube from the neural plate. (A–D) Cross sections of a frog neurula at successive stages during the formation of the neural tube and neural crest. Unlike terrestrial vertebrates, closure of the amphibian neural tube occurs synchronously along its length rather than progressively from head to tail. (E) Cross section of a chick embryo, showing the relation of the neural tube to other structures that form during neurulation. (After Saunders, 1970.)*

plate has distinct ridges at its margins: the neural folds. These folds gradually become more pronounced and bend toward the midline, where they meet and fuse from anterior to posterior. This process is called neurulation and gives rise to the neural tube (Figure 8). Some mesodermal structures also develop during neurulation. The most prominent of these are the notochord along the rostrocaudal axis in the midline and the masses of mesoderm lateral to the notochord called somites (see Figures 7 and 8). The notochord is a longitudinal rod of cells that in vertebrates is eventually incorporated into the spinal column. The somites, which provide the first indication of segmentation in the embryo, give rise to the vertebrae, the ribs, skeletal muscle, and the dermis (the deeper part of the skin). The neural tube and its anterior widening eventually form the brain and spinal cord (i.e., the central nervous system).

The peripheral nervous system originates from a distinct group of precursor cells called the neural crest. The neural crest arises from the neural plate but separates from it to form a band running the length of the neural plate at the dorsolateral border of the neural folds (Figure 8). As the neural tube closes, the crest comes to lie just dorsal and lateral to it. Neural crest cells give rise to the spinal and autonomic ganglia; to the glial cells of the peripheral nervous system; to a variety of nonneural tissues including melanocytes, chromaffin cells of the adrenal medulla, cartilage, blood-forming cells, the connective tissue cells covering the brain and spinal cord; and to parts of the facial bones (making the point, incidentally, that some adult tissues such as bone and connective tissue arise from more than one embryonic germ layer). Because of the relative accessibility of the neural crest to experimental manipulations, this part of the developing nervous system has been the object of numerous studies detailed in subsequent chapters.

A final source of neural tissue (in addition to neural tube and neural crest) is the epidermal (sensory) placodes, which arise from separate thickenings of the ectoderm in the head region. There are 9 or 10 pairs of placodes in vertebrates; these are divided into groups called lens, otic, nasal, epibranchial, and dorsolateral. Together with neural crest, the placodes give rise to the central ganglia of the relevant cranial nerves and the cranial sense organs.

Throughout neurulation, the neural ectoderm is only one or two cells thick. A wide range of explanations involving pushing, pulling, and changes of density or adhesion have been proposed to explain neurulation (His, 1874; Trinkhaus, 1969; Jacobson, 1978, 1981; Edelman, 1984). In fact, it seems that several mechanisms are involved. Analyses of cell shape and position in time-lapse movies of the neural plate in amphibian embryos indicate that the marked changes that occur in neurulation are correlated with a decrease in the apical surface of cells and an increase in their height (Figure 9) (Burnside and Jacobson, 1968). At the same time, the area that overlies the notochord elongates, thereby causing cells to converge and relocate along the midline. Finally, changes in the distribution and types of cell adhesion molecules on cell surfaces during this period are likely to be important in regulating cell movement (Edelman, 1984). Because there is relatively little cell division in the neural plate at this stage, proliferation is probably not a major factor in neurulation.

The subsequent formation of the neural tube also involves changes in cell shape and adhesive forces that further alter the topology of the

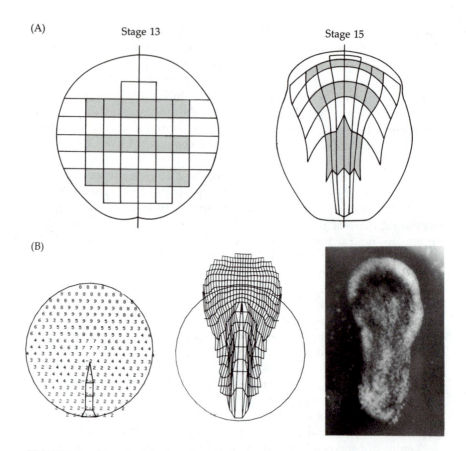

FIGURE 9. *Neural plate formation in an amphibian embryo studied by time-lapse cinematography. (A) Fifty grid divisions on the surface of a newt neurula (stage 13) were followed by noting variations of pigment and other landmarks. At a somewhat later stage (15), the shape of the grid has changed markedly; part of this transformation is due to a reduction in the apical surface area of ectodermal cells while their height is increasing (see Figure 10). (B) Computer simulation shows that these cellular changes, together with midline elongation, produce a change in shape that closely matches the change in the embryo during neurulation. Numbered diagram on left is an idealized stage 13 embryo and indicates the degree of apical shrinking postulated in each region. Computer simulation of this effect is shown in the center, and a photomicrograph of an actual newt neurula (stage 15) is shown on the right. (A after Jacobson, 1981; B after Jacobson, 1978.)*

neural plate. The continued contraction of the apical surfaces of the neural plate cells causes the basal ends of the cells to become progressively broader than the apices (i.e., they become flask-shaped; Figure 10). This evidently makes the neural plate curve in on itself. The continued extension of the neural plate along the midline may provide a second force that promotes the formation of a tube (Jacobson, 1981). However, even this relatively simple orchestration of cellular events to produce a change in embryonic shape is not well understood.

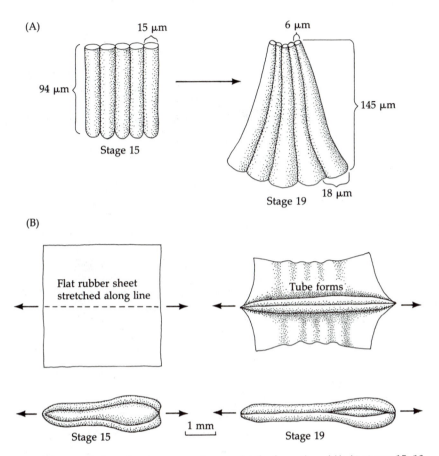

(A)

15 μm

6 μm

94 μm

145 μm

Stage 15

18 μm

Stage 19

(B)

Flat rubber sheet
stretched along line

Tube forms

1 mm

Stage 15

Stage 19

FIGURE 10. *Factors that may promote neural tube formation. (A) At stages 15–19, the shape of neuroectodermal cells in a newt embryo continues to change so that the cells become increasingly flask-shaped. This change throughout the sheet presumably promotes an inward curvature of the neural plate. (B) The continued elongation of the neural plate in the midline may also contribute to neural tube formation, as suggested by the effect of pulling an elastic rubber sheet—as the sheet is pulled, it tends to form a tube. (After Jacobson, 1981.)*

When neurulation is complete, the primordia of most adult structures in vertebrates are apparent and the developing organism is simply referred to as an embryo (rather than as a blastula, gastrula, or neurula).

Emergence of the vertebrate brain

A further specialization of the neural tube begins in the neurula stage: three distinct swellings appear at the rostral end of the tube and are called the forebrain vesicle (prosencephalon), the midbrain vesicle (mesencephalon), and the hindbrain vesicle (rhombencephalon) (Cowan, 1978, 1979). The forebrain vesicle ultimately gives rise to the cerebral hemispheres, the midbrain vesicle to the adult midbrain, and the hind-

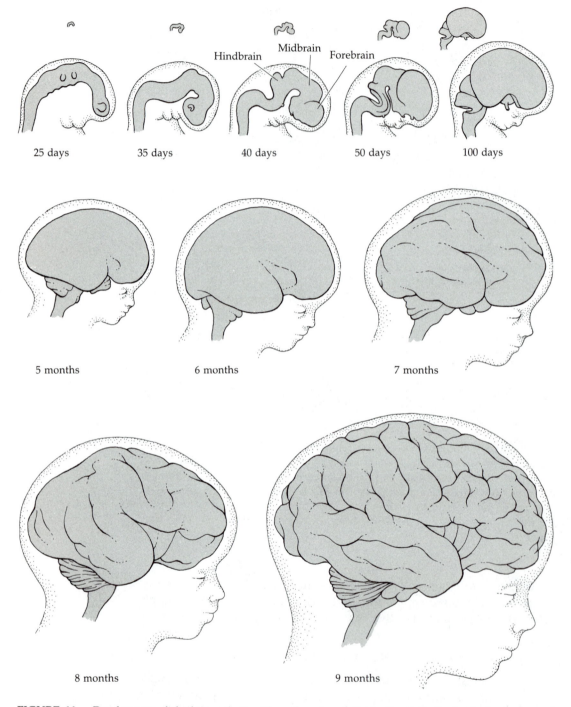

FIGURE 11. *Development of the human brain. The diagrams in this sequence are about four-fifths life-size; the lower diagrams in the first row are enlarged for clarity. Assuming that the fully developed human brain contains approximately 100 billion neurons and that these do not divide after birth, the developing brain must add an average of 250,000 neurons per minute of early development. Note the exceptional growth of the forebrain rudiment, which gives rise to the cerebral hemispheres. (After Cowan, 1978.)*

brain vesicle to the lower brain stem (pons and medulla) and cerebellum (Figure 11). Thus, growth along the length of the neural tube is regionally diverse from the earliest stages.

These swellings are largely the result of rapid and disproportionate cell proliferation along the neural tube. Most of the proliferation of nerve cell precursors occurs at the inner surface of the neural tube (Sauer, 1935; Fujita, 1963; Rakic, 1974). Because this layer is the wall of the lumen that will eventually form the ventricles of the brain and the central canal of the spinal cord, it is called the ventricular zone (Figure 12). The concentric layers of the expanding neural tube superficial to this are called, respectively, the intermediate zone and the marginal zone. As cells proliferate in the ventricular zone and migrate locally to more superficial layers (Chapter 4), a longitudinal indentation appears in the neural tube of many vertebrate embryos and divides it into dorsal (alar) and ventral (basal) plates. These plates give rise to the dorsal and ventral horns of the gray matter of the spinal cord.

There is a rostrocaudal progression of maturation in the development of the neural tube (and other embryonic structures), as well as a ventral-to-dorsal gradient of proliferation (Figure 13) (Hamburger, 1948).

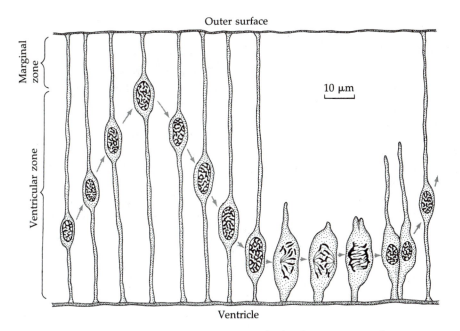

FIGURE 12. *Cell division in the wall of the neural tube. For many years the arrangement of dividing cells in the neural epithelium was a matter of controversy. It is now clear that at early stages this layer is a pseudostratified epithelium in which the processes of neuron and glial cell precursors extend from the inner to the outer surface. However, nuclei divide only at the inner surface of the epithelium, for reasons that are obscure. This diagram shows the normal cycle of events during cell division in this tissue. After nerve cell precursors finish dividing, they migrate away from this epithelium to form other layers of the central nervous system (Chapter 4). (After Sauer, 1935.)*

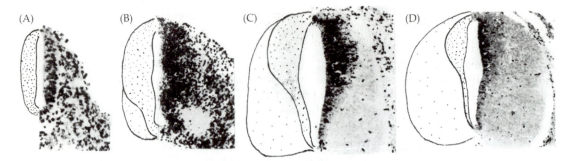

FIGURE 13. *Evidence for a ventral to dorsal progression of cell proliferation in the developing nervous system. These pictures show autoradiograms and corresponding cross-sectional diagrams of the spinal cords of rat embryos given tritiated thymidine on embryonic day 11 (A), 12 (B), 14 (C), or 15 (D) and sacrificed 12 hours later. Dark cells indicate dividing precursors that have incorporated the label into their DNA. As development proceeds, proliferation diminishes in the ventral cord, and by day 15 of gestation only the most dorsal portion of the ventricular zone remains active. (From Nornes and Das, 1974.)*

As a result, the motor system, which is located in the ventral cord, develops earlier than the dorsal sensory system does.

INITIAL FORMATION OF NEURAL STRUCTURES IN INVERTEBRATES

Although the invertebrate nervous system also arises primarily from the ectoderm of the early embryo, there are major differences between neurogenesis in vertebrates and neurogenesis in invertebrates (Slack, 1983).

The nervous systems of annelids, arthropods and mollusks usually occupy a ventral rather than a dorsal position in the embryo and are organized into a series of ganglia (often segmental) rather than into brain, spinal cord, and peripheral ganglia. The nervous system of the leech provides a good example (Figure 14) (Fernandez and Stent, 1980; Weisblat, 1981). It consists of a chain of 32 segmental ganglia with fused ganglia at the head and the tail (euphemistically called brains). A distinct feature in the neural development of the leech (and some other invertebrates) is the presence of a germinal band. The fifth-generation cells that ultimately give rise to all of the ectoderm and the mesoderm are called teloblasts; in the course of development they undergo a series of asymmetrical divisions that produce a single column of stem cells (Figure 14). These parallel germinal bandlets zip up to form a central band called the germinal plate along the ventral midline. Ectodermal cell masses form along the germinal plate in register with mesodermal blocks, similar to somites. These right- and left-sided ectodermal masses then fuse to form the ganglionic primordia.

There are, of course, major differences in the neural development of various invertebrates, which makes generalization difficult. This is

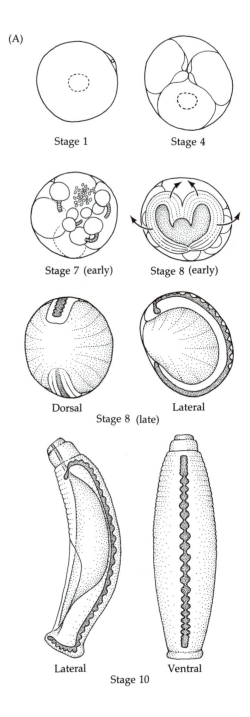

(A)

Stage 1   Stage 4

Stage 7 (early)   Stage 8 (early)

Dorsal   Lateral
Stage 8 (late)

Lateral   Ventral
Stage 10

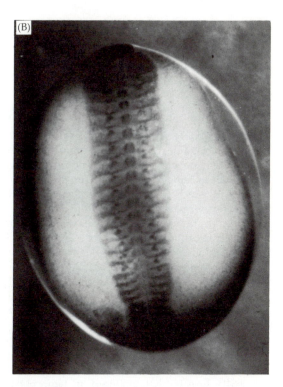

(B)

FIGURE 14.   *Neurogenesis in an invertebrate embryo. (A) Diagram of the development of the leech (Helobdella triserialis). The diameter of the uncleaved egg (stage 1) is about 0.5 mm. Germinal bandlets begin to form at stage 7; by early stage 8 the germinal bands (dotted lines) begin to fuse in the midline (arrows). The developing chain of segmental ganglia is shown in heavy stipple in stages 8 and 10. This sequence of neural development is very different in style from that of vertebrates. (B) Photomicrograph of a stage 9 leech embryo (Haementaria), comparable to late stage 8 in A. The preparation has been stained with hematoxylin. The segmental arrangement of the developing midline ganglia on the ventral surface of the embryo is obvious. Note that, as in vertebrates, there is a rostrocaudal gradient of maturation (rostral is up). (A after Weisblat et al., 1980; B from a photograph by R. T. Sawyer, reprinted in Weisblat, 1981.)*

not surprising since invertebrates are extremely diverse and comprise the vast majority of the species in the animal kingdom. Perhaps it is enough at this point to emphasize that nature has evidently devised a number of ways to build nervous systems.

Metamorphosis

Some invertebrates (as well as some vertebrates) undergo dramatic changes at relatively late stages of development. Perhaps because of our own development, we tend to think of growth as being a more or less progressive process in which the remarkable changes of the first few weeks and months of life are followed by only gradual transition. The phenomenon of metamorphosis serves as a useful antidote to the idea that development is always smoothly progressive and limited to early life.

Although some insects develop in a simple continuous manner (examples are springtails and bristletails—such insects are called ametabolous), most insects undergo some form of metamorphosis, that is, a more or less radical change in form after initial (larval) "development" is complete (Schneiderman and Gilbert, 1964). Insects that undergo metamorphosis more or less gradually are called hemimetabolous. Holometabolous insects, on the other hand, have a distinctive larval form: maggots are larval flies and caterpillars are larval butterflies. In these animals, many parts of the adult form (the imago) are actually contained within the larva in undifferentiated structures called imaginal disks (Chapter 3).

Insect metamorphosis is controlled by the interaction of two hormones: ecdysone, which is produced by the prothoracic gland and which sets in motion the molting process, and juvenile hormone, which is secreted by organs called the corpora allata that act to keep insects in the larval stage (Schneiderman and Gilbert, 1964). Many insect tissues are competent to respond to these hormones, as might be expected from the coordinated nature of metamorphosis. These effects, which involve both the involution of tissues and the initiation of

tissue growth, are mediated through influences on genes. Evidence for this idea has come from studies of the giant chromosomes in some organs of insects such as *Drosophila* or the midge *Chironomous*; extensive duplication of DNA renders these chromosomes easily visible. Giant chromosomes are punctuated by bands (called Balbiani rings) that probably represent the spacing of different genes. Treatment of such insects with ecdysone causes enlargement (puffing) of specific regions of the chromosome, a phenomenon thought to signify selective gene activation (Beermann and Clever, 1964).

Metamorphosis is, of course, not limited to insects but occurs in many other animals. In anurans (frogs and toads), metamorphosis of tadpoles into adults often occurs in only a few days (Etkin, 1964). Internal changes in such animals are every bit as profound as the changes in external form. In frogs, for example, the animal's entire excretory machinery shifts as the tadpole's ability to excrete ammonia into the surrounding water is lost. In urodeles (salamanders), metamorphosis is less striking and more gradual. Although the gills of the aquatic form are lost and a variety of other morphological changes occur, the larval and the adult forms are recognizable as variants of the same animal. These metamorphic changes in amphibians are also under hormonal control (in this case, thyroid hormone; Allen, 1918, 1938).

The significance of these events for neural development is both practical and general. From the practical point of view, the occurrence of "developmental" events in larger larvae provides a technically easier context for performing many kinds of experiments. An example is the study of developing neurons in tadpole larvae described in Chapter 2. Similarly, the presence

CONCLUSIONS

Until the end of the nineteenth century, the approach to development was more philosophical than experimental. The direct attack on the proximate causes of developmental events that began in the late nine-

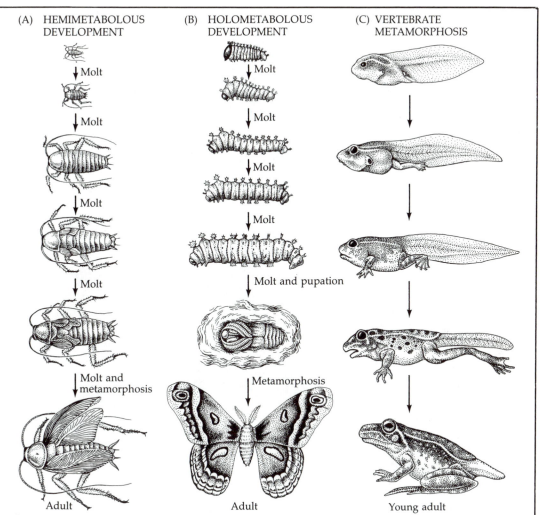

(A) HEMIMETABOLOUS DEVELOPMENT

(B) HOLOMETABOLOUS DEVELOPMENT

(C) VERTEBRATE METAMORPHOSIS

↓ Molt

↓ Molt

↓ Molt

↓ Molt

↓ Molt and metamorphosis

↓ Molt

↓ Molt

↓ Molt

↓ Molt

↓ Molt and pupation

↓ Metamorphosis

Adult

Adult

Young adult

Metamorphosis in different animals. (A) Gradual metamorphosis of a hemimetabolous insect, the cockroach. (B) Holometabolous metamorphosis in the development of the giant silkworm moth. (C) Metamorphosis in a frog. (A,B after Turner and Bagnara, 1971; C after Balinsky, 1975.)

of cryptic body parts in the imaginal disks of larval insects has been important in establishing several rules of insect development (Chapter 3).

On a more general level, metamorphic events show that many tissues, nervous tissues included, are capable of profound changes even at relatively late developmental stages. The morphological and behavioral changes of puberty in mammals are similar examples of the hormonal control of later developmental events.

teenth century continues unabated. In spite of considerable progress, many developmental issues debated in earlier times are still unsettled; preeminent among these are differentiation and morphogenesis, the topics of the following two chapters.

Neuronal Differentiation

INTRODUCTION

Generation of specialized cells from less specialized ancestors is perhaps the central feature of development. Understanding this phenomenon, however, is complicated by the fact that the phenotype of developing cells is influenced by both genes and the local environment. To make matters worse, the distinction between genetic and epigenetic influences is often cloudy. Indirectly, genes affect the cellular environment, and the environment affects gene expression. Because there is no obvious way to open this loop, assessing the genetic and epigenetic contributions to phenotype is difficult at best. Although the proximate causes of differentiation first sought by W. Roux have remained elusive, modern descriptions of differentiation at the cellular and molecular level have given considerable insight into the way cells become specialized.

INFLUENCES ON CELL DIFFERENTIATION

Differentiative events are influenced by at least three categories of instructions: instructions contained within the nucleus, instructions from the cytoplasm of the developing cell, and instructions arising from other developing cells and the extracellular environment.

Influence of the nucleus

Perhaps the simplest scheme to explain differentiation was proposed in the 1890s by A. Weismann who envisioned a progressive loss of genetic material from the nucleus as the basis of specialization (Barth, 1964; Karp and Berrill, 1981). In fact, DNA loss does occur in the development of some insects and nematodes. For example, some invertebrates show a large-scale (50 percent) reduction in the DNA content of all but one blastomere during cleavage (Gurdon and Woodland, 1968; Beermann, 1977). In accord with Weismann's original suggestion, the only blastomere that retains its full complement of DNA gives rise to the germ line.

On the other hand, a variety of experiments in vertebrates indicate that simple loss of genetic material is not a general explanation for differentiation. For a long period during development, and perhaps throughout the life of some cells, the entire set of genetic instructions is retained. This conclusion is based on experiments that involve transplantation of nuclei, in the simplest cases from cells of progressively later stages of development into uncleaved eggs from which the nucleus

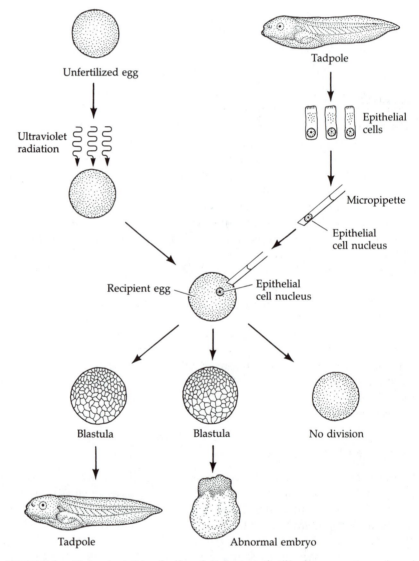

FIGURE 1.   *Transplantation of cell nuclei into an unfertilized egg sometimes gives rise to a normal tadpole. An unfertilized frog egg is irradiated to kill its nucleus, and an epithelial cell nucleus from a tadpole or an adult frog is then introduced through a micropipette. Although development is abortive in most instances, occasionally a normal tadpole (or even an adult frog) develops. To rule out persistence of the original egg nucleus, two different strains of frogs are used. (After Gurdon, 1968.)*

has been removed (Figure 1). R. Briggs and T. J. King (1952) found that nuclei from frog blastomeres, when inserted into enucleated eggs, gave rise to normal tadpoles. This result, incidentally, was anticipated by H. Spemann, who showed that a blastomere that received a nucleus from a 16-cell zygote sometimes developed normally (Spemann, 1938). Thus nuclear instructions can remain quite complete, at least until a stage when there are already many cells in the embryo (see also Illmensee, 1973). On the other hand, at later stages eggs with transplanted nuclei give rise to increasing numbers of abnormal embryos; by the neurula stage nuclear transplantation is usually unsuccessful in producing a normal frog larva. Occasionally, however, nuclear transplantation from an adult epithelial cell to an oocyte does give rise to a normal tadpole (Gurdon, 1968; 1974; Gurdon et al., 1975). Moreover, even in those cases in which normal embryos are not forthcoming, adult nuclei transplanted into an enucleated egg cause the development of structures with a variety of specialized cells (Danielli and Di Berardino, 1979). It seems likely, then, that the nuclei of differentiated cells can, in at least some circumstances, be reactivated by the egg cytoplasm to a state of "totipotency." In confirmation of this view, DNA hybridization studies show that the genes present in differentiated cells are capable of producing enzymes and proteins that the cell never uses; for example, the instructions for making hemoglobin can be demonstrated in liver cells (Packman et al., 1972; DeRobertis et al., 1977). Finally, the dissociation and reassociation of mammalian blastulae to produce chimeras that go on to develop normally (as well as the ability of some tumor cells to incorporate into blastulae) further demonstrates the broad developmental potential of early embryonic cells (Mintz and Illmensee, 1975; Kelly, 1977).

The general view of differentiation at present is that particular phenotypes are generated by selective gene expression. Indeed, qualitative change in gene expression, whether elicited by intrinsic or extrinsic factors, is really the modern definition of differentiation. There are a number of points at which gene expression could be controlled. Genes themselves could be altered by diminution, amplification, rearrangement, or modification; or gene expression could be changed at the transcriptional, posttranscriptional, translational, or posttranslational control levels (Brown, 1981); any or all of these effects could have lasting consequences on cell phenotype.

The view that cellular differentiation is largely the result of selective gene expression raises fundamental questions. Are phenotypic features explicitly related to genetic instructions, or are these features so remote from genetic causes that understanding genes per se will reveal relatively little about the development of phenotype (see Box A)? A related question is whether there are genes dedicated solely to developmental strategies and events. Some genes in invertebrates do appear to control decisions about alternative fates of specific cells or body parts (Lewis, 1978; Chalfie et al., 1981; Greenwald et al., 1983; see also Chapter 3). Nonetheless, the way that genes regulate development is not yet clear.

What is the relation of genes to development?

One of the most perplexing problems in development is how ontogenetic events are related to genetic instructions. On the face of it, the problem seems straightforward. The discovery that genes are first and foremost a repository of information leads naturally to the supposition that developmental events are, in some fairly strict way, based on genetic instructions. It would then follow that the fundamental task of developmental biologists is to discover those genes or parts of genes that control development (see, for instance, Benzer, 1971; Brenner, 1973). The situation, however, is unlikely to be so simple.

A provocative analysis of the strengths and weaknesses of the genetic approach to development has been provided by G. S. Stent (1977, 1981). Stent invites us to consider the situation outlined by astronomer C. Sagan in which earthlings transmit the complete DNA sequence of a cat's genome to a distant supercivilization. The question that Stent poses is whether the aliens, whatever their level of sophistication, would be able to reconstruct a cat from the base sequence of its DNA. The reasons for his negative appraisal are important for anyone interested in development. In order to make a cat, Stent argues, the aliens would also need to know about the environment in which the genome operated. Divorced from biology and evolution on earth, the information in cat genes is relatively meaningless. For example, the aliens would need to know about amino acids and the conformation of proteins. Because this information is not in the genes, the aliens would not get very far.

A more mundane problem discussed by Stent is understanding neural development through an analysis of neurological mutants. An example is albinism. The defect in albinos is quite clear at the genetic level: albino animals are unable to catalyze the conversion of tyrosine to melanin at body temperature because of a defect in the enzyme tyrosinase. This deficiency is accompanied by an abnormality of neural development that has been most clearly described in cats. In Siamese cats (which have a form of albinism), the crossing of retinal axons at the optic chiasm is abnormal and some optic fibers from each eye reach the wrong side of the brain. This finding, described in a series of experiments by R. W. Guillery and his collaborators (Guillery, 1974; Guillery et al., 1974), presents a puzzle. What is the relationship between a defect in tyrosinase and the misrouting of axons? Stent suggests some plausible links but emphasizes that various explanations do not concern genetic information but rather cellular interactions based on events that genetic instructions only set in motion.

The general problem, as Stent puts it, is that "in view of their general remoteness from the primary action of the genes, the great majority of epigenetic algorithms are unlikely to refer to any gene at all" (Stent, 1977, p. 143).

Influence of the cytoplasm

The ability of enucleated eggs to stimulate transplanted nuclei to initiate development argues that extranuclear (epigenetic) factors regulate gene expression. H. Spemann was perhaps the first to demonstrate directly an influence of the cytoplasm on differentiation. Thus, when he divided an amphibian egg in the dorsoventral plane so that the gray crescent was apportioned to both halves (see Figures 2 and 3 in Chapter 1), each cell could develop into a normal embryo (Spemann, 1938). However, when he placed a ligature in the equatorial plane, only the cell with the gray crescent developed normally; the other half gave rise to a disorganized ball of liver, gut, and other endodermal organs [Spemann called this ball *bauchstück* (roughly, "belly-piece")]. The influence of the cytoplasm on gene expression has been amply confirmed (Fankhauser, 1955). For example, somatic cells synthesize mainly RNA. However, when the nucleus of a somatic cell is transplanted to an enucleated but fertilized egg, the hybrid cell synthesizes primarily DNA; only at later stages of development does it resume RNA synthesis (Gurdon and Woodland, 1968).

Influences arising from other cells

The specialization of cells also depends on signals arising from nearby tissues. This phenomenon is called induction. Induction of ectoderm by the underlying mesoderm produces a variety of ectodermal specializations (Figure 2) (Spemann, 1938; Cairns and Saunders, 1954; Jacob-

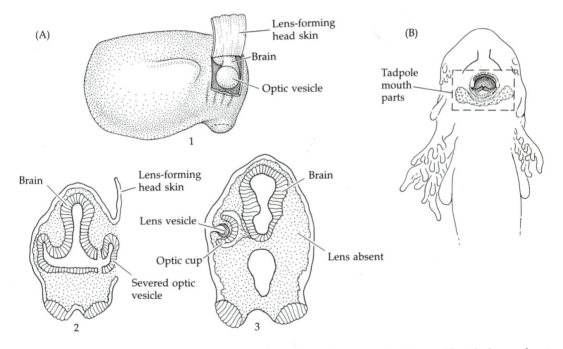

FIGURE 2. *Differentiation can be induced by neighboring cells. (A) This diagram shows an experiment demonstrating the dependence of lens formation on the presence of the underlying optic vesicle. A flap of epidermis containing the lens-forming area of an amphibian embryo is deflected with a glass needle (1) and the optic vesicle is cut off at its base, as shown in the cross section labeled (2). In the majority of frog species tested, no lens formed in the absence of the optic vesicle (3). Such experiments indicate that ectodermal specialization can be induced by the underlying mesoderm. (B) Ventral view of a salamander larva with tadpole mouthparts following transplantation of ectoderm from a frog gastrula to the prospective mouth region of a salamander gastrula. The horny jaws, horn stumps, and suckers typical of tadpoles are evident in the mouth region of the salamander. This striking result confirms the importance of mesodermal induction in ectodermal differentiation and indicates that the inductive signals have been highly conserved in evolution. (A from Hamburger, 1963; B after Spemann, 1938.)*

son, 1966; Sengal, 1975). Perhaps the best-studied example is the induction of the lens in the ectoderm overlying the optic vesicle (Spemann, 1938; Karkinen-Jääskeläinen, 1978). When the optic vesicle is removed at an early embryonic stage, the lens fails to develop. Conversely, when the optic vesicle is transplanted to another part of the organism, a lens is induced in the overlying ectoderm. Although these results show that inductive phenomena occur, the underlying mechanism is unknown and is probably quite complicated. For example, the ability of the optic vesicle to induce a lens depends on the species (Karp and Berrill, 1981). In some frog species, only the normal overlying ectoderm can respond to the optic vesicle, whereas in other species any ectoderm is competent. In yet other species, the lens develops in its normal position with or without the underlying optic vesicle (Karp and Berrill, 1981; Karkinen-Jääskeläinen, 1978). Unrelated tissues can also induce lens differentiation (Jacobson, 1966; Karp and Berrill, 1981).

The most dramatic examples of induction come from experiments in which tissue from one species is transplanted to another. When undifferentiated ectoderm of a frog gastrula is transplanted to the prospective mouth region of a salamander gastrula, some of the resulting salamanders had the unmistakable horny jaws and horn stumps of a tadpole (Figure 2B) (Spemann, 1938). Similarly, chick ectoderm can be induced to form dentine (and even an occasional tooth) by exposure to mesoderm taken from the mouth region of mouse embryos (Kollar and Fisher, 1980)! Evidently mesoderm induces region-specific differentiation of ectoderm which then expresses its fate according to the species from which it derives.

In sum, differentiation as a result of induction by signals from other cells certainly occurs in vertebrates (see also Chapter 3). The phenomenon, however, is poorly understood and its mechanism unclear. In some simpler systems such as slime molds, the inductive signal for differentiation is well established (Kay and Jermyn, 1983).

FATE MAPPING AND CELL DETERMINATION

Differentiation refers to the visible (or otherwise measurable) differences between cells that emerge as the embryo matures. This idea must be distinguished from the related concept of determination, which refers to the transition of cells from totipotency to a more limited fate. A cell is said to be determined when changing its situation in the embryo (or manipulating it in some other way) no longer influences what it becomes.

Studies of cell fate have depended largely on marking methods that allow the same cells to be followed over time. Classical fate-mapping studies were carried out by staining small patches of embryonic cells with vital dyes (Vogt, 1925, 1929). More recently, a variety of other techniques have been used for the same purpose. One such method is the creation of embryonic chimeras by mixing blastomeres of two strains that can be distinguished histologically. Studies of chimeras show that the progeny of particular mammalian blastomeres contribute in a patchy way to most tissues and organs (Kelly, 1977). Another way of marking cells over time is by the injection of blastomeres with markers, such as the enzyme horseradish peroxidase or a fluorescent dye, which are then carried into the descendants of the injected progenitor. This technique was developed by G. S. Stent and his colleagues for analysis of development in the leech (Weisblat et al., 1978; Stent et al., 1982) and has been used extensively by M. Jacobson to map the fate of the progeny of *Xenopus* blastomeres (Figure 3) (Jacobson, 1978, 1982; see Chapter 3).

Because following the progeny of labeled cells tells only what the descendants *normally* become, but not what they *can* become, a good deal of confusion has arisen over the interpretation of fate mapping. Although fate maps may imply something about the state of determination, the test of commitment must be a challenge that shows that the cells are irrevocably set on a particular course of differentiation. In practice, this is a difficult business. "In my opinion," wrote R. G. Harrison in 1937, "this expression ["determined"] were best dropped from the language of embryology, for there is no criterion for finding out when this condition is reached, if indeed it ever is. It is never

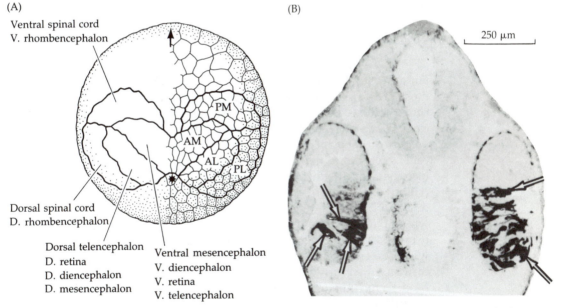

(A)

Ventral spinal cord
V. rhombencephalon

PM

AM

AL

PL

Dorsal spinal cord
D. rhombencephalon

Dorsal telencephalon
D. retina
D. diencephalon
D. mesencephalon

Ventral mesencephalon
V. diencephalon
V. retina
V. telencephalon

(B)

250 μm

FIGURE 3. *Occupation of discrete regions at later embryonic stages by the progeny of individual blastomeres labeled with horseradish peroxidase in* Xenopus. *(A) Diagram of a 512-cell stage blastula; injection of any of the blastomeres in the outlined regions (right) consistently yields labeled progeny that contribute to the structures indicated on the left-hand side of the diagram. PM, Posteromedial cell group; AM, anteromedial; AL, anterolateral; PL, posterolateral. The star indicates the* animal pole, and the arrow the vegetal pole; the diameter of the blastula is about 1.5 mm. (B) Coronal section through a Xenopus larva (stage 34) showing the location of the progeny of a single blastomere of the anteromedial group injected with horseradish peroxidase (HRP) at the 512-cell stage. The HRP-labeled progeny (arrows) go to stereotyped locations, in this case the ventral retinas. (A after Jacobson, 1980; B after Jacobson, 1983.)

possible to know whether some new set of conditions to which a developing part may be subjected may not undo what seems to have been already done irrevocably" (Harrison, 1937, p. 373).

DIFFERENTIATION OF NERVE CELLS

Given that human neurons may live for a century or more, the few weeks in which nerve cells become specialized in embryonic life represents a miniscule fraction of their lifetime. Nerve cells, of course, must continue to change; the ability of the nervous system to learn and remember throughout life makes this point. But whereas many other systems retain some differentiative potential, the remarkable abilities of the nervous system are based largely on relatively subtle changes in synaptic connections and neural function (Chapters 13 and 14). Although these changes modify neuronal phenotype, to call this differentiation goes beyond the usual meaning of the word. Indeed, the reversible nature of many of these changes suggests quite different mechanisms. In short, some aspects of neuronal phenotype are based on qualitative changes in gene expression, whereas others appear to depend purely on extrinsic influences (e.g., experience). Because there is often no clear way to distinguish these categories, this problem must be borne in mind when neuronal differentiation is discussed.

Early attempts to define the origin of nerve and glial cells

For at least a hundred years, neuroembryologists have recognized that most of the cells in the vertebrate central nervous system arise from active mitosis in the portion of the neural tube that lines its central canal (Chapter 1). A number of early embryologists, W. His in particular, imagined that a special subpopulation of these epithelial cells (germinal cells) gave rise to neurons and that supporting (glial) cells arose from a histologically distinct population of precursors (called spongioblasts) (His, 1887). One of the few things that is generally accepted about the origin of nerve and glial cells at present is that this initial view was wrong (Figure 4). Both neurons and glia arise from the same epithelium (Cowan, 1978). What remains very much a question is the point at which precursor cells begin to follow separate pathways and the extent to which they are determined as they proceed toward different fates. Modern techniques have enabled investigators to study these questions in fairly sophisticated ways. For instance, cell-specific markers can distinguish neurons and glia (Raff et al., 1978; see also Raff et al., 1983). An example of a glial-specific marker is glial fibrillary acidic protein (GFAP). This protein is characteristic of mature glial cells, and antibodies to it can be tagged with a fluorescent label and used to mark glial cells. The point in development at which some cells of the neuroepithelium become positive for this molecule can then be assessed. Glial fibrillary acidic protein is already present in some of the dividing cells of the ventricular zone (Levitt and Rakic, 1980; Levitt et al., 1981). If

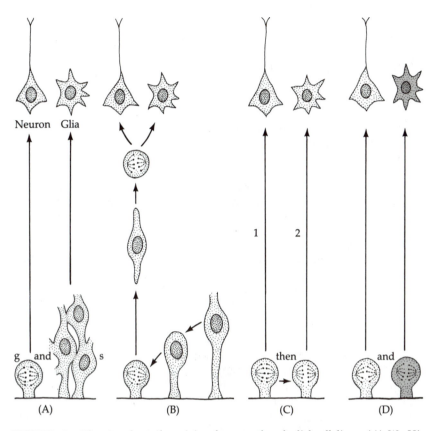

FIGURE 4. *Theories about the origin of neuronal and glial cell lines. (A) W. His originally proposed about a century ago that neural and glial lines were entirely separate. g, Germinal cell; s, spongioblast. (B) An alternative view, suggested by A. Schaper, was that these two cell types arise from a single class of precursors that divide after migrating away from the ventricular zone. (C) The introduction of thymidine autoradiography led S. Fujita to conclude in the 1960s that dividing cells first give rise to neurons (1) and then, after neurogenesis has ceased, produce glial cells (2). (D) The ability to demonstrate glial fibrillary acidic protein, a specific glial marker, provides evidence for the current view that nerve and glial cell precursors coexist in the ventricular zone from very early stages. (After Rakic, 1981.)*

one assumes that GFAP is not transiently present in neuronal precursors, it follows that glial and neuronal cell lines are already different at the peak of neurogenesis, before migration from the neuroepithelium begins. This probably means that the differentiation of neurons and glia begins at a very early time in development.

Modern studies of nerve cell lineage

A more direct way of gaining insight into neuronal differentiation is to follow the descendants of identified precursors. This approach is similar to fate mapping, but focuses on individual cells rather than on groups

BOX

B

Molecular Biologists Captivated by Neurobiology

In spite of the immense success of molecular biology in the last three decades, many of its brightest exponents were attracted to neurobiology in the 1960s. Preeminent among these mavericks were Sydney Brenner, Seymour Benzer, Gunther Stent, Cyrus Levinthal, Marshall Nirenberg, and Francis Crick. Although not all these individuals have been entirely loyal to neurobiology (Crick, for example, ranges widely over biological problems, and Brenner's work has perhaps said as much about development generally as about the development of the nervous system), in the aggregate the efforts of these defectors have substantially changed the neurobiological landscape. Perhaps their major effect was to introduce the imaginative style of molecular biology to a discipline that had been dominated by a largely biophysical and anatomical approach to the nervous system. Some account of the work of each of these men in their adopted field can be found in various chapters—the efforts of Brenner, Stent, and Levinthal, in particular, are relevant to neural differentiation.

of cells. Such studies require special circumstances in which an individual precursor cell and its progeny can be followed continuously in a living embryo. This is feasible only in a system in which the number of cells is small and in which individual cells can be seen in the microscope from more or less the beginning of development. Several invertebrates meet these requirements. Preeminent is the tiny roundworm *Caenorhabditis elegans*. The small number of cells in the nervous systems of some nematodes was first described by D. Goldschmidt in the 1940s (Chitwood and Chitwood, 1974); the detailed development of *C. elegans* has been pursued by S. Brenner and colleagues (Box B).

Caenorhabditis elegans is a free-living soil organism consisting, in maturity, of 959 somatic cells; some 302 of these cells make up the animal's nervous system (Figure 5). About 550 somatic cells arise during embryogenesis (i.e., from fertilization to hatching). The remainder develop during the larval stage; thus, workers in this field refer to embryonic and postembryonic lineages. Given these small numbers, it has been possible to make a complete library of the animal's construction (including the wiring of the nervous system) by cutting serial electron microscopical sections through the worm and indexing each cell. This herculean task was undertaken by Brenner and a series of colleagues and assistants in the 1960s and 1970s and is now virtually complete (White et al., 1976). A second advantage of this animal is that the embryo is translucent; therefore the divisions of individual cells and their subsequent fates can be followed continuously in the intact organism (Sulston and Horvitz, 1977; Horvitz, 1981). This job has also been largely completed, and the lineage of virtually every somatic cell can now be traced back to the zygote (Figures 5 and 6) (Sulston et al., 1983).

Several aspects of lineage studies in the nematode are probably of

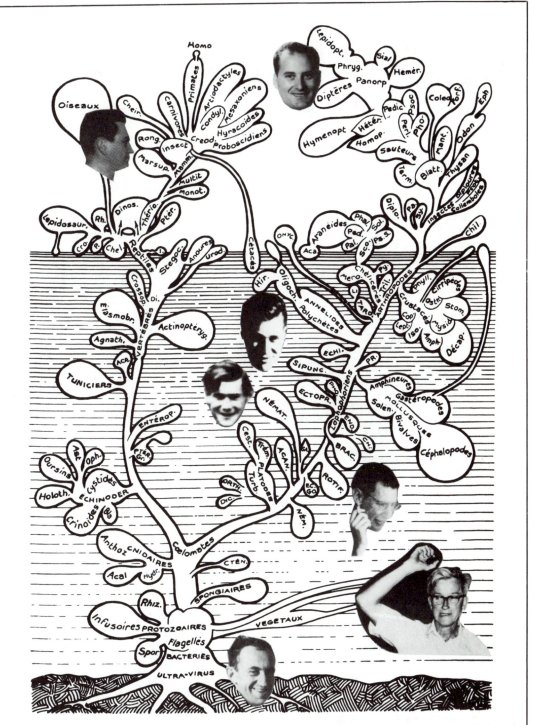

Phyletic tree of molecular biologists. The faces, from top to bottom, are S. Benzer, M. Nirenberg, G. Stent, S. Brenner, M. Delbrück, C. Levinthal, and J. Adler. (Courtesy of S. Benzer.)

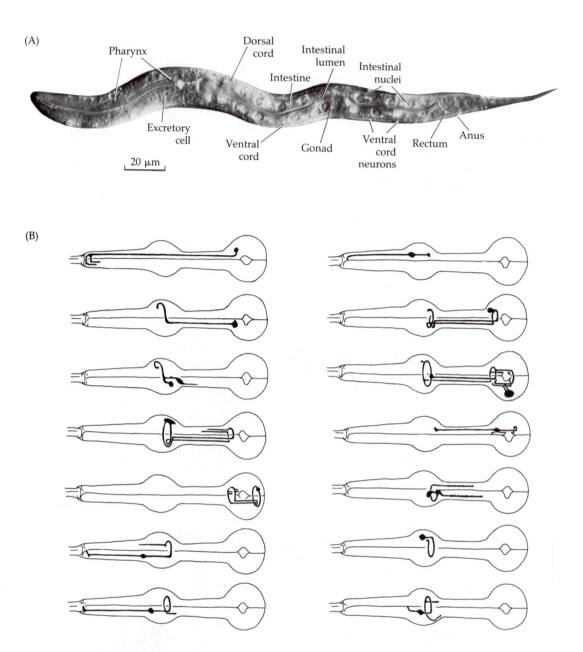

(A)

Pharynx

Dorsal
cord

Intestinal
lumen

Intestinal
nuclei

Intestine

Excretory
cell

Ventral
cord

Gonad

Ventral
cord
neurons

Rectum

Anus

20 μm

(B)

FIGURE 5. *Cell by cell reconstruction of the round-worm* Caenorhabditis elegans. *(A) Photomontage of a young worm seen with Nomarski optics. The advantage of* C. elegans *for detailed developmental studies is that individual cells can be identified and followed directly under the microscope. (B) Serial reconstructions at the electron microscopic level have shown the struc-ture and connectivity of the entire nervous system. This series of drawings provides reconstructions of all the neurons in the region of the pharynx. The outline is the pharynx (cf. A); each diagram shows a different nerve cell. (A from Sulston and Horvitz, 1977; B after Albertson and Thompson, 1976.)*

general significance. First, the early development of the animal, and of its nervous system in particular, is highly stereotyped at the cellular level (Sulston and Horvitz, 1977; Deppe et al., 1978; Kimble and Hirsh, 1979). In every animal, identified precursors undergo the same sequence of divisions with the same consequences (an exception is the germ line, which seems to obey somewhat different rules; see Kimble, 1981). These divisions are easy to keep track of because each dividing cell gives rise to daughters that line up side by side, usually in the anterior–posterior axis (Figure 6). A second feature of these lineages is the predictable death of certain progeny (Sulston and Horvitz, 1977; Kimble et al., 1979; see also Chalfie et al., 1981, and Chapter 6).

One might expect that cells having a common function in maturity would arise from the same progenitor. However, in *C. elegans*, cells with similar functions share a common lineage (genealogy) rather than a common precursor (Sulston and Horvitz, 1977). To take a specific example, the primary neuroblasts, which are the ancestors of all the nerve cells in the nematode, are located at equally spaced intervals in two rows along the rostrocaudal axis of the worm, one row on each side of the body. In the course of development each neuroblast divides into two daughter cells, one of which is rostral and the other caudal; this process is repeated for their daughters and their daughter's daughters and so on. Cells that have the same function in two different parts of the worm are generally descendants of different cells. However, they have the same lineage. For instance, the functionally homologous cells might be the posterior daughters of the anterior daughters of the anterior daughters of the anterior daughters of the primary neuroblasts (this is actually the lineage of one of the classes of motor neurons that innervate the ventral musculature of the worm; see Figure 6). Thus, to generate similar cells, the same general lineage scheme is played out in each part of the worm.

Worms are, of course, specialized at the head and the tail; and other regions are specialized for sexual function. How does development in these portions of the animal differ from the standard program? The way in which these differences come about seems to be partly by the selective survival or death of particular cells in the stereotyped lineage histories. Thus, a cell line that would have died out in a "standard" lineage is retained in the gonadal regions and contributes to the sex organs (Sulston and Horvitz, 1977).

An important test of the rigidity of such apparently programmatic events is to destroy a particular cell and observe how the fates of its neighbors are affected by the deletion. This can be done with a small laser beam (Sulston and White, 1980). In most cases, the deletion of an individual cell has little effect on the further development of its neighbors, a finding that supports the view that the early developmental program of the worm is highly determined (Sulston and Horvitz, 1977; see also White et al., 1982). In some instances, however, ablation of one cell does alter the fate of its neighbors (Kimble et al., 1979; Sulston and White, 1980; see also Blair, 1983; Taghert et al., 1984). For instance, in

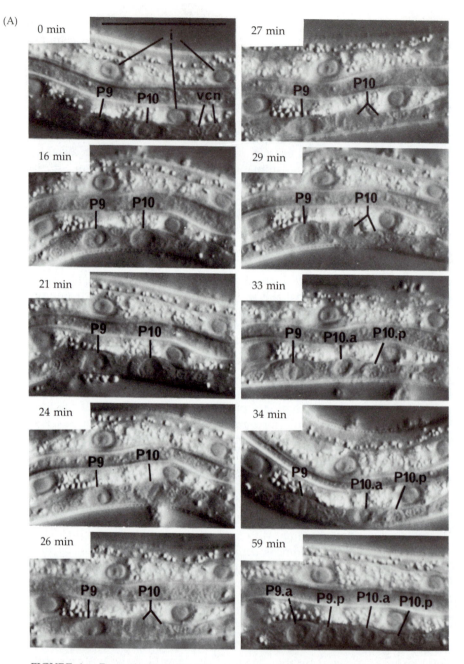

FIGURE 6. *Determination of cell lineages in* C. elegans. *(A) Higher magnification view of a living worm showing, in sequential photomicrographs, cell division of some of the precursor cells that form the ventral nerve cord. The cells labeled P9 and P10 are two neuronal precursor cells that are in the process of division. The daughter cells are designated "a" or "p" according to whether they lie more anteriorly or posteriorly in the worm. i, Intestinal nuclei; vcn, ventral cord nuclei. (B) The entire embryonic lineage of the worm, determined by observing the sequential divisions of individual cells. Labels omitted for clarity. (A from Sulston and Horvitz, 1977; B after Sulston et al., 1983.)*

(B)

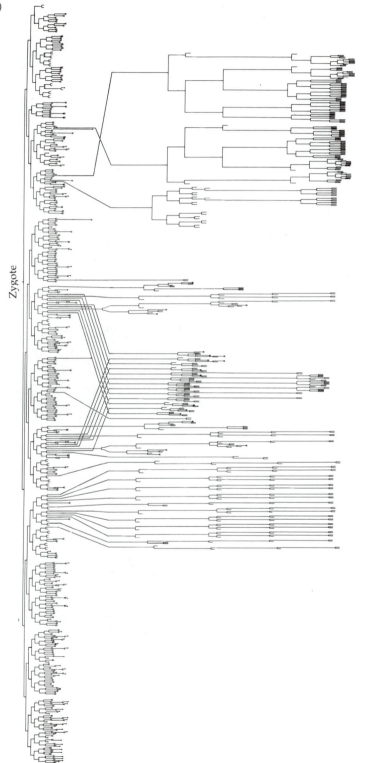

Zygote

some parts of the worm, ablation of a given cell is followed by recruitment of a neighboring cell which adopts the missing cell's fate (the progeny of the original lineage are simply missing in these animals). In these cases there appears to be a hierarchy such that cell Y can replace cell X, but X cannot replace Y. This phenomenon defines so-called equivalence groups in the worm (Kimble, 1981). Interestingly, cells that can replace one another (i.e., equivalence groups) have similar lineages (Kimble et al., 1979). In other instances, ablation of several cells gives rise to proliferation of neighboring cells, even though these do not necessarily replace the missing cell's function (Sulston and Horvitz, 1981). Finally, in at least one case ablation causes the remaining cells to change the polarity of their divisions (e.g., from anterior–posterior to medial–lateral). All this suggests that, even in worms, developing cells have some flexibility.

Lineage studies have also been carried out in a number of other invertebrates, notably the grasshopper (Figure 7) (Goodman and Spitzer, 1979) and the leech (Weisblat et al., 1980; Weisblat, 1981). In both instances, the neurons and their precursors have the additional advantage of being large enough to be impaled with microelectrodes

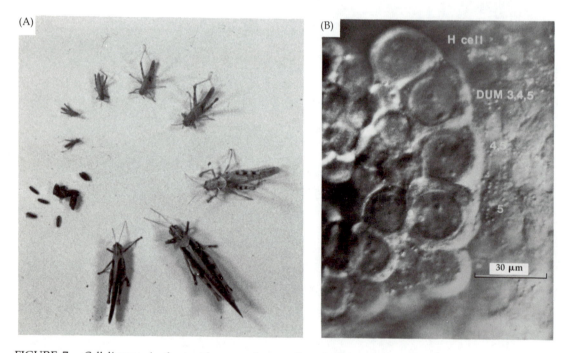

FIGURE 7. *Cell lineages in the grasshopper embryo* (Schistocerca nitens). *(A) Development of the grasshopper egg to hatching takes approximately 20 days; there are then 5 larval instars. Adults (bottom) are sexually dimorphic (the smaller insect is the male). (B) Nomarski photomicrograph of the cell bodies of several identified neurons (DUM, H) in the metathoracic ganglion of a living 14-day-old embryo. These neurons arise from a series of asymmetric mitoses of a single neuroblast, a style that is different from cell division in C. elegans. Unlike neurons in the worm, the grasshopper neural cells are large enough to be impaled with microelectrodes. (A courtesy of N. Spitzer; B from Goodman and Spitzer, 1980.)*

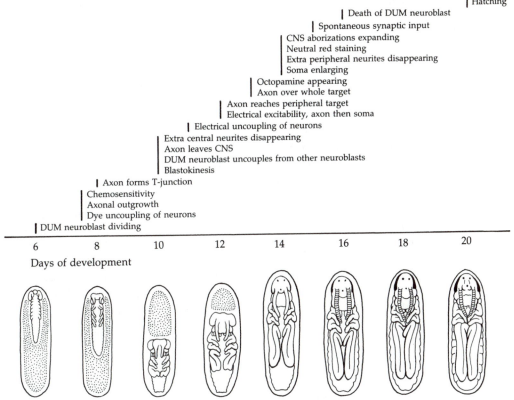

| Death of DUM neuroblast
| Spontaneous synaptic input
| CNS aborizations expanding
| Neutral red staining
| Extra peripheral neurites disappearing
| Soma enlarging
| Octopamine appearing
| Axon over whole target
| Axon reaches peripheral target
| Electrical excitability, axon then soma
| Electrical uncoupling of neurons
| Extra central neurites disappearing
| Axon leaves CNS
| DUM neuroblast uncouples from other neuroblasts
| Blastokinesis
| Axon forms T-junction
| Chemosensitivity
| Axonal outgrowth
| Dye uncoupling of neurons
| DUM neuroblast dividing

| | | | | | | | |
| 6 | 8 | 10 | 12 | 14 | 16 | 18 | 20 |

Days of development

FIGURE 8. *Developmental timetable for the dorsal unpaired median (DUM) neurons in the grasshopper. The first appearance of a phenotypic feature in these neurons is indicated by a vertical bar. (After Goodman and Spitzer, 1979.)*

(this is not possible in *C. elegans*). In the grasshopper, the size of developing neurons has facilitated studies of developmental events such as electrical coupling, electrical excitability, and chemosensitivity in both precursor cells and their descendants (Figure 8) (Spitzer, 1979, 1982; Goodman and Spitzer, 1980, 1981a–c; Goodman, 1982a; see also following sections). It has been possible to determine when these changes occur and whether they are correlated with any particular stage or phenonomen during development.

In general, these studies of lineage underscore the relatively stereotyped and programmatic development of invertebrates. Invertebrate cells seem to differentiate nearly immediately—after all, they have only a few divisions in which to create the finished product (see Figure 6B). Consistent with rapid differentiation is the obvious mosaicism of invertebrate eggs (Chapter 1) and the limited ability of invertebrate embryos to replace missing cell lines following ablation. A variety of experiments and observations on developing vertebrates (e.g., egg ligation, nuclear transplantation, induction, the creation of chimeras) indicate that cells at early stages have a much broader range of potential fates. This raises the interesting question of whether vertebrates and invertebrates are fundamentally different in this respect.

Acquisition of transmitter properties

A number of differentiated neuronal properties are sufficiently important for the function of mature nerve cells to have become the objects of study in their own right.

One series of such studies has focused on the factors that influence the choice of neuronal transmitter. That the local environment can affect the differentiation of neurons in this respect was shown in experiments carried out by N. LeDouarin and her colleagues in the early 1970s (LeDouarin and Teillet, 1974; LeDouarin, 1980, 1982). These workers took advantage of the fact that the neural crest cells of quail and chick can be distinguished by differences in nucleolar size and staining properties (Figure 9). LeDouarin and M.-A. Teillet transplanted portions of neural crest from one rostrocaudal level of quail to a different level in a chick host; they then determined the fate of the heterotopic transplants at later developmental times and compared them to control (homotopic) transplants (Figure 10). Neural crest cells give rise to a number of neural and nonneural derivatives, including sympathetic and parasympathetic autonomic ganglia (Chapter 1). Although these broad divisions of the

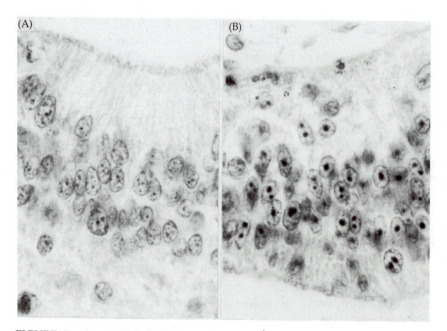

FIGURE 9. *Morphological differences between chick and quail cells can be used to asssess the fate of interspecies neural crest transplants. Chick cells (A) have less prominent nucleoli than quail cells (B) when stained by the Feulgen technique. These photomicrographs were made from the mesencephalon of 7-day-old embryos. ×720. (Courtesy of N. LeDouarin.)*

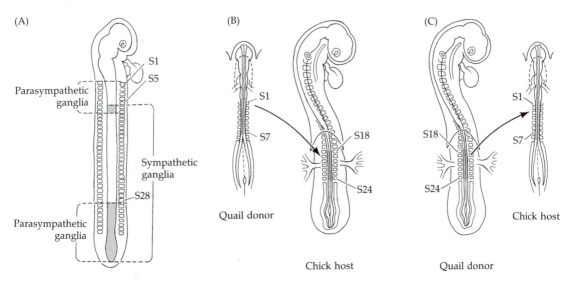

FIGURE 10. *Diagram of transplantation experiments between quail donors and chick embryo hosts to determine the influence of the local environment on neural crest development. (A) Diagram of the origins of different groups of autonomic neurons from the neural crest. The upper (vagal) levels of the crest (somites 1–5) give rise only to parasympathetic (cholinergic) gut ganglia. Intermediate levels of crest (somites 8–28) generate only sympathetic (adrenergic) ganglia. The filled in regions of crest give rise to both sympathetic and parasympathetic ganglia. (B) The cephalic neural primordium from a quail donor can be transplanted heterotopically to the adrenal medullary level of the chick neural axis. (C)*

Conversely, the adrenal medullary neural primordium of a quail can be transplanted to the vagal region of a chick host. Because crest cells destined to form autonomic ganglia from cephalic and adrenomedullary regions normally elaborate different neurotransmitters, such experiments test whether neural crest from different levels is preordained to differentiate in a certain way, or whether the environment influences transmitter choice. The different sizes of donor and host reflect embryonic age; because development proceeds rostrocaudally, the adrenal crest develops later than the vagal crest. S, Somite. (After LeDouarin, 1980.)

autonomic system do not bear very close scrutiny, one general rule is that most sympathetic ganglion cells are adrenergic (and therefore contain the synthetic enzymes for norepinephrine), whereas parasympathetic ganglion cells are cholinergic and thus have a different set of transmitter enzymes. Because these two neuronal classes come from the same tissue (the neural crest), a natural question is whether different parts of the crest are regionally differentiated from an early stage or whether the differentiation of crest cells into sympathetic and parasympathetic neurons is influenced by destination or migratory route. In both chick and quail, the so-called vagal region (the first seven somites) gives rise to the parasympathetic ganglia of the gut, which are cholinergic. The ganglion cells of the sympathetic chain, on the other hand, arise from trunk neural crest and are adrenergic in maturity. When sympathetic trunk crest from the quail is transplanted to the vagal region of a chick host (Figure 10C), the transplanted crest gives rise to cholinergic ganglia that arrive at their destination by a migratory route characteristic of the vagal neural crest. Thus, crest that would ordinarily have generated sympathetic (adrenergic) ganglia now forms parasympathetic (cholinergic) ganglia; conversely, when vagal crest from the quail is transplanted to the chick trunk, the tranplanted neural crest gives rise to adrenergic ganglion cells.

These results from surgically constructed chick–quail chimeras could be interpreted in two ways. One possibility is that the environment of relatively undifferentiated precursor cells instructs the developing neuron regarding its future transmitter; alternatively, neural crest might comprise different classes of precursor cells whose survival is differentially affected by the respective environments after transplantation. In this case the effect would be permissive rather than instructive: the environment would not have influenced the differentiation of individual cells but rather would have selected among previously determined populations.

Experiments in tissue culture carried out in several laboratories have made clear that environmental factors can influence the differentiation of individual ganglion cells or their precursors (Patterson, 1978; Bunge et al., 1978). The work in tissue culture depended on a series of technical advances in the early 1970s that allowed sympathetic ganglion cells from late embryos to be dissociated and grown for several weeks or longer in vitro (Mains and Patterson, 1973). That transmitter choice might be malleable in relatively late stage (postmitotic) nerve cells was suggested by the observation that the cholinergic–adrenergic balance in neuronal cultures could be shifted without changing the number of nerve cells present (Patterson and Chun, 1974, 1977; see also Johnson et al., 1976). Different stimuli can initiate this switching: the cholinergic–adrenergic balance of cells in culture can be shifted by changing the concentration of serum added to the culture medium and by adding culture medium derived from fluid that has been in contact with several types of nonneuronal cells (Patterson and Chun, 1977; Patterson, 1978). For example, medium from a culture of heart cells has a dose-dependent effect on the transmitter content of cultured sympathetic neurons (Figure 11). Morphological observations also indicate that cultured neurons can undergo a transition in transmitter synthesis (Figure 12) (Landis, 1976, 1980; Bunge et al., 1978).

Unimpeachable evidence that transmitter choice occurs in individual neurons was provided by actually following this cellular decision over time in single cultured neurons (Furshpan et al., 1976; Reichardt and Patterson, 1977; Potter et al., 1981). In these experiments, very small numbers of ganglion cells were cultured in microwells or on islands of heart cells (Figure 13). In some of these cases, a single neuron survived and was able to innervate the heart cells. E. J. Furshpan, D. D. Potter, and their colleagues could then study the transmitter function of these solitary cells over several weeks by means of intracellular recording and various pharmacological tests. They observed a number of instances in which isolated neurons switched from adrenergic to cholinergic transmission under the influence of medium conditioned by heart cells; individual cells actually passed through a stage in which both acetyl-

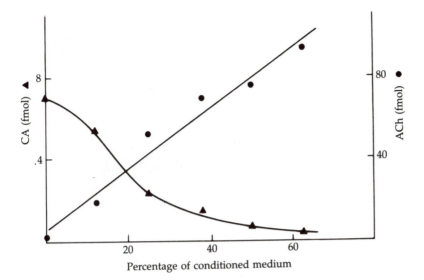

FIGURE 11.   *The effect of heart-conditioned medium on the choice of neurotransmitter in sympathetic neurons maintained in culture. Sympathetic ganglion cells from late embryonic rats were maintained in culture for 20 days. On the second day, and every second day thereafter, fresh medium was added to the cultures. The amount of conditioned medium mixed with fresh medium varied from about 10 to about 62 percent (as indicated on the abscissa). On day 20, the cultures were incubated with labeled choline and tyrosine to determine their ability to synthesize radioactive acetylcholine (ACh) and catecholamines (CA). Those cultures maintained in high concentrations of conditioned medium synthesized smaller amounts of catecholamines (▲) and larger amounts of acetylcholine (●) than cultures maintained in lower concentrations of conditioned medium. The number of surviving cells does not vary as a function of the amount of conditioned medium supplied. (After Patterson and Chun, 1977.)*

choline and norepinephrine were released (Figure 13). This noradrenergic to cholinergic transition appears to be the usual life history of the relatively few neurons in sympathetic ganglia that are cholinergic in maturity (Landis and Keefe, 1983; see also Jonakait et al., 1979). Thus these neurons not only have the capacity to change phenotypes but at least some of them use this ability in normal development.

Although a variety of stimuli can influence autonomic transmitter choice, the fact that certain nonneural cells such as cardiac myocytes induce cholinergic expression presents a prima facie case for the influence of normal target cells on the transmitter choice of the neurons that innervate them (Patterson and Chun, 1977; Hawrot, 1980). The circumstances of culture provide a better chance of determining the signals that influence this choice than does the in vivo circumstance of chick–quail chimeras. A major effort is underway to characterize the relevant molecule from cardiac myocytes; so far, a 45-kilodalton protein has been purified approximately a million fold from serum-free conditioned medium (Fukada, 1983; see also Weber, 1981; Weber and Le Van Thai, 1982).

Whatever the outcome of studies aimed at further defining the

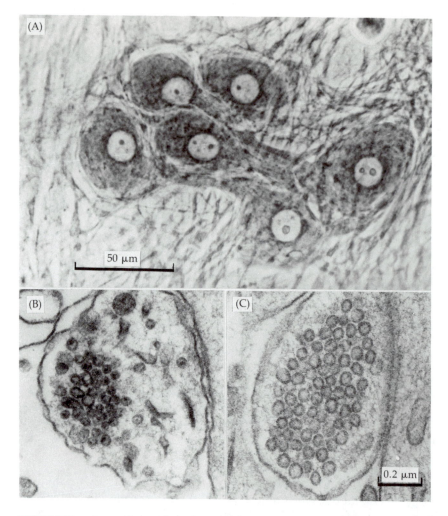

FIGURE 12. *Anatomical evidence for a shift from adrenergic to cholinergic transmitter function in cultures of neonatal rat sympathetic neurons. (A) Light micrograph of a cluster of six sympathetic neurons after 1 month in culture. (B) Electron micrograph of synaptic vesicles in a similar preparation after 1 week in culture; the cells were incubated in norepinephrine and fixed with potassium permanganate. When treated in this way, most vesicles contain dense cores indicative of adrenergic transmission. (C) Synaptic vesicles in another preparation after 4 weeks in culture; the neurons were treated in the same manner as the cells in B. These vesicles lack dense cores and are typical of vesicles found in cholinergic nerve endings. (Courtesy of R. Bunge.)*

agents in conditioned medium that influence transmitter choice, in normal development a number of other factors almost certainly operate in this decision. For example, electrical activity in cultured sympathetic neurons exerts a stabilizing influence on the initial noradrenergic phenotype: neurons made active in culture are less susceptible to the cholinergic switching influence of heart-conditioned medium (Walicke et

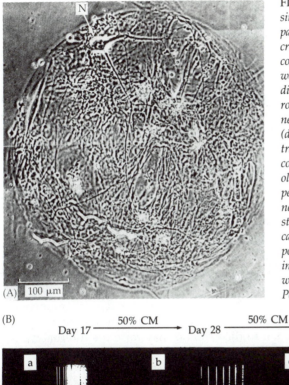

FIGURE 13. *Electrophysiological evidence for a transition of transmitter function in an individual rat sympathetic neuron in microculture. (A) Phase-contrast micrograph of a microculture of cardiac myocytes containing a single sympathetic neuron (N) after 2–3 weeks. (B) Repeated electrophysiologic records from cardiac myocytes contacted by the processes of such a neuron indicate a transition from the secretion of norepinephrine (day 17) to the secretion of acetylcholine alone (day 62). At the outset, stimulation of the neuron (lower trace) excites the cardiac myocytes (a), an effect that is completely blocked by the adrenergic inhibitor propranolol (not shown). The neuron was then cultured in 50 percent conditioned medium (CM) to induce a cholinergic transition. At 28 days in culture, intracellular stimulation of the neuron produces a dual effect on cardiac myocytes, first inhibiting them (slight hyperpolarization) and then exciting them (b). After 62 days in culture, stimulation of the neuron inhibited myocytes without evidence of subsequent excitation (c). (A from Potter et al., 1980; B after Potter et al., 1981.)*

(B)

Day 17 $\xrightarrow{\text{50\% CM}}$ Day 28 $\xrightarrow{\text{50\% CM}}$ Day 62

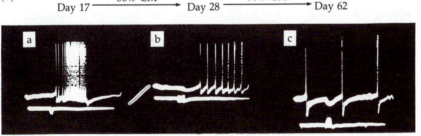

al., 1977). The role of electrical activity in the normal development of sympathetic ganglia remains uncertain. Another factor that is likely to have an influence on normal transmitter choice, at least to judge from effects in tissue culture, is the prescence of glucocorticoid hormones. These hormones affect transmitter choice indirectly by inhibiting the synthesis and/or release of the putative cholinergic factor produced by heart cells (Fukada, 1980; see also McLennan et al., 1980; Jonakait et al., 1980). Another remarkable effect of glucocorticoid hormones on developing autonomic ganglia is their ability to increase the numbers of small intensely fluorescent (SIF) cells in sympathetic ganglia (Eränkö et al., 1972; Doupe and Patterson, 1984a,b). Depending on the concentration of glucocorticoids, SIF cells secrete different transmitters; this observation provides further evidence for the importance of hormones in the determination of neuronal phenotype.

The evidence on transmitter choice argues persuasively for an epigenetic influence on at least this aspect of neuronal differentiation. On the other hand, the interplay of activity, hormonal influences, and factors elaborated by neuronal targets suggest a complex regulatory scheme. The most important lesson of this work is that some aspects of neuronal fate are clearly regulated by the cell's environment.

Differentiation of electrical excitability

Another aspect of neuronal differentiation that has been studied in some detail is the acquisition of the characteristic ion channels that support signaling. This issue has been explored by a number of people, perhaps most thoroughly by N. C. Spitzer and his colleagues who have focused on the Rohon-Beard cells of amphibian embryos (Spitzer, 1979, 1981, 1982). These sensory neurons are present in the spinal cords of a variety of lower vertebrate larvae but disappear after metamorphosis. A particular advantage of Rohon-Beard cells is that they arise in the gastrula and can be easily recognized in the early neurula (Lamborghini, 1980).

Rohon-Beard cells are initially electrically inexcitable but generate a peculiar form of electrical response during the early tailbud stage (Figure 14): depolarization of the cell body gives rise to a prolonged overshooting plateau, which may last several hundred milliseconds (Spitzer, 1979, 1981, 1982). The inward current responsible for this phenomenon is carried by calcium. Because of the prolonged plateau, a relatively large amount of calcium gets into the cell and may raise the internal calcium concentration by as much as a hundredfold (from about 10^{-7} to 10^{-5} M). However, between the early tailbud and the early larval stages, the action potential changes so that the plateau is preceded by an initial spike that lasts only a few milliseconds (Figure 14). This spike is produced by a sodium current. In the end, the cells have an action potential that is wholly Na^+-dependent. Because the Rohon-Beard cells ultimately disappear in amphibian larvae, the observations necessarily end at this stage. Nonetheless, they show that these nerve cells are initially activated by voltage-sensitive Ca^{2+} channels; this early property is then gradually replaced by the sodium conductance mechanisms characteristic of most mature nerve cells. Studies of vertebrate neurons in culture confirm this view (Spitzer and Lamborghini, 1976; Spitzer, 1979; Willard, 1980).

Similar studies of developing skeletal and cardiac muscles suggest that a gradual transition from calcium-dependent to sodium-dependent action potentials may be a rather general feature of excitable cells during development (Kano, 1975; Spitzer, 1979, 1982). The purpose of this transition is not clear, although some evidence suggests that long-lasting depolarization can effectively uncouple embryonic cells for short periods (Spitzer, 1982). Because Ca^{2+} often serves as an intracellular messenger or activator, prolonged action potentials may play a role in modifying the metabolism of embryonic neurons. Whatever its significance, the transition from calcium to sodium is not universal. For example, action potentials in developing grasshopper neurons are initially supported by either Ca^{2+} or Na^+ but later require both ions (Goodman and Spitzer, 1979, 1981a-c; see also Bader et al., 1983).

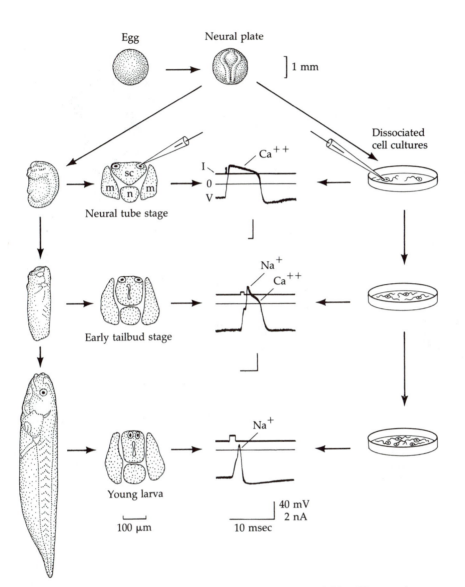

FIGURE 14. *The development of the action potential in amphibian* (Xenopus) *neurons. Intracellular records from cultured neurons prepared from the neural plate stage (right) show a gradual change in the ionic dependence of the impulse from calcium to sodium. Similar records from Rohon-Beard neurons in intact* Xenopus *larvae (left) show the same transition over time. I, Current injection; 0, 0 membrane potential level; V, intracellular recording of membrane voltage; sc, spinal cord; m, myotome; n, notochord. (After Spitzer, 1981.)*

Differentiation of neuronal form

One of the most striking characteristics of differentiated neurons is the immense diversity of their dendritic branching patterns. Indeed, much of the work of classical anatomists involved categorizing neurons ac-

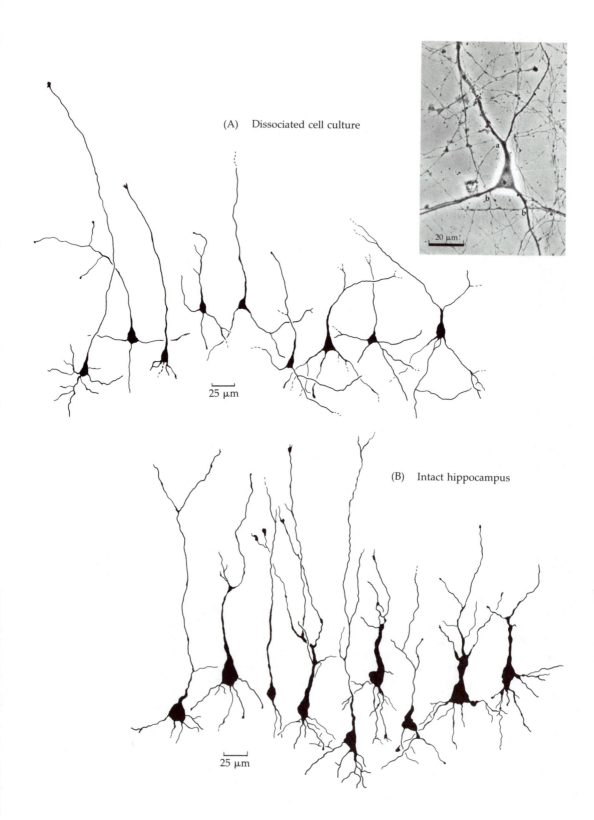

(A) Dissociated cell culture

20 μm

25 μm

(B) Intact hippocampus

25 μm

◄ FIGURE 15. *Evidence for some intrinsic determination of neuronal shape. Camera lucida drawings of cultured hippocampal neurons after 1 week in culture (A) compared to similar drawings of Golgi-impregnated neurons from the hippocampus of 4-day-old rats (B). Upon dissociation, the branches of the neurons are amputated; moreover, these neurons in 18-day fetuses (the time of removal for culture) have only begun to send out processes. Nonetheless, in culture the cells grow to resemble a normal hippocampal pyramidal neuron with a triangular soma, one large process extending from the apex of the cell body (analogous to the apical dendrite), and several smaller processes that emerge from the opposite pole and resemble the basal dendrites. Inset is a phase-contrast photomicrograph of one such cultured neuron (a, putative apical dendrite; b, putative basal dendrites). Because the cultured neurons were taken from 18-day fetuses, the age of the cells in vitro and in vivo are roughly the same. (From Banker and Cowan, 1979.)*

cording to their shape. Although each neuron has a unique branching pattern (think of individual trees), different classes of neurons tend to have similar geometries (think of oaks and maples). Are class-specific differences in neuronal geometry the result of systematically different extrinsic influences, or does neuronal geometry reflect some intrinsic similarity of the neurons in a given class?

One sort of experiment designed to test an intrinsic basis for branching patterns involves placing developing neurons in tissue culture to ask whether they then elaborate branches typical of their geometry in vivo. Neurons do elaborate, even in the limited circumstances of a two-dimensional culture dish, processes that have some of the characteristics of their in vivo morphology. When neurons are dissociated in preparation for culture, most or all of their processes are lost. In spite of this, sensory ganglion cells become largely unipolar in culture (Scott et al., 1969), motor neurons become multipolar (Fischbach, 1970), and pyramidal cells from cerebral cortex and hippocampus elaborate processes typical of pyramidal cells (Figure 15) (Dichter, 1978; Banker and Cowan, 1979; Kriegstein and Dichter, 1983). Another approach to the genesis of neuronal form is to examine the shapes of neurons with the same genotype. The geometries of equivalent neurons from isogenic animals are very similar but are not identical (Figure 16) (Levinthal et al., 1975; Goodman, 1982b).

On the face of it, these several results suggest that neuronal shape is the product of both intrinsic and extrinsic influences. Nerve cells that are nominally from the same class show broad similarities of shape when challenged in tissue culture; on the other hand, neurons with identical genotypes are not isomorphic. This is not surprising. Maples and oaks show obvious class-specific differences that are presumably intrinsic; yet the shape of individual trees varies widely as a function of nutrition, available moisture, sunlight, and so on. There is no reason to believe that neurons are much different.

CONCLUSIONS

The progressive specialization of cell types arises from complex interactions between genetic instructions, influences arising from the cell cytoplasm, and influences from the extracellular environment. Dissect-

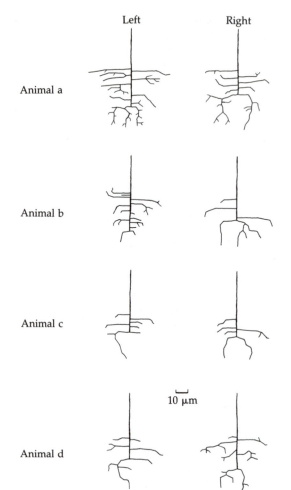

Left   Right

Animal a

Animal b

Animal c

10 μm

Animal d

FIGURE 16. *Dendritic branching patterns of the homologous neurons on the left and right sides of the optic ganglion neuropil in four water fleas (Daphnia magna). Because these fleas were produced by parthenogenesis, the genetic compositions of all of the animals are presumably the same. The variability in pattern between the left and right sides of the same animal, and between the same neuron among isogenic animals (a–d), indicates that the detailed branching pattern of individual neurons is not under strict genetic control. (After Levinthal et al., 1975.)*

ing the relative contributions from each of these categories for any particular feature is a difficult business. An important generalization is that for a long period during development, and perhaps throughout life, differentiating cells retain the entire set of genetic instructions. Normally, however, a gradual restriction of gene expression causes cells to become more and more specialized. As far as one knows, these ideas about cell differentiation apply equally to developing neurons.

In vertebrates, the phenomenon of induction shows that neighboring cells and tissues are important determinants of cell fate. Changing the environment of a cell (by transplantation, for example) often alters what it becomes. In invertebrates, on the other hand, studies of cell lineage indicate that cell fate depends much more heavily on mitotic history. Perhaps this difference between invertebrates and vertebrates reflects a more rigid developmental strategy appropriate to the generation of relatively simple animals, and a more flexible strategy appropriate to more complex animals.

Pattern and Positional Information

INTRODUCTION

Many features of development—regional differentiation of tissues, stereotyped movements of cells, emergence of the characteristic shape of various parts of the embryo, the highly organized outgrowth of nerves to targets—suggest that cellular information about position dictates pattern. Because morphogenesis and neurogenesis are inextricably linked, the influences of such information probably apply equally to neural and nonneural tissues. The purpose of this chapter is to review the evidence for the existence of positional information during development, and to consider its effect on differentiation.

QUEST FOR AN ORGANIZING
PRINCIPLE IN EMBRYONIC DEVELOPMENT

The quest for the principles that dictate embryonic form goes back at least a century. H. Driesch's demonstration that separated blastomeres can develop into complete embryos (Chapter 1) suggested that a cell's fate depends on its context. Although Driesch abandoned research, H. Spemann and others took up the challenge of how embryonic cells influence one another as the centerpiece of their scientific careers (see Box A). Spemann began studying development in amphibians just after the turn of the century by separating blastomeres with a human hair cinched around one of the first cleavage furrows (see Figure 2 in Chapter 1). When the tie was made in a cleavage furrow in the median plane each cell gave rise to a full embryo, as Driesch had described in the sea urchin. When, however, the ligature coincided with the dorsoventral plane of the embryo, only the dorsal cell developed into a whole animal (Chapter 2). The determinant of embryogenesis or involution was evidently the inclusion of the gray crescent. Because the gray crescent defines the future position of the dorsal lip of the blastopore, Spemann supposed that this region might be particularly important for the formation of a complete embryo. He suggested that these results signified the action of a "center of differentiation" that organized embryonic form in surrounding tissues (Willier and Oppenheimer, 1974). In apparent

Hans Spemann (1869–1941)

Hans Spemann was born in Stuttgart in 1869 and studied medicine at Heidelberg and Munich before he abandoned this career for zoology. He graduated from the University of Würzburg in 1895, and in 1898 he became a lecturer in the zoology department. He remained at Würzburg until 1909, when he accepted a job as chairman of zoology at Rostock. In 1914 he was named associate director of the Kaiser Wilhelm Institute of Biology in the Berlin suburb of Dahlem; finally he became chairman of zoology at the University of Freiburg, where he worked from 1919 until his retirement in 1937.

Spemann, who felt that "my strongest inclination and talents are a combination of inquiry into general problems and technical invention" (Hamburger, 1969), worked on three issues united by the theme of early embryonic organization (Hamburger, 1981). His experiments began around the turn of the century in a rather derivative way: he pursued the egg constriction experiments that had nominally settled the famous Roux–Driesch controversy (Chapter 1). However, his more complete observations on the actual events of egg cleavage went far beyond earlier studies and contributed importantly to several embryological issues (Chapters 1, 2, and 3). This work laid the foundation for understanding embryonic duplications and led to the realization that the formation of a normal embryo depends initially on the dorsal region of the egg and its organizing potential. At the same time, Spemann developed a variety of difficult microsurgical methods, which became his technical trademark.

The second phase of his work occupied the period 1904–1912, during which he turned to a series of experiments on lens induction (Chapter 2). This work established another important principle: certain tissues will not differentiate by themselves but require a stimulus from adjacent tissues.

The third period of Spemann's work, generally regarded as his most important, involved investigations of the "organizer." The crucial experiments in these years were carried out by Hilde Proescholdt, a doctoral student. In this work a small piece of the upper blastoporal lip of a salamander gastrula was transplanted into a relatively indifferent region of another embryo. The remarkable ability of this tissue to

confirmation of this idea, Spemann discovered that most pieces of newt embryos, when transplanted at the early gastrula stage, integrated into their surroundings and developed according to their new position in the host. An exception, however, was the dorsal lip of the blastopore. In this case, a variety of unexpected tissues such as neural plate, neural tube, notochord, and somites were induced in the region of the transplant. Some of these evidently came from the host and some from the donor (Spemann, 1938). Clearly, the transplanted dorsal lip of the blastopore had the capacity to cause considerable deviation from the normal developmental plan (Figure 1).

The use of a pigmented donor and an unpigmented host allowed Spemann and his graduate student H. Mangold to identify the origin of the tissues in the secondary embryos that sometimes arose after transplantation of the dorsal lip (Spemann and Mangold, 1924; see also Gimlich and Cooke, 1983; Smith and Slack, 1983; Jacobson, 1984). In

induce reasonably well formed parts of a second embryo was taken as a dramatic demonstration of the organizational powers of a developmental "center." Unfortunately, Hilde Proescholdt (who subsequently married and published under the name of Mangold) died in an accident (an explosion in her kitchen) at the age of 26, at about the time of the publication of her classic paper with Spemann (Spemann and Mangold, 1924). Although Spemann's name precedes Mangold's, the paper was essentially her doctoral thesis.

The understanding of embryonic organization in the general sense that Spemann sought is little more advanced today than it was 50 years ago when Spemann was awarded the Nobel prize for this work in 1935. In spite of this lack of progress, Spemann's contributions were of the greatest importance. The appreciation of regulation and induction in embryonic development grew directly out of his work; these remain important principles, which are now being explored at the cellular level. Equally important, Spemann taught his microsurgical techniques to a series of zealous students including V. Hamburger, the Mangolds, J. Holtfreter, O. Schotté, and others, thus providing the next generation of experimental embryologists. His precise technical and intellectual style made this field one of the most exciting areas of biology in the early twentieth century.

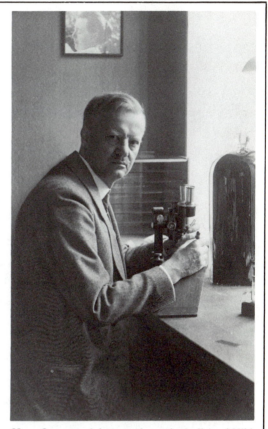

Hans Spemann (photograph on the wall is of Hilde Mangold). (Courtesy of V. Hamburger.)

general, some of the tissues in the secondary embryos were derived from the host and others from the graft; in particular, the mesoderm around the notochord was often grafted tissue, whereas the nervous system usually arose from the host. From these observations, Spemann and Mangold (1924) generalized that the dorsal lip of the blastopore was "the region of the embryo that has preceded the other parts in determination and thereupon emanates determination effects of a certain quantity in certain directions." In short, they saw this bit of tissue as having special properties that were in some way capable of organizing embryonic form.

Although this work was the basis of Spemann's Nobel prize in 1935, the mechanism of the organizing effects of the dorsal lip is still not clear. J. F. K. Holtfreter, a student of Spemann's and subsequently a central figure in his own right (see Box A in Chapter 4), later found that other tissues were just as good "organizers" as the lip of the

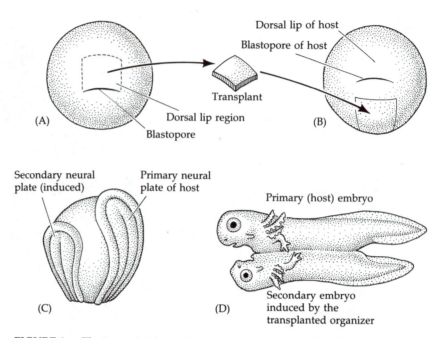

FIGURE 1. *The "organizer" experiment carried out in the early 1920s by H. Spemann and H. Mangold. Transplantation of the upper lip of the blastopore from one amphibian gastrula to another (A,B) often led to the induction of a second neural plate (C). In some instances an entire secondary embryo formed on the flank of the host (D). The ability of the upper lip of the blastopore to induce the formation of a secondary embryo suggested that this piece of tissue organized development in some fairly general way. (After Hamburger, 1963.)*

blastopore. Thus, a number of tissues from both vertebrates and invertebrates can induce complex structures, even after they are boiled or fixed (Holtfreter, 1933); indeed, steroids (Needham et al., 1934), organic acids (Lehmann, 1938), RNA (Niu, 1958), other organic compounds (Saxen and Toivonen, 1962) and even cotton plugs soaked in turpentine (Holtfreter, 1933) are all capable of "organizer" effects in early embryos.

In spite of this lack of specificity, groups in Finland, Japan, and Germany have obtained results that may reflect some aspects of the normal chemical signals that influence early embryonic form. The Finnish group, led by S. Toivonen, concluded that two factors (a "neuralizing" and a "mesodermalizing" agent isolated from bone marrow) are involved in producing inductive effects (Nakamura and Toivonen, 1978). H. Tiedemann and his group in Germany have purified from chick embryos a protein that induces complex mesodermal structures (notochord, somites) and another that induces cephalic structures (forebrain, eyes) (Tiedemann, 1968). Together these two agents stimulate the formation of posterior brain parts and spinal cord. However, no consensus about the nature of normal inducers has yet emerged (Nakamura and Toivonen, 1978).

Because of the failure of his successors to unravel the molecular biology of the "organizer," Spemann is sometimes accused of having advocated an organizational principle where none exists (at least in any simple sense). However, Spemann was well aware that the development of embryonic form is the result of complex interactive phenomena that can be perturbed in a variety of ways. "For the moment it is of little significance," he wrote in his paper with Mangold in 1924, "whether the concept of 'organizer' or 'organization center' will still be appropriate with more advanced analysis, or whether [these terms] should be replaced by others." In retrospect, the organizer experiment established the importance of the epigenetic influences on embryonic development and extended the concept of induction from cellular differentiation to the genesis of supracellular pattern.

COMPENSATORY PHENOMENA IN THE GENESIS OF EMBRYONIC FORM: REGULATION AND MORPHOGENETIC FIELDS

Even if transplantation of the dorsal lip of the blastopore did not yield the organizing principle that some embryologists envisioned, these and related microsurgical experiments carried out in the early part of the century did lead to a further conclusion that is central to modern conceptions of morphogenesis. Following the removal of an embryonic part in vertebrates (for example, excision of part of the neural plate), there is a marked tendency for the surrounding intact portions of the embryo to replace the structures that would have arisen from the excised tissue. For example, O. Mangold (1929; H. Mangold's husband) and later R. G. Harrison (1947) showed that early removal of the portion of the neural plate destined to become the eye and related parts of the amphibian brain is completely compensated for as development proceeds: both eyes and both sides of the brain are normal in late-stage embryos after this surgery. This sort of compensation is called regulation.

Underlying regulation is the notion of morphogenetic fields. A morphogenetic field is defined operationally as an embryonic region, any part of which can give rise to the whole structure later on. For example, the neural plate is the morphogenetic field of the nervous system because removal of the entire neural plate eliminates the nervous system, whereas extirpation of any portion of the neural plate is followed by regulation (i.e., the nervous system develops normally). Similarly, the limb field is the embryonic region that, when extirpated, causes the limb to be missing; any part of the field, however, is capable of forming a whole limb (Figure 2).

As development proceeds, the size of morphogenetic fields decreases in relation to the embryo as a whole. Thus, at the 2-cell stage, as Driesch and Spemann showed, half of the sea urchin or amphibian embryo can sometimes regulate to form an entire animal. Subsequently, more restricted regions of the embryo (such as the neural plate or limb field) constitute morphogenetic fields. At still later embryonic stages,

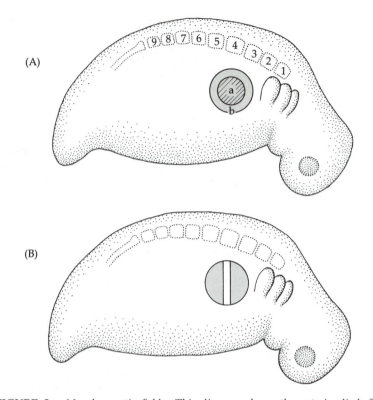

FIGURE 2. *Morphogenetic fields. This diagram shows the anterior limb field of a salamander* (Ambystoma) *embryo. (A) The circle marked b circumscribes the field—if this tissue is removed, the limb will fail to develop. On the other hand, if a part of the field (a) is removed, the remaining tissue will regulate to form a normal limb (numbers indicate somites). (B) If the limb field is split and the two parts are prevented from refusing, each half will regulate so that two limbs develop. Thus, any part of the field is capable of generating the entire structure. As the embryo matures, morphogenetic fields become progressively restricted in the sense that what they give rise to is ever more limited. (After Karp and Berrill, 1981.)*

an early field like the neural plate becomes divided into subfields (such as the forebrain–eye field) (Mangold, 1929; Jacobson, 1959). An ablation within the subfield will be compensated by regulation, but removal of the entire subfield, by definition, will leave a permanent defect (the forebrain and eye will be missing). Conversely, when half the forebrain–eye field is transplanted to another embryo, the eyes and forebrain are duplicated (Alderman, 1935).

In most adult vertebrates, morphogenetic fields become very restrictive indeed. For example, in adult mammals the tips of fingers will regenerate completely, but only if the amputation is distal to the last interphalangeal joint (Borgens, 1982). In man, such regeneration is successful only up to about 11 years of age (Illingworth, 1974; Rosenthal et al., 1979). In general, adult mammals are capable of healing only small defects and then only with limited and imperfect regeneration of the missing structures (see also Chapter 8).

The cellular basis of regulation is not clear. Compensation for missing embryonic parts might occur because the fate of remaining cells is altered or because the remaining cells normally contribute progeny to the entire morphogenetic field. Thus, in cellular terms, a field might simply be a collection of cells that in some mysterious way can substitute for one another; or a field might be a collection of cells that *each* contribute to all of the classes of differentiated cells that will arise from the field. If the latter idea were true, the remaining part of a partially excised morphogenetic field would still differentiate into all the tissues of the field, although the resulting structure might be abnormally small because of the reduced number of progenitors. In fact, the products of regulation (twin embryos induced by ligation of the developing egg, for example) *are* smaller than normal. The prevailing view, however, is that regulation involves altered cell fate as a result of an altered local environment. Whatever the cellular basis of regulation turns out to be, it seems likely that morphogenetic fields become restricted as development continues because of the limited number of cell types that can be generated from progressively more differentiated cells (Chapter 2).

POSITIONAL INFORMATION

The effects of dorsal lip transplantation, evidence for regulation, and the nature of morphogenetic fields all argue for mechanisms that influence differentiation in a coordinated way as a function of cell position. Many recent efforts to understand this phenomenon are based on an analysis of pattern in relatively simple systems. The outcome of these experiments supports in various ways the general idea that developing tissues—the nervous system included—possess information about position that influences the fate of constituent cells. The way in which information about position is encoded and interpreted is a central (and controversial) issue in modern biology.

Evidence for positional information in a one-dimensional system

The reality of positional information is most apparent in simple one- or two-dimensional systems in which cells clearly behave differently as a function of location. Perhaps the simplest of these cases is the blue-green alga *Anabaena*, the cells of which are strung together like beads on a necklace (Wilcox et al., 1973; Mitchison et al., 1976). Although most of the cells along these chains are identical, every fourth or fifth cell is distinct in shape and function (Figure 3). These nondividing cells are called heterocysts and are thought to be important in nitrogen fixation. Simply by observing algal chains, G. J. Mitchison and his collaborators found that heterocysts rarely arise when the daughters of a cell division are within two or three cells of a preexisting heterocyst.

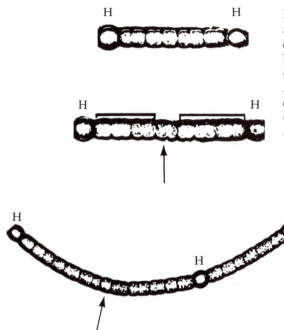

FIGURE 3. *Positional information along a one-dimensional line of cells. Phase-contrast photomicrographs of a growing filament of the blue-green algae Anabaena. The larger cells at intervals are the heterocysts (H); the smaller intervening cells are the vegetative cells. New heterocysts (arrows) are generated from vegetative cell divisions only at a prescribed minimum distance (brackets) from preexisting heterocysts. ×750. (Courtesy of M. Wilcox.)*

This finding implies an inhibitory influence emanating from the heterocysts and extending along the chain. By microsurgical ablation of cells or by breaking the chains into smaller units, Mitchison and his colleagues confirmed this idea. The upshot was a model of heterocyst spacing that involves secretion of an inhibitor that acts on the nearby cells (as well as on the heterocyst itself). Although the model and the arguments for it are somewhat complicated, the observations make a strong case for positional information in this one-dimensional system: the daughters of cells in the chain are somehow informed about their distance from a heterocyst and behave accordingly.

Evidence for positional information in two-dimensional systems

A number of relatively simple two-dimensional systems, such as insect cuticle, also provide fairly direct evidence for the importance of positional information. Many species of insects have striking cuticular patterns. Particularly conspicuous are the familiar eyespots on the wings of some moths and butterflies (Figure 4). B. N. Schwanwitsch in Russia and F. Süffert and A. Kühn in Germany addressed the biological basis of this colorful display early in this century (Schwanwitsch, 1924; Sondhi, 1963). Experiments carried out by H. F. Nijhout suggest that these patterns are best explained by a chemical signal from the eyespot center, a signal that determines the pigment elaborated by surrounding cells as a function of local concentration (i.e., distance from the center of the spot) (Nijhout, 1978, 1980a,b, 1981). In support of this idea, excision of the eyespot center in early pupal stages results in the absence of eyespot pigmentation from the corresponding wing segment. Conversely, transplantation of the eyespot center to an ectopic locus stimulates the development of an eyespot in the surrounding tissue.

Another example of positional information in two dimensions comes from work on the cuticular pattern of the blood-sucking insect *Rhodnius prolixus* (Wigglesworth, 1940). In the 1950s, M. Locke took advantage of the fact that the abdominal segments (tergites) of *Rhodnius* have an array of transverse lines in the adult (Locke, 1959, 1967). By rotating rectangular bits of the cuticle in larvae, Locke showed that there is a local signal in each segment that determines this pattern (this evidence is described later in the section on gradients).

Evidence for positional information in a simple three-dimensional system

Of course one could argue that these examples of positional information in algae or in the cuticle of insects are special cases that do not apply to the more complex topology of developing embryos. Another simple

(A)

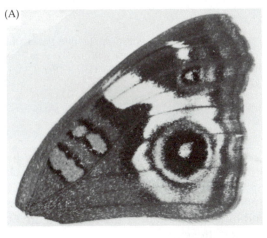

(B)

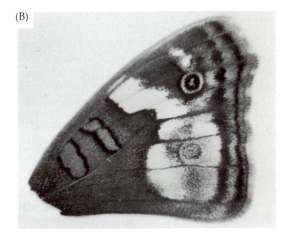

(C)

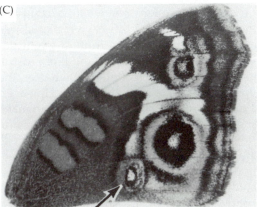

FIGURE 4. *Evidence for positional information in the generation of eyespots on butterfly wings. (A) Eyespots on the dorsal surface of the fore wing of an adult Buckeye butterfly* (Precis coenia). *(B) Ablation of about 300 cells at the presumptive center of the spot in the early pupa inhibits subsequent development of the spot. (C) Transplantation of an extra eyespot focus onto an otherwise intact wing induces the formation of an extra eyespot (arrow). (From Nijhout, 1980b.)*

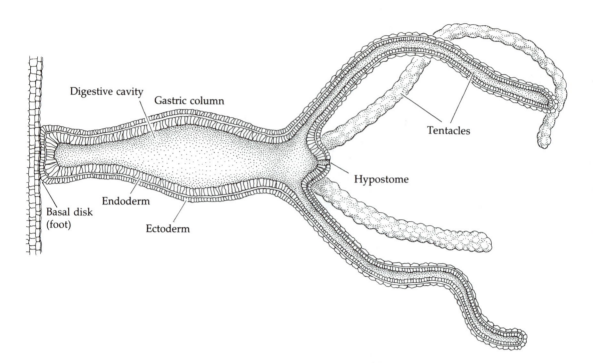

Digestive cavity

Gastric column

Tentacles

Hypostome

Endoderm

Basal disk
(foot)

Ectoderm

FIGURE 5.   *Positional information in a simple three-dimensional system, the freshwater coelenterate called hydra. One end of the hydra is specialized for attachment to a substrate, and the other end is easily distinguished by tentacles. The entire animal comprises only about a dozen cell types. If the animal is cut into pieces, the most rostral part of a fragment will make a new head and the most caudal part a new foot. (After Gierer, 1974.)*

example, the behavior of the coelenterate hydra, provides evidence for positional information in three dimensions and seems in many respects a reasonable analogy for embryonic morphogenesis.

Hydra is a freshwater animal that is basically a tube with a tentacle-ringed mouth at one end and an adhesive foot at the other (Figure 5). Experiments on hydra date back to the eighteenth century, when it was noted that small pieces of the animal rapidly regenerate a complete organism. A. Gierer and others (Gierer, 1974, 1977) have explored this phenomenon in some detail. Pieces of hydra taken from different positions along the body have polarity in the sense that the most rostral portion of a hydra fragment regenerates the rostral end, whereas the foot of the animal develops from the caudal end of the pieces. However, the same piece of tissue that makes a foot in one circumstance can make a head in another, depending on whether it is at the caudal or rostral end of the excised piece. Evidently, the way in which regenerating cells differentiate is determined by their relative position.

The molecular basis of positional information in hydra has been explored by H. C. Schaller and her colleagues, who have separated and partially purified four "morphogens" from a large number of cultured hydra (about 100,000) (Schaller et al., 1979). Two of these activate or inhibit head formation, whereas the others activate or inhibit foot formation. More recently, the amino acid sequence of the head activator has been determined (Schaller and Bodenmüller, 1981). The characterization of this substance depended on the chance discovery that a sea anemone, which is about 10,000 times larger than hydra, contains the same molecule. Even so, 200 kg of anemones were required to isolate 20 μg of activator. Curiously, this 11-amino acid peptide is also produced by the mammalian hypothalamus and intestine (Schaller, 1975; Bodenmüller et al., 1980).

Evidence for positional information in a more complex three-dimensional system: morphogenesis of the vertebrate limb

Obviously, morphogenesis in vertebrate embryos must be a much more complicated affair than differentiation according to position in algae, insect cuticle, or even hydra. In an attempt to simplify these issues in vertebrate development, a great deal of interest has been focused on the morphogenesis of the limb (Figure 6) (Ede et al., 1977; Hinchliffe

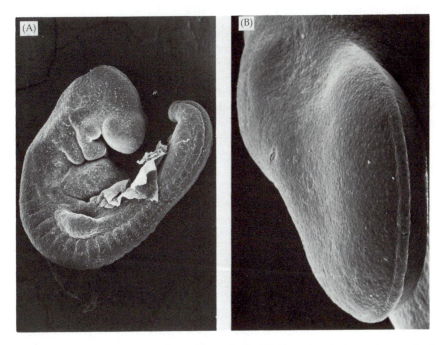

FIGURE 6.   *Development of the vertebrate limb. (A) Scanning electron micrograph of a hamster embryo; the limb bud is the bulge just ventral to the row of somites on the right flank. ×100. (B) As development proceeds, the limb bud becomes more prominent. In this higher power view, the apical ectodermal ridge is evident along the anterior–posterior axis of the limb bud tip. ×300. Excision of this region stops further development of the limb. (From Kelly and Fallon, 1981.)*

and Johnson, 1980; Wallace, 1981; Kelley et al., 1983; Fallon and Caplan, 1983).

The idea that the shape of the limb is regulated by positional information is suggested by the finding that cells in a small region on the posterior margin of the developing limb of chicks control limb polarity in the anteroposterior axis (i.e., the axis of the thumb and little finger in a human hand) (Saunders and Gasseling, 1968; Wolpert, 1978; Summerbell, 1979; see, however, Saunders and Gasseling, 1983). This region is called the zone of polarizing activity, or ZPA. When the ZPA is transplanted from the normal posterior position to an anterior position on another limb bud, the resulting limb is abnormal: the limb is duplicated as a mirror image (Figure 7) (Tickle et al., 1975; Shellswell and Wolpert, 1977). In general, workers in this field have taken these results to mean that the ZPA is the source of a diffusible positional signal (morphogen). In support of this contention, the results of X irradiation to the ZPA suggest that there is a signal that can be attenuated in a graded manner. Thus, when an irradiated ZPA is grafted onto the anterior margin of the limb bud, the most anterior new digit formed falls from digit 4 to 3 to digit 2 as the amount of radiation (and, presumably, damage to the ZPA) increases (Smith et al., 1978).

The zone of polarizing activity at the base of the limb does not seem to influence the proximodistal axis. In this dimension, morphogenesis appears to be dictated by the time that cells spend in the apex of the growing limb bud just beneath the apical ectodermal ridge, a region called the progress zone (see Figures 6 and 7) (Saunders, 1948; Summerbell et al., 1973; Summerbell, 1979). Although the evidence is indirect, the general idea is that cells that leave the progress zone last acquire the most distal positional values. Perhaps the most impressive evidence in this regard is that grafting a young progress zone in place of an older one results in a tandem duplication of distal limb structures (wrist and digits). Similarly, when an older progress zone is grafted onto a younger stump, deletions occur (Summerbell et al., 1973).

As with other highly interactive developmental phenomena, untangling the cellular and molecular basis of limb morphogenesis will be difficult at best. The story has some of the same qualities as the history of the attempts to unravel the "organizer" experiment in amphibian embryos. Experimental manipulations on limb buds systematically alter the normal sequence of developmental events; although the conventional wisdom is that such results reveal the physiological basis of limb morphogenesis, this interpretation is by no means certain. J. W. Saunders and M. T. Gasseling, who initially described the zone of polarizing activity in 1968, have more recently reported that other nonlimb tissues can produce similar effects (shades of Holtfreter!) (Saunders and Gasseling, 1983). Moreover, exogenous agents such as retinoic acid can mimic the effects of the ZPA (Tickle et al., 1982; see also Maden, 1982, 1983). To paraphrase J. Cooke (1982), these results must be telling us something about the biochemistry and cell biology of limb morphogenesis, but no one has yet discovered what.

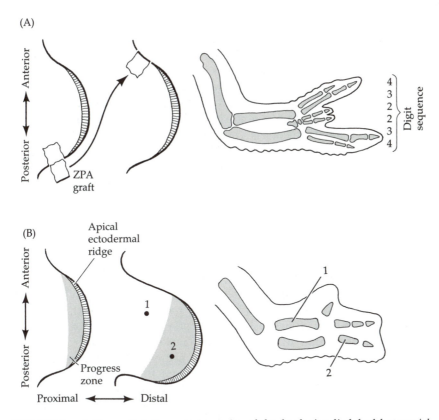

FIGURE 7. *Evidence that the posterior region of the developing limb bud has special properties with respect to limb morphogenesis. (A) When this region (called the zone of polarizing activity—ZPA) is transplanted from one limb bud to the anterior region of another, the resulting limb (right) is duplicated in the anterior–posterior axis. Numbers indicate digits. (B) Mechanism for the assignment of morphogenetic values to the tissues of a developing limb bud, suggested by L. Wolpert and his colleagues. Cells are hypothesized to receive information about their proximodistal position in the limb by virtue of time spent in the so-called progress zone, which is just beneath the apical ectodermal ridge (see also Figure 6). Thus point 1, which is outside the progress zone, has already had its positional information specified, whereas point 2 has not. At a later stage (right), the cells at both these points have interpreted their position and formed a part of the radius and a digit, respectively. (A after Summerbell, 1981; B after Tickle et al., 1975.)*

HOW POSITIONAL INFORMATION MIGHT OPERATE

Gradients

Many of the experiments described in the preceding sections suggest that morphogenetic events are influenced by gradients of a chemical signal. Over the years a number of people have favored the idea of gradients on general principles (see, for example, Boveri, 1901; Weiss,

1939; Child, 1941; see also Baltzer, 1967); recent advocates are F. H. C. Crick and H. Meinhardt, who have suggested that concentration differences of morphogens could account for a number of developmental phenomena (Crick, 1970; Meinhardt, 1978, 1982). The common denominator of these schemes is a morphogen which diffuses from its source toward a sink, thus establishing a continuous range of concentration values in the intervening space. Theoretically, such gradients can only operate over small distances (perhaps 50–100 cell diameters) (Crick, 1970). Positional information conveyed by a gradient could explain a number of observations, including the differentiation of heterocysts along an algal chain, patterns on insect cuticle, regeneration of hydra, and perhaps even some aspects of limb morphogenesis.

Good evidence for a gradient of positional information in insect cuticle was provided by M. Locke's experiments on *Rhodnius* (Locke, 1959; see also Lawrence, 1966). By transplanting small pieces of cuticle in larvae, Locke showed that disturbances in the linear pattern observed in adults could be nicely explained by an anterior–posterior gradient of a positional signal within each segment (Figure 8). Thus, when Locke rotated the transplant 180°, an abnormal pattern resulted, thereby suggesting a disturbance in an anterior–posterior gradient. Anterior–posterior transplantation within a segment also caused an altered pattern, whereas isotopic transplantations from segment to segment did not. These results are consistent with a gradient that is reiterated in each segment. H. F. Nijhout has argued that the generation of eyespots and other aspects of wing pattern in moths and butterflies are also explained by a gradient of diffusible chemical signals (Figure 9) (Nijhout, 1981).

Gradients of a chemical signal are an attractive way of thinking about how positional information is mediated, particularly in one- or two-dimensional systems in which the evidence for gradients is fairly straightforward. In more complex situations, such as the development of the vertebrate limb, the existence of gradients is inferential and one can argue whether or not it is useful to discuss the development of the limb in terms of positional information (see Box B).

FIGURE 8. *Evidence for an anterior–posterior gradient of positional information in the cuticle of the kissing bug,* Rhodnius. *(A) Transverse lines in the adult cuticle form a distinct pattern, which can be easily observed. When a small patch of tissue is rotated 90° in a segment from a fifth instar larva, the cuticular lines remain orthogonal in the adult. (B) When, however, the patch is rotated 180°, as shown in the diagram here, the lines are dramatically disturbed. (C) This disturbance is probably the result of an anterior–posterior gradient, because two pieces transposed in the anterior–posterior axis within a segment also result in a disturbance of the adult pattern. (D) Evidently the gradient is iterated from segment to segment as transplantation of a patch from one segment to an adjacent one causes no disturbance in the cuticular pattern. (A from Locke, 1967; B–D after Locke, 1959.)*

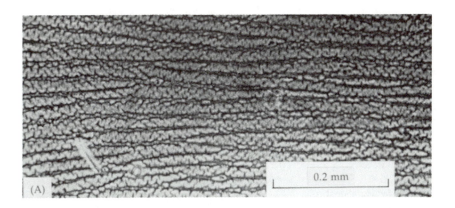

(A)

0.2 mm

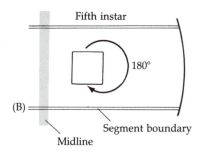

Fifth instar

180°

(B)

Midline

Segment boundary

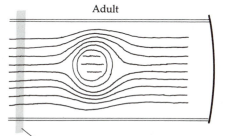

Adult

Midline

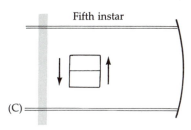

Fifth instar

(C)

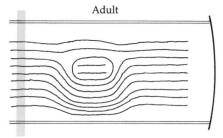

Adult

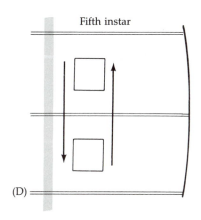

Fifth instar

(D)

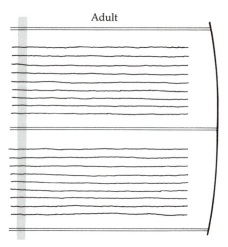

Adult

Propriety of Positional Information in Limb Morphogenesis

[This exchange between S. Brenner, J. H. Lewis, and L. Wolpert followed a presentation by Wolpert and his colleagues at a CIBA Symposium in 1975 (Wolpert et al., *CIBA Symposium* 29: 123ff, 1975). The heated argument shows that the meaning of positional information can be difficult to agree upon, especially when applied to developing systems as complex as the vertebrate limb. Evidently the interpretation of positional information is less problematic for animals than it is for the biologists who study them.]

BRENNER: I take very strong objection to Professor Wolpert's interpretation of the development of the chick limb in terms of the idea of positional value. After all, in a trivial sense, because an organism is stuck together in space, everything has a positional value. The terms positional information, positional value, and so on, should be reserved for cases where specification is a function of spatial relations, and should not be used when structures have trivial positional values but are generated by a completely different mechanism, such as a clock or a lineage. It is important to make the distinction. . . .

WOLPERT: We are saying that the positional value determines the behaviour of the cells, such as their growth programme, which varies along the axis. It is these properties that give rise to humerus, radius, etc. . . . One of the virtues of calling it positional information is that you raise specific questions such as whether there are interactions involving averaging and where the boundary regions are. It can emphasize that there may be common mechanisms for example between the chick limb, the amphibian limb and the insect. If you simply call it regional specification, you lose the possibility of there being mechanisms in common. . . . If you move out of the positional information framework, you are left in a vacuum.

BRENNER: We could have eliminated all this talk of position and discussed it in terms of turning the pages of a book. At each cell division a page is turned, and the cells peeled off from the zone have one open page in front of them and, according to Wolpert, the capacity to read the rest of the book, but not what has been read already. That would account for all your results, but it has nothing to do with position, and conceptually it is very different.

LEWIS: But you need a generic term: you cannot reel off the whole dictionary of parts of the body every time you want to refer to this type of specification.

BRENNER: Maybe not, but I think you have gone too far the other way when you say that positional value is the big thing and not any other property. Let us be clear on this issue. We make external descriptions of organisms, whether we band messenger RNA in sucrose or draw pictures of wings, and we classify these descriptions often in quite arbitrary ways. There is no guarantee that the internal description matches any of the distinctions we make; the important thing is to get hold of the internal description. If the internal description does not use position as a device for computation, the fact that position is part of the external description is incidental, like hair colour or anything else that we consider trivial. It is important to know what is inside the organism and when you use the term positional value, especially with a model that has nothing to do with positional computation, this seems to me to be misleading at the very least. Some objects have a positional value, of course, but they may have lots of other values that we do not know.

WOLPERT: I say that is fudging the issue; just saying it happens because it happens. We are being specific and suggesting a mechanism.

BRENNER: No. Everything happens because it happens, but what is really happening may be something different from what you think is happening!

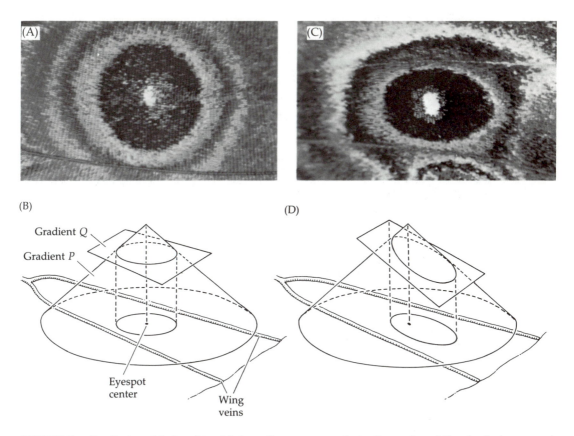

FIGURE 9. *Gradient model of positional information proposed to explain the establishment of markings on butterfly wings. (A) Photograph of the eyespot on the wing of the butterfly* Morpho peleides. *(B) Diagram of a two-gradient model that might explain the way in which the eyespot is generated. The three-dimensional shape of a linear gradient (that is, a chemical diffusing equally in all directions) is a cone (gradient P), the height of which reflects the concentration of the signal. The origin of the signal is the apex of the cone, which* corresponds to the center of the developing eyespot. *Concentration Q represents the level of chemical necessary to reach the threshold sensitivity for the formation of a color in the cells of the wing. If that sensitivity level is the same throughout the wing, it will cut the cone orthogonally, resulting in a circular eyespot. (C) In other species, in this case* Smyrna blomfildia, *the eyespots are elliptical. (D) Different orientations of the sensitivity gradient Q could result in such elliptical eyespot patterns. (After Nijhout, 1981.)*

French flag model

Several people have proposed specific models of the way gradients of positional information might actually work. Perhaps the best known of these schemes has been put forward by L. Wolpert and is called the "French flag model" (Wolpert, 1969, 1978). In this model Wolpert attempts to explain how different qualities represented by the three colors of the French flag could be established in a sheet of tissue (Figure 10). The scheme involves a source of a putative morphogen, which diffuses across a sheet of cells. By virtue of the concentration of this molecule

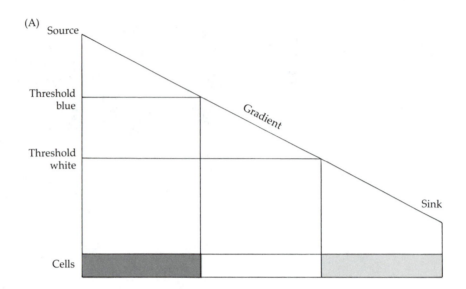

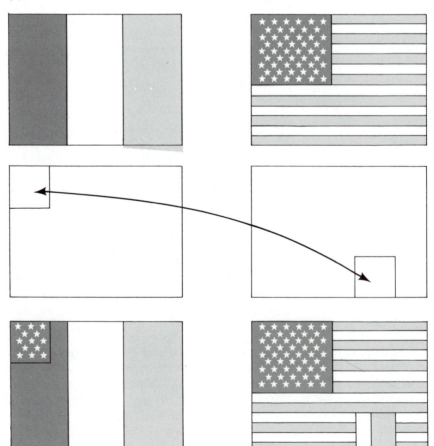

FIGURE 10. *French flag analogy for a possible mechanism of operation of a gradient of positional information. (A) In L. Wolpert's model, information is delivered by a gradient of a diffusible morphogen from a source toward a sink. The thresholds indicated on the left are cellular properties that enable the gradient to be interpreted; for example, a cell sensitive to one threshold becomes white, and another blue. The result in this case is a pattern of three colors (therefore, the epithet "French flag"). (B) An important feature of the model is that a piece of tissue transplanted from one region to another retains its identity but differentiates appropriately according to its new positional instructions. This is indicated schematically here by "grafts" from one country's flag to another. An example of this sort of phenomenon is the* antennapedia *mutation in fruitflies, in which structures in abnormal positions differentiate appropriately according to positional cues in the new location (see Figure 16). (After Wolpert, 1978.)*

at various points in the sheet, cells at different positions react in a systematically different way. Their reaction is considered to be a result of their intrinsic properties and their position in the gradient.

Polar coordinate model

A different conception of the way in which positional information might be encoded and interpreted has been put forward to explain a variety of puzzling experimental results in studies of both development in insects and limb regeneration of lower vertebrates and invertebrates (Bohn, 1976; French et al., 1976). For example, removing part of an imaginal disk (see below) or a limb may, quite paradoxically, give rise to supernumerary parts. These observations led S. French, V. French, and P. J. Bryant to suggest a polar coordinate scheme of positional information (French et al., 1976; Bryant et al., 1977, 1981; see also Bohn, 1976). In this model, each cell in the imaginal disk or in a limb is considered to be labeled with a circumferential and a radial (proximodistal) positional value (Figure 11). The operation of two simple rules within this scheme appears to account for the peculiar experimental results observed. In general, the idea is that a cell that finds itself among other cells that are out of order in the sequence of polar coordinate values will continue to proliferate until its descendants interpolate all the missing values between themselves and the cells that they were initially next to. This rule is called intercalation. A second rule, called the rule of distal regeneration, states that if at a cut surface all positional values are present, then the distal part will regenerate. The basic idea of both these rules is that cells are stimulated to divide by the absence of adjacent cells with proper positional labels. In certain well-defined circumstances, supernumerary parts are predicted as a direct consequence of intercalation and distal regeneration (see Bryant et al., 1977). Although these observations on duplicated structures had been in the literature for a long time, no one had suggested a set of morphogenetic rules to explain them.

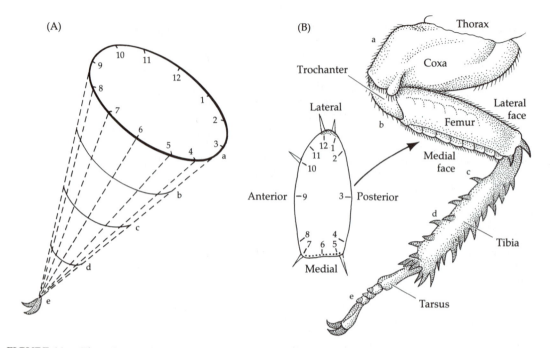

FIGURE 11. *The polar coordinate model of positional information as applied to a limb. (A) Diagram of the model. Each position on the leg of an insect such as the cockroach is envisioned as having two sorts of positional information: a proximodistal value (indicated by the letters a–e) and a circumferential value (indicated by the clockface numbers around each circle). (B) Diagram showing polar coordinate values as they would be applied to an actual cockroach leg. The left metathoracic leg is shown in anterior view (schematic cross-section shows circumferential values at mid-femur). On the basis of this model, a number of regenerative and developmental results can be explained by the operation of two basic principles. First, if two circumferential values are juxtaposed, any missing positional values will be intercalated by cell proliferation. If there is an option between going the long way around or the short way, the short way will always be taken. The second rule is that missing distal values will be regenerated only if the full set of circumferential values is present at the amputation stump. (After French, 1981.)*

Compartments

Positional information based on gradients is only one way in which a sense of location could be imparted to cells. Studies of the development of the fruitfly *Drosophila* suggest an alternative (or perhaps additional) way in which positional information can influence developmental events. Although this work has been carried out in a number of laboratories, many of the basic observations were made by A. Garcia-Bellido and his pupils in the 1970s (Garcia-Bellido, 1975; Garcia-Bellido et al., 1979; see also Crick and Lawrence, 1975).

Much of the adult fruitfly (although not the nervous system) arises from about 20 isolated groups of cells in the larva that take little or no part in larval function; these are called imaginal disks (Hadorn, 1968). Each of these disks contributes to a different portion of the adult insect (Figure 12).

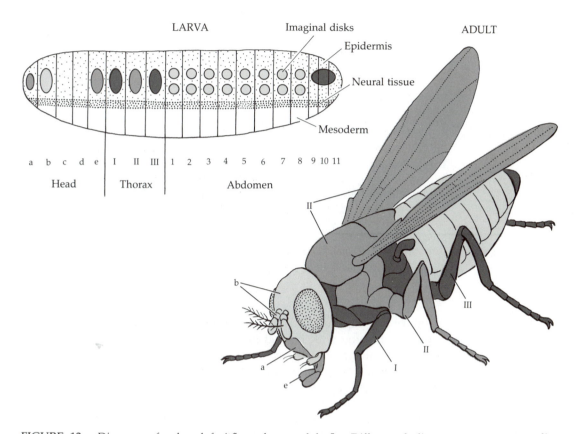

FIGURE 12. *Diagrams of a larval fruitfly and an adult fruitfly* (Drosophila melanogaster). *The larva is divided into segments, each of which contains imaginal disks. The disks of the larval segments give rise to many structures of the corresponding segments of the adult fly. Different shading represents corresponding larval and adult regions. a–e, Head structures; I–III, thoracic segments; 1–8, abdominal segments; 9–11, genitalia. (After Garcia-Bellido et al., 1979.)*

A larval fly can be irradiated to induce recombination during mitosis, thus producing cells that are homozygous for some phenotypically distinct feature; commonly used markers are abnormal wing hairs or cell color. The progeny of a single mutant cell (a clone) can thus be localized in the adult. Mutant cells produced at an early stage of development, when a great deal of cell proliferation still lies ahead, give rise to large clones that are not distinctive in either their shape or their position in the adult (Figure 13A). However, the shapes of clones produced at later stages are quite different. Garcia-Bellido and his collaborators found that such clones tended to form remarkably straight borders along boundary lines that were otherwise invisible (Figure 13B and C). Moreover these straight-line boundaries form predictably from one fly to another.

The analysis of these boundaries was greatly facilitated by the use of a mutant fly called *Minute*, in which cells proliferate more slowly

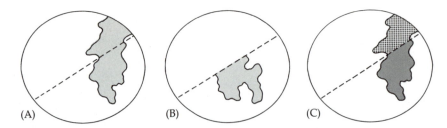

(A)   (B)   (C)

FIGURE 13.   *Compartments in insect development. This diagram represents an arbitrary part of the surface of a developing fruitfly. A clone derived from a cell marked prior to the formation of the compartment border (dotted line) does not respect any obvious boundary but extends rather formlessly over a large area (A). A clone descended from a cell marked* after *the formation of a compartment border, however, is straight along that border but convoluted elsewhere (B). Thus, progeny of two daughter cells of the clone shown in (A) will not mingle across the compartment border if they arise after a certain early stage of development (C). The invisible boundary respected by the descendants of a few founder cells defines the compartment. (After Crick and Lawrence, 1975.)*

than normal (Figure 14). When a phenotypically distinct clone in such a fly is wild type with respect to the *Minute* gene, that clone occupies a much greater territory because of the slow proliferation of the background cells. In spite of their much larger size, clones of wild-type cells in *Minute* flies respected the same straight-line boundaries. Evidently, after some developmental stage clones stay strictly on one side or the other of a line that splits the wing, for example, into anterior and posterior parts. The location of this line does not coincide with the wing veins or any other anatomical structure (Figure 14). Indeed, the boundaries are often in completely unexpected locations. In other parts of the fly, and in other insects such as the milkweed bug (*Oncopeltus*), the boundaries respected by proliferating clones are often segmental (Figure 15) (Lawrence, 1973; 1975). Just as in the wing, however, the boundary

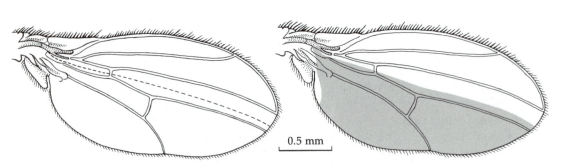

0.5 mm

FIGURE 14.   *Definition of the anterior–posterior compartment border in the* Drosophila *wing using* Minute *mutants. On the left, the compartment border is shown by a dotted line. On the right, the dark area represents a clone of wild-type cells in a* Minute *fly wing. The rapid growth of the wild-type cells in the background of slowly growing* Minute *cells entirely fills the compartment, thus facilitating the definition of compartment boundaries. (After Crick and Lawrence, 1975.)*

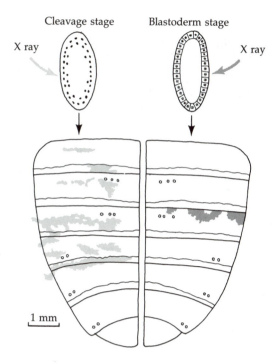

Cleavage stage   Blastoderm stage

X ray   X ray

1 mm

FIGURE 15.   *The coincidence of compartment and segment boundaries in the milkweed bug* Oncopeltus. *X irradiation of embryos at either the cleavage stage (left) or the blastoderm stage (right) generates mutant clones that, at a much later larval stage (below), are visible as patches of differently colored cells. Early irradiation results in colored clones that often cross segmental boundaries (as well as the dorsoventral compartment boundary). On the other hand, clones produced at the blastoderm stage respect the compartment boundaries that coincide with the segment (and dorsoventral) border. (After Lawrence, 1981a.)*

between segments is not mechanical: the segment border harbors no obvious barrier to the mixing of cells from one segment with those of another.

These observations define developmental *compartments*. Compartments are thus regions to which clones are restricted, even though the borders of the region present no gross impediment to movement of cells across the boundary. Each compartment comprises a set of clones that represent the descendants of a small group of founder cells that appear to have held some positional quality in common. Although each compartment is made up of a number of different clones, all of the clones within a compartment (a polyclone) respect its boundaries. As development proceeds, compartments are progressively subdivided. In the wing, for example, the anterior–posterior boundary forms in the embryonic imaginal disk; in later larvae, proximodistal and dorsoventral boundaries subsequently emerge (Garcia-Bellido, 1975). Each of these subdivisions affects all of the existing compartments, much like sequentially slicing an orange along its three major axes.

Although the nature of compartment boundaries is not understood, it is clear that compartmentalization is under genetic control (Morata and Lawrence, 1975, 1977; Garcia-Bellido et al., 1979). This is apparent in homeotic mutants in which one part of the body is characteristically transformed into another (Figure 16). For example, whereas wild-type flies have a pair of wings and a pair of balancing organs called halteres, in the homeotic mutant called *bithorax* the anterior half of the haltere is

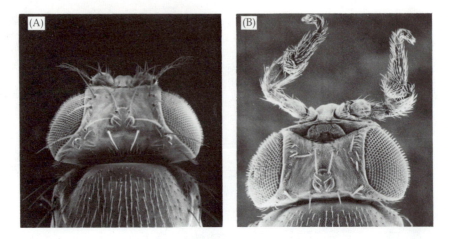

FIGURE 16. *A homeotic mutation in* Drosophila. *(A) Scanning electron micrograph of the head of a normal fly (dorsal view). (B) Similar view of the head of a mutant* antennapedia *fly. In this mutation, well-formed mesothoracic legs replace the antennae, although the fly also has normal mesothoracic legs in the usual position. This is an extreme example of this mutation; usually only parts of the antennae are changed into leg structures. (From Palka, 1982.)*

transformed into an anterior wing. According to G. Morata and P. A. Lawrence (1977), this mutation suggests that "there is at least one moment in normal development of the haltere in which the alternative—haltere or wing—is open." In their view, homeotic genes are single loci that determine which of these (or other) developmental pathways is taken by particular groups of cells. Especially noteworthy is that these mutations obey compartmental boundaries. Perhaps these genes are involved in establishing the distinctive qualities of the founder cells that provide the common denominator of the compartmental polyclone. Although other explanations are possible, this common denominator appears to be a cellular mechanism (e.g., preferential adhesion, contact inhibition, polarity of cell division) that prevents the cells of one compartment from mingling with those of another.

Homeotic mutants are relevant to the notion of positional information in other ways as well. Most homeotic mutations transform compartments incompletely; nonetheless, the mutant structure is appropriately integrated in terms of its position. For instance, when only the distal parts of the antennae are transformed into legs in the mutant called *antennapedia* (Figure 16), the mutant elements are distal leg parts (Postlethwait and Schneiderman, 1971). Conversely, when the proximal parts of the antennae are transformed, the mutant elements are proximal leg parts. This finding suggests that the means by which position influences differentiation are the same for leg and antenna (and presumably for the rest of the fly).

Whether compartments exist in other invertebrates is unclear. Because many animals show a striking segmental organization, it would be surprising if there were not some similarity in the control of this process in flies and other invertebrates (see Box C). The clones that make up a segment in insects appear to have some quality imposed on them by their position at the blastula stage. In the development of the leech, on the other hand, the position of cells is determined by lineage (Weisblat et al., 1978; Weisblat, 1981; Stent et al., 1982; Zackson, 1982). In consequence, segmentation in the leech can be explained by ancestry without recourse to positional information.

In vertebrates, the situation is even more uncertain. M. Jacobson (1982) has carried out experiments in which individual *Xenopus* blastomeres are marked with horseradish peroxidase in order to follow the progeny (see Chapter 2). On the basis of these results, Jacobson has made an explicit case for compartmental development in vertebrates. Before the 512-cell stage, the progeny of any particular blastomere are interspersed with other cells. However, when injected at the 512-cell stage, individual blastomeres give rise to clones that later occupy a discrete region (see Figure 3 in Chapter 2) (Hirose and Jacobson, 1979; Jacobson and Hirose, 1981; Jacobson, 1980, 1982, 1983). Each of these regions appears to be populated by the progeny of several different blastomeres (like polyclones in the fly). On the other hand, these observations on amphibians do not really address either of the major criteria for compartmentalization in *Drosophila*: (1) that the cells of one compartment do not mingle with the cells of another across straight line boundaries, and (2) that the compartment represents a genetic unit in the sense that mutations of homeotic genes reorganize structures along compartmental lines. Because these basic features have not been assessed in vertebrate embryos, it is premature (and confusing) to use the term *compartment* when discussing the development of vertebrates (see also Cooke, 1980).

CONCLUSIONS

The experimental investigation of form and pattern in embryonic development began with the work of H. Spemann and his students on the amphibian gastrula. These experiments showed that inductive and regulative phenomena are prominent features of early vertebrate development and gave rise to the realization that the behavior of developing cells in vertebrates is somehow influenced by their position.

More recently, developmental biologists have approached the issue of embryonic pattern largely from the vantage of positional information generated by chemical signals. Examples ranging from simple one-dimensional animals such as algae to complex three-dimensional structures such as hydra indicate that cells differentiate according to their position in the organism. These observations imply a means of providing information about position, and cellular mechanisms that interpret

BOX

C

Segmentation

Segmentation is a fundamental part of the morphogenetic plan of many animals, including primates, presumably because iteration simplifies a number of developmental problems. In the simplest cases—consider a tapeworm—segmentation joins nearly identical modules, which have only limited interaction with each other and, therefore, limited significance in the integrative behavior of the animal. In more complex animals, segmentation is increasingly overridden by integrative aspects of organization that cut across segmental limitations in a variety of important ways.

In the insect epidermis, segmental boundaries are coextensive with compartment boundaries (see text), although segments often comprise several compartments. Additional evidence for a close relationship between compartments and segments is the occurrence of mutations that interfere with segmentation in insects (Nusslein-Volhard and Wieschaus, 1980). One mutation, for example, removes the segment boundary in *Drosophila* along with some of the neighboring cuticular pattern. The result is a duplication of the remaining pattern with reversed orientation. Interestingly, reversed orientation also occurs through regulation when the segmental boundary is surgically removed in insects (Wright and Lawrence, 1981a,b). A variety of additional manipulations in *Oncopeltus* suggest that the segment boundary results from differences in cell affinities that arise from lineage. Because this is the presumptive reason for compartmental boundaries generally, some relationship between segments and compartments in insects is again implied.

The diversification of thoracic and abdominal segments in *Drosophila* is apparently under the control of a complex of genes (at least eight) called *bithorax* (Lewis, 1978). Each of these genes normally acts on only a subset of segments. When this complex is missing, embryonic flies develop a series of identical segments all of which look like the mesothoracic segment

this information and act upon it. The ways in which positional information is laid down and interpreted are, at best, unclear. In some instances (the cuticle of *Rhodnius*, the butterfly wing), gradients of a chemical signal appear to be the basis for positional information. Such gradients have also been postulated as the basis of limb morphogenesis in vertebrates, but in this case the argument is more speculative.

A different aspect of the way cells are influenced by position is the compartmental development of some insects. Polyclones in the fruitfly (see figure). Remarkably, the sequence of *bithorax* genes is ordered along the chromosome in the same sequence as the segments on which the genes act (Lewis, 1978; Struhl, 1981). E. B. Lewis has suggested that the control mechanism for segmentation has phylogenetic as well as ontogenetic significance (Lewis, 1978). Because flies apparently arose from ancestors with four wings instead of two (and many legs), the additional wings and legs must have been suppressed in the course of evolution. It is also clear that other genes are necessary for the normal operation of the *bithorax* complex (Lewis, 1978; Struhl, 1981). For example, when the locus called *engrailed* is inactivated, the fly seems incapable of keeping cells in anterior and posterior compartments from mixing with one another, or indeed from mixing between segments (Morata and Lawrence, 1975; Lawrence and Morata, 1976; Kornberg, 1981).

Sorting out these gene effects (which is now proceeding at the level of characterizing the structure of the genes involved and their products; see Bender et al., 1983) may provide some insight into the control of this basic morphogenetic arrangement.

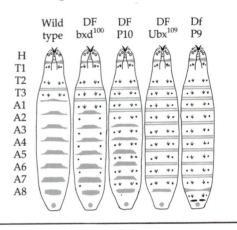

Genetic control of segmentation in the fruitfly. A normal Drosophila *larva (wild type, left), showing distinctions between various segments. Mutant larvae (right) that lack part or all of the* bithorax *gene complex. Although the number of segments is normal, there are increasing degrees of reiteration of the mesothoracic segments with increasing inactivation of the* bithorax *complex (left to right). The symbols in the diagram are various cuticular structures that identify each segment. H, head; T, thorax; A, abdomen. The genotypes of the mutants are shown above. (After Struhl, 1981.)*

evidently share some positional property that keeps them from intermingling across invisible boundaries. The additional finding that some genes affect development according to these units has underscored the significance of compartmental organization in *Drosophila*. Whether compartmentalization is an organizing principle in the development of other invertebrates and of vertebrates is, at present, a matter of debate.

Whatever the outcome of particular controversies in this field, it is clear that cell position is a major determinant of early development.

Movement and Migration of Neurons

INTRODUCTION

A cell's position in the embryo is important because differentiation is often dictated by location (Chapter 3). The final location of nerve cells is particularly important because neural function depends on the precision of connections between neurons and their targets: the presynaptic and postsynaptic elements must be in the right place at the right time. Because appropriate position is a criterion that every cell in the embryo must meet, the way this is achieved in the nervous system is only a special case. In simpler invertebrates, the unfolding of stereotyped cell lineages may be a sufficient explanation of final location; in vertebrates, however, developing cells often actively migrate to their proper place.

MECHANISMS OF CELL MOVEMENT

The majority of early embryonic cell movements occur as migrations of populations in which individual cells retain their approximate neighbor relationships. The movement of most of the cells is actually passive: they are pulled by actively moving cells on the margin of the sheet or by other forces. Examples of this kind of movement occur during gastrulation and neurulation (Chapter 1).

Most information about the mechanisms of such mass movements has been gained by observing epithelial cells during wound healing or in cell culture (Abercrombie and Middleton, 1968). As a rule, epithelial sheets move when there is a substratum to which the sheet can adhere along a free margin (Vaughan and Trinkaus, 1966). In wound healing, for example, the force is generated by prime movers that pull the other cells in the sheet (Radice, 1980).

As the body plan becomes increasingly organized, active movements of individual cells become more obvious. Movements of cells as individuals can be categorized as ameboid translocation, creeping across surfaces, or translocation by means of cilia or flagella. Ameboid movement is achieved by active extension of a pseudopodium into which the cytoplasm flows (Allen and Taylor, 1975; Taylor and Condeelis, 1979). This mechanism of motion occurs in only a few cell types in higher animals, such as macrophages. Nor do ciliary or flagellar movements

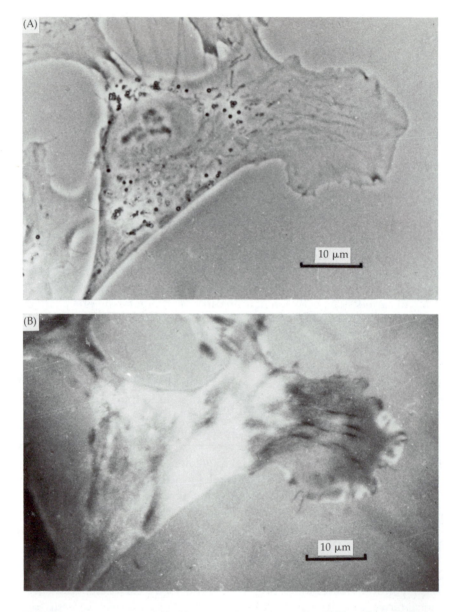

FIGURE 1. *Movement of fibroblasts in culture. (A) A prominent ruffling membrane is apparent on the right side of this chick-heart fibroblast; the ruffling membrane moves by extending lamellipodia and filopodia. The cell nucleus, mitochondria, and microfilaments are also apparent. (The direction of movement is left to right; phase-contrast micrograph.) (B) An interference-reflection photomicrograph of the same cell shows that the ruffling membrane has a number of attachments to the substrate, which appear as dark streaks with this method. (From Abercrombie, 1980.)*

figure prominently in developmental cell movements (other than in fertilization).

The cell movements that seem particularly important in embryogenesis are those that occur by gliding or crawling along surfaces (Figure 1). Cultured fibroblasts and other cells that creep have delicate sheetlike extensions (lamellipodia) which tend to arise from their shortest side (Lewis, 1934; Abercrombie, 1961; Abercrombie et al., 1970). Although the movements of the lamellipodia are too slow to discern in real time, their vigorous activity is apparent with time-lapse photography. W. H. Lewis coined the term "ruffling membrane" to describe moving lamellipodia, which he likened to "the ruffles of a dress in a slight breeze."

The way that the ruffling membrane leads to cell movement is by extension, attachment to the substrate, and subsequent traction. A useful tool for studying the sites of adhesion between cell and substrate is interference-reflection microscopy (Figure 1) (Curtis, 1964). This light microscopical technique (in which differences in brightness represent the distance between the cell and the substrate) shows that the initial sites of adhesion are near the leading edge of the ruffled membrane (Izzard and Lochner, 1976). These contact points remain stationary as the bulk of the cell moves forward. When the cell moves over the contact sites (called plaques), new adhesion sites form at the leading edge. Some plaques are so adhesive that they are left behind; these remain attached by long fibers, which eventually break when the distance becomes too great (Lazarides and Revel, 1979).

Movement requires not only adhesion to a substrate but generation of force. With fluorescent antibody techniques, musclelike proteins such as actin, myosin, tropomyosin, and α-actinin have been found in many motile cells (Abercrombie, 1982). In general, these proteins are associated with bundles of microfilaments, many of which are oriented in the direction of cell movement (Figure 2). These contractile proteins are certainly the best candidates for generating the force that pulls cells along surfaces (Isenberg et al., 1976; Abercrombie, 1982).

CUES FOR THE INITIATION, DIRECTION, AND CESSATION OF CELL MOVEMENT

Although cell movements in tissue culture may seem rather aimless, cell movements in vivo are highly directional. What are the signals that tell cells where to go and when to stop?

Inherent directional preferences

A possibility that seems improbable a priori is that cells have a directional predilection apart from various environmental cues. In spite of this prejudice, observations on fibroblasts made by G. Albrecht-Buehler (1977, 1978) indicate that cells are not entirely without such predispositions. Albrecht-Buehler watched cultured cells divide; he then fol-

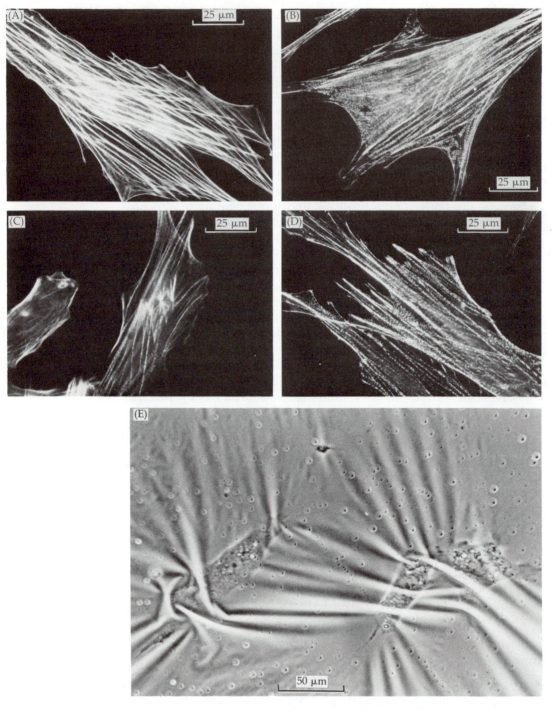

FIGURE 2. *Cultured fibroblasts stained with fluorescent antibodies to various contractile proteins. (A) Actin. (B) Myosin. (C) Tropomyosin. (D) α-Actinin. (E) Fibroblasts cultured on a thin film of silicone rubber demonstrate directly the traction generated during cell movement; note the wrinkles produced in the rubber film. (A–D from Abercrombie, 1982; courtesy of M. Osborne; E from Harris, 1982.)*

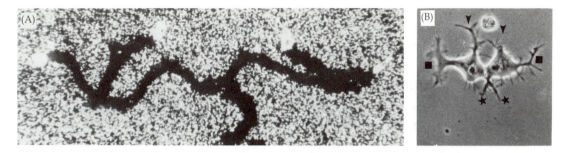

FIGURE 3. *Intrinsic determinants of cell movement and neurite outgrowth. (A) Progeny of a dividing fibroblast leave tracks on the surface of a culture dish plated with particles of colloidal gold. In this photomicrograph, the tracks of the two daughter cells (which begin at the branch point in the middle) and four granddaughter cells (secondary branches), are mirror-symmetrical. (B) Pairs of neuroblastoma cells shortly after division tend to have symmetrically oriented neurites. The mechanisms underlying these phenomena may be important in establishing some aspects of early embryonic pattern. Symbols indicate homologous neurites of the two daughters. (A courtesy of G. Albrecht-Buehler; B from Solomon, 1979.)*

lowed the movements of the two daughter cells on a culture dish plated with colloidal gold. Because the cells take up the gold particles, their movements leave tracks (Figure 3A). These trails leave little doubt that two daughter cells often move apart in mirror-image patterns. Albrecht-Buehler proposed that because cell division duplicates, and therefore polarizes, cell organelles, the motility apparatus in daughter cells is often at opposite poles. Thus, the motility of daughters in an otherwise homogeneous environment would tend to be mirror-symmetric. Such inherent directional propensities may be important in early embryonic events such as the development of bilateral symmetry, and in directing the initial extension of neurites (Figure 3B).

Chemotaxis

Another influence on the direction of cell movement is diffusible agents which establish chemical gradients (see also Chapter 5). Such gradients play a central role in the movement of prokaryotes and simple eukaryotes like slime molds. Responses to gradients (either positive or negative) are remarkable in that they require discrimination of concentration differences over approximately the diameter of a cell, or a "memory" that allows cells to compare a gradient at more widely separated points. In fact, bacteria and other prokaryotes appear to use both these strategies (Adler, 1976; MacNab, 1980; Koshland, 1981; Boyd and Simon, 1982).

Chemotaxis is also characteristic of some vertebrate cells. For example, polymorphonuclear leukocytes actively migrate up concentration gradients of several substances (Zigmond, 1978; Schiffmann, 1982). Specific receptors cause the cells to orient toward the attractant by redistributing microtubules and microfilaments, which in turn change the direction of movement (Gallin et al., 1978).

In spite of the importance of chemotaxis in various biological systems, the role of this phenomenon in developmental cell movements is uncertain.

Differential adhesion

R. G. Harrison (see Box B) was the first person to study the relationship between cell movement and substrate in a systematic way. The observation that cultured amphibian neuroblasts prefer surfaces to liquid media led Harrison to the notion of "thigmotaxis," a propensity of cells to cling to solid surfaces and move along them (Figure 4) (Harrison, 1914; see also Loeb and Fleisher, 1917). P. Weiss coined the term "contact guidance" after noting that cells oriented themselves on a protein film by adhering selectively to micelles of colloidal material (Weiss, 1939). Weiss also found that when embryonic epithelial cells are cultured on a glass plate scored with fine grooves, the cells confine themselves to the grooves and tend to move along them (Weiss, 1941, 1961; see also Rovensky et al., 1971; Rovensky and Slavnaya, 1974). Thus, rather than simply being guided by *any* solid surface in their vicinity, cells choose a "directional response to directional properties within a solid" (Weiss, 1961). Although Weiss argued for a rather complex chemical basis for this phenomenon (a mechanism involving cellular secretion of specific macromolecules that ran down the grooves and tended to orient the cells), it is now accepted that cells conform to different surfaces during movement because of differential adhesiveness (Letourneau et al., 1980; Dunn, 1982).

That cell movement can actually be directed in culture by gradients of adhesiveness has been shown in a variety of ways. Perhaps most instructive is the creation of a relatively adhesive pathway upon which cells move preferentially (Figure 5) (Rovasio et al., 1983; see also Chapter 5). Although there is only fragmentary evidence that similar gradients or pathways actually exist in embryonic life, this seems likely. Certainly a number of migratory phenomena that occur in development—the

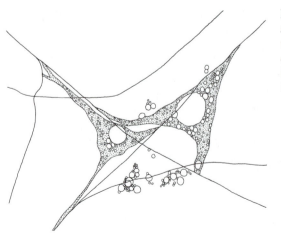

FIGURE 4. *The tendency of cells to cling to solid surfaces and move along them. Drawing by R. G. Harrison of frog spinal cord cells grown in hanging drop culture with filaments of spider web. The cells attach to the web filaments and send fine processes along them. (After Harrison, 1914.)*

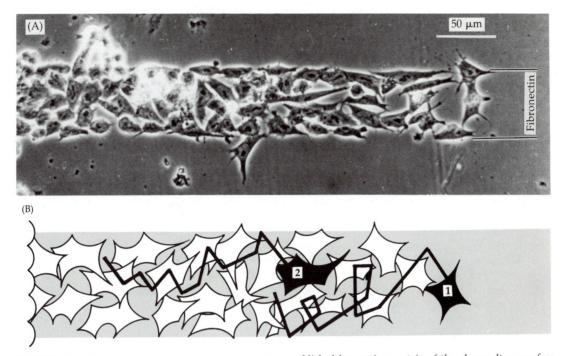

FIGURE 5. *The movement of populations of cells along an adhesive pathway in vitro. (A) After 24 hours in culture, these chick neural crest cells have migrated along a rectilinear path of preferential adhesiveness es-* *tablished by coating a strip of the glass culture surface with fibronectin. (B) Video analysis indicates the trajectory of individual cells (1,2) along the adhesive strip (gray area). (From Rovasio et al., 1983.)*

migration of melanocytes along blood vessels, the movement of lateral-line rudiments in teleosts, and the movement of the cells that make up the amphibian pronephric ducts—provide examples that might be explained in this way (see, for instance, Poole and Steinberg, 1982).

Another indication that differential adhesiveness is important in embryogenesis can be traced to the provocative experiments of H. V. Wilson in the early part of the century on the aggregation of marine sponges (Wilson, 1907; Wilson and Penney, 1930). Wilson dissociated the cells of a species of sponge that is bright red; when he pressed the cells through a fine cloth into seawater, he found that clusters of individual cells slowly reaggregated to form a complete sponge. Moreover, when he used two species that were colored differently, he found that reaggregation was species specific (see also Humphreys, 1963; Moscona, 1962, 1963). In the 1930s and 1940s, J. F. K. Holtfreter (see Box A) studied cell sorting in vertebrate embryogenesis (Holtfreter, 1939, 1944; Townes and Holtfreter, 1955). He found that the tissues of amphibian embryos could be dissociated at high pH. Remarkably, the cells reaggregated selectively when the pH was returned to normal (Figure 6). Dissociated organ rudiments from chick embryos also reassociate in vitro into recognizable tissues and continue to develop (Moscona and Moscona, 1952; Steinberg, 1978).

Cell sorting according to adhesive properties seems likely to play a

Johannes Friedrich Karl Holtfreter (b.1901)

Johannes Holtfreter was born in Richtenberg, Germany. He was educated at the University of Freiberg, where he received his Ph.D. in 1924 under the supervision of H. Spemann (see Box A in Chapter 3). In 1928 he became an associate at the Kaiser Wilhelm Institute in Berlin and in 1933 advanced to associate professor in the zoology department at the University of Munich. Discouraged with academic life in Germany, he left in the 1930s. Holtfreter became a Rockefeller Fellow at McGill, and subsequently a Guggenheim Fellow during the war years. From 1946 until his retirement in 1968 he was professor in the zoology department at the University of Rochester.

Holtfreter is generally acknowledged to be one of the most inventive and original thinkers in experimental embryology. In a series of experiments carried out in Berlin, he showed that fixed tissues, and even nonbiological materials, could produce the same effects as dorsal lip transplantation (Chapter 2). The discovery that dead tissues can induce organized structures led to two important conclusions: (1) that induction is probably the result of a chemical agent and (2) that the embryo has considerable "self-organizing" ability that can be triggered by a variety of stimuli. Holtfreter's student H. H. Chuang (1939) found that different sorts of tissues induced region-specific parts of the neural tube; this discovery led to the isolation of various region-specific inducers by later workers. In short, Holtfreter's work moved this field toward an understanding of embryonic events on a cellular and molecular level.

Holtfreter was one of the first embryologists after Harrison to use the tissue culture method to good purpose, and he provided extensive descriptions of the differentiation of various parts of amphibian gastrulas in vitro (Holtfreter, 1938). It was finally this methodology that led him to study recombinations of cells from gastrulas and neurulas isolated in vitro (Holtfreter, 1939). This initiated a series of investigations, which culminated in a classic paper with P. L. Townes in 1955, showing that embryonic cells of the different germ layers have a strong tendency to reaggregate in a tissue-specific manner (Townes and Holtfreter, 1955). This result stimulated a variety of work by others ranging from detailed analyses of cell sorting to investigations of differential adhesion in axon outgrowth and in selective synapse formation (Chapters 5 and 11). These areas remain intensely active and, although much current work no longer cites Holtfreter's investigations, most modern efforts can be traced to his initial studies of selective aggregation and adhesion.

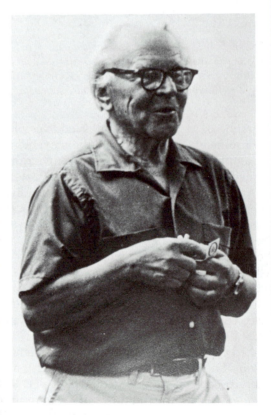

Johannes F. K. Holtfreter. (Courtesy of V. Hamburger.)

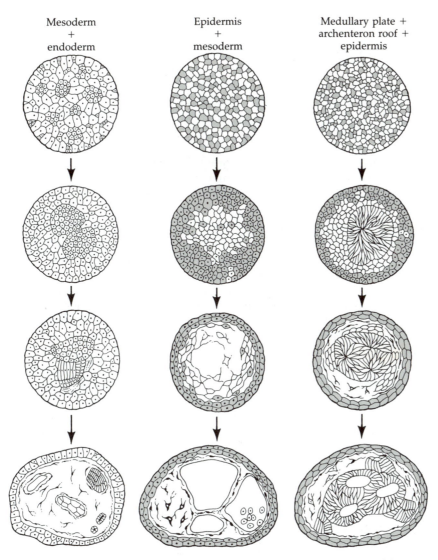

| Mesoderm
+
endoderm | Epidermis
+
mesoderm | Medullary plate +
archenteron roof +
epidermis |

FIGURE 6. *Selective segregation of various combinations of tissues in vitro following dissociation of amphibian embryos. Randomly arranged cell masses of different tissue types (top) sort themselves out with remarkable efficiency and continue to develop (bottom). (After Townes and Holtfreter, 1955.)*

major part in the cellular movements of the early embryo (e.g., gastrulation and neurulation; see Chapter 1). A reasonable scenario would be systematic changes in the adhesiveness of various cells as a function of developmental age; such programmed changes might then regulate morphogenetic changes at different developmental stages (see Johnson, 1969, 1970; Edelman, 1983; Edelman et al., 1983; Edelman, 1984). Aggregation of cells to form organs might be explained by the inhibition of cell movement that occurs when adhesive cells contact one another (contact inhibition) (Abercrombie and Heaysman, 1954).

Like other cells, neuronal precursors in vertebrates migrate extensively during early life. Peripheral neurons migrate long distances from their origin in neural crest; central nervous system neurons also migrate to their definitive locations.

Migration of neurons in the peripheral nervous system

Many studies of nerve cell migration have examined the vertebrate neural crest, the embryological source of peripheral nerve cells (Chapter 1) (LeDouarin, 1980b, 1982; LeDouarin et al., 1984). This neural tissue is remarkable for a variety of reasons. First, it provides precursors to an unusually large assortment of cell types which colonize different regions of the embryo; the progeny of neural crest cells include autonomic ganglion cells, glia, pigment cells, and cartilage (Chapter 1). Second, because these cells migrate long distances from their origin along predictable trajectories, they can be manipulated to explore the mechanisms involved. For example, patterns of skin pigmentation reflect crest migration and have been studied in detail (Rawles, 1948). Third, neural crest cell movement during embryonic life is particularly robust and still occurs after a variety of perturbations (Weston, 1982).

Prior to migration, neural crest cells are located at the margins of the neural plate and remain as a distinct group just dorsal and lateral to the neural tube (Figure 7; see also Figure 8 in Chapter 1). The crest cells usually migrate laterally in two streams, one stream proceeding dorsolaterally and the other ventrolaterally (Weston, 1963). The dorsal stream migrates more or less directly into the ectoderm and gives rise

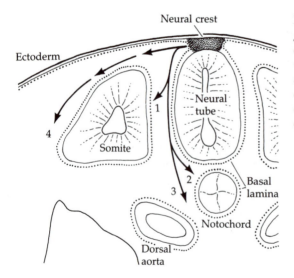

FIGURE 7. *Migration of neural crest cells. This diagram represents a cross section through the trunk region of a chick embryo at the time of neural crest migration. Crest cell migration occurs in two main streams: a superficial pathway just beneath the ectoderm, and a deeper, more ventral pathway. The ventral stream forms dorsal root ganglia (1), sympathetic ganglia (2), and adrenal medulla (3); the dorsally migrating cells enter the dermis to become melanocytes (4). (After Sanes, 1983.)*

to pigment epithelium. The ventral stream moves through the mesenchyme between the neural tube and the developing somites and eventually gives rise to autonomic and sensory ganglia, glial cells, adrenomedullary cells, and some of the cartilaginous structures of the head and neck.

The mechanism of the initial splitting into two migratory streams is not clear; this division might be imposed on the crest cells by intrinsic properties, local mechanical features or by the qualities of the extracellular matrix near the origin of the migration (Löfberg et al., 1980). Whatever dictates the initial route, their subsequent course is clearly under environmental control. This has been demonstrated by transplantation experiments. In the chick, parasympathetic neurons originating from the crest at levels corresponding to somites 1 through 7 colonize the entire gut; crest cells migrating from caudal regions (somites 28 and more caudally) give rise only to the ganglia of the postumbilical gut (see Figure 10 in Chapter 2). Neural crest cells from the intervening regions (somites 8 to 27) do not normally contribute to the enteric ganglia at all, but rather colonize the adrenal medulla and form the sympathetic chain ganglia (LeDouarin and Teillet, 1973; LeDouarin, 1980a). When segments of neural crest are transplanted from one level to another, the transplanted cells adopt the route characteristic of their new location (Noden, 1975). Thus, the migratory patterns of developing crest cells are apparently imposed by the environment through which they move.

Therefore the structure and composition of the matrix that neural crest cells traverse is of great interest (Figure 8). These areas are rich in glycosaminoglycans, chondroitin sulfate, fibronectin, and collagen (Pratt et al., 1975; Toole, 1976; Ebendal, 1977; Derby, 1978; Pintar, 1978; Newgreen and Thiery, 1980; Löfberg et al., 1980; Newgreen et al., 1982; Rovasio et al., 1983). Which, if any, of these molecules is important in directing neural crest migration is largely a matter of speculation (Sanes, 1983), although some evidence has implicated fibronectin in movements associated with gastrulation (Boucaut et al., 1984).

Migration of neuronal precursors in the developing central nervous system

The movement of developing neurons in the central nervous system appears different from the migration of neural crest cells. Following mitosis at the ventricular lining, neuronal precursors migrate to more superficial layers. In the cerebral cortex, the cells that undergo their last mitotic division relatively early in development end up in the deepest layers of the cortex, whereas neurons produced somewhat later migrate to the superficial layers (Figure 9) (Rakic, 1972; see also LaVail and Cowan, 1971; Caviness et al., 1981). Because all these cells proliferate in the ventricular zone, younger neurons must migrate through regions of older cells. In some cases more complex secondary migrations also

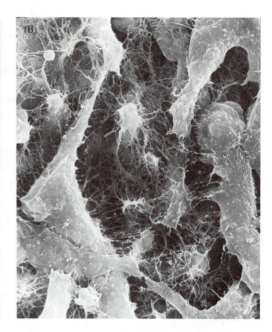

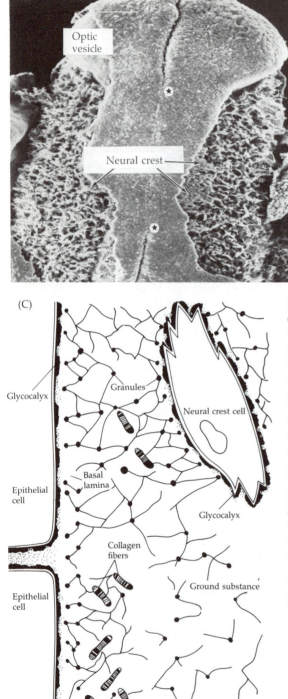

FIGURE 8. *Scanning electron micrographs of neural crest and the tissue through which neural crest cells migrate. (A) Dorsal view of a chick embryo (stage 8) (rostral above); the surface ectoderm lateral to the midline has been removed from both sides. The region where the neural tube has fused is indicated with stars. Arrows point to the mesencephalic neural crest. ×110. (B) Higher power scanning electron micrograph of individual neural crest cells (arrows) in a 10-day-old axolotl, which are migrating through a thicket of filamentous material (extracellular matrix). ×1,155. (C) Arrangement of cell surface and extracellular matrix elements that may influence migrating neural crest cells. The plasma membrane of cells is usually covered with a glycocalyx; superficial to this, many cell types (epithelial cells are shown here) have a basal lamina composed of collagen and other molecules. Beyond this is a tangle of collagen fibers and other fibrous elements embedded in an amorphous ground substance containing granules rich in glycosaminoglycans and other molecules. (A from Anderson and Meier, 1981; B from Alberts et al., 1983; courtesy of J. Löfberg; C after Sanes, 1983.)*

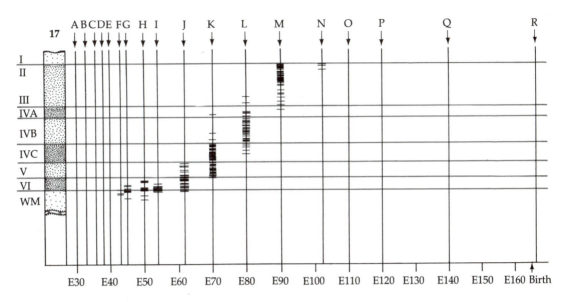

FIGURE 9. *The final position of neurons in the monkey visual cortex (area 17) born at different embryonic times. On the left is a diagram of the cortical layers; the abscissa represents embryonic age (e.g., E30 is 30 days gestation). The vertical lines (A–R) indicate the time of thymidine injection; the short horizontal lines indicate the position of labeled neurons. Because all neurons are produced in the ventricular and subventricular zones, the progressively more superficial position of neurons generated late in development indicates that cells born at later stages must migrate through regions of older cells. This is referred to as the "inside-out" pattern of cortical development. WM, white matter. (After Rakic, 1974.)*

occur. Among the more striking examples are the secondary migrations of the column of Terni cells in the chick spinal cord (Figure 10) (Levi-Montalcini, 1950), the migration of granule cells in the mammalian cerebellar cortex (Rakic, 1971b), and the secondary migration of neurons in the avian optic tectum (LaVail and Cowan, 1971).

Migrating neuronal precursors in some regions of the cortex evidently move along the surface of a particular cell type (usually called radial glia), which tends to guide them to their destination, or at least to limit the routes that they might otherwise take (Figure 11) (Rakic, 1971a,b, 1972). Several aspects of these glial elements are consistent with a role in neuronal migration. First, they have an orientation appropriate for radially migrating neurons: they extend from the ventricular to the pial surface of the developing cortex. Second, they are present in the developing central nervous system at appropriate times (Levitt and Rakic, 1980). Indeed, in many areas of the cortex radial glia are transitory elements and disappear after the period of migration is over (possibly becoming astrocytes; Ramón y Cajal, 1911; Levitt and Rakic, 1980). Third, and perhaps most important, migrating neurons are intimately associated with the processes of these radial glial cells (Figure 11) (Rakic, 1971b; Rakic et al., 1974). There is, in addition, some

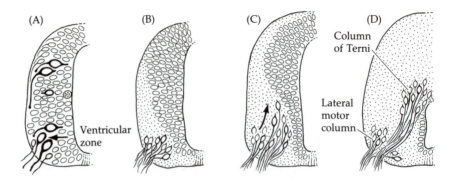

FIGURE 10. *Secondary migration of neurons in the chick spinal cord. A uniform column of motor cells first forms ventrolaterally by an initial migration of neuronal precursors from the ventricular zone (A,B). In the thoracolumbar region (shown here in cross section), some of these cells undergo a secondary migration in a mediodorsal direction to form the preganglionic visceral motor nucleus (the column of Terni). This secondary migration takes place from about the fifth to the eighth days of incubation (C,D). (After Hamburger and Levi-Montalcini, 1950.)*

experimental evidence for a causal relationship between radial glia and appropriate migration of cortical neurons. Thus, in the mutant mouse called *weaver*, abnormal radial glia are associated with a failure of granule cells to migrate to their correct location in the cerebellum (Rakic and Sidman, 1973a,b). On the other hand, studies of chimeric mice suggest that the defect in *weaver* is intrinsic to the granule cells (Goldowitz and Mullen, 1982; see also Sotelo and Rio, 1980). Of course, if radial glia do provide guides for the early migration of cortical neurons, there must be other cues in the local environment that signal these cells to stop at the appropriate layer. Moreover, such guidance by glial fibers cannot be a general mechanism of directed neuronal migration because other neuronal classes (e.g., neural crest cells) migrate without benefit of associated glia.

NERVE CELL GROWTH CONES
AND THEIR MECHANISM OF MOVEMENT

In addition to migrating in their entirety, developing nerve cells have the unique ability to place parts of themselves in strategic positions by extending processes substantial distances. This form of neuronal movement occurs at structures called growth cones at the tips of the elongating neurites. In spite of their specialized appearance, growth cone extension is probably similar to other forms of cell movement.

Structure of growth cones

That nerve cell processes (both axons and dendrites) grow at specialized terminations was recognized by S. Ramón y Cajal in 1890 who called

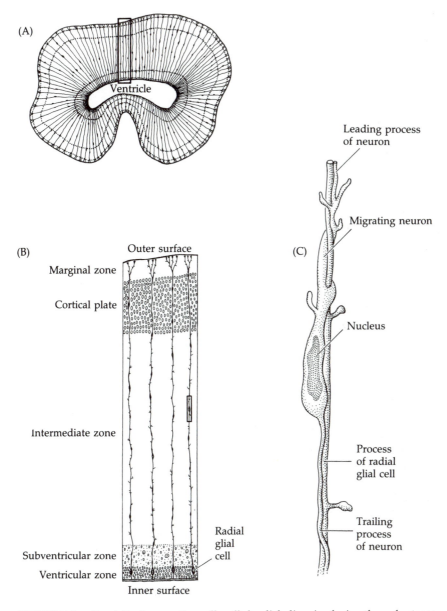

(A)

Ventricle

(B)

Outer surface

Marginal zone

Cortical plate

Intermediate zone

Subventricular zone

Ventricular zone

Inner surface

Radial glial cell

(C)

Leading process of neuron

Migrating neuron

Nucleus

Process of radial glial cell

Trailing process of neuron

FIGURE 11. *Specialized supporting cells called radial glia arise during the early stages of development in the primate cortex. The processes of these cells span the entire thickness of the wall of the neural tube and its derivative structures. (A) Radial glial cells in a Golgi-stained preparation of a thick transverse section through the wall of the cerebral hemisphere of a fetal rhesus monkey. The cell bodies lie in the ventricular zone and their processes extend to the outer surface of the surrounding layers, where they appear to form expanded terminal attachments. (B) An enlarged view of the boxed region in A. (C) The small portion of tissue inside the rectangle in B is further magnified in this detailed three-dimensional view. In most parts of the developing brain, there is a close relation between the processes of the radial glial cells and migrating cortical neurons. (After Rakic, 1972, 1978.)*

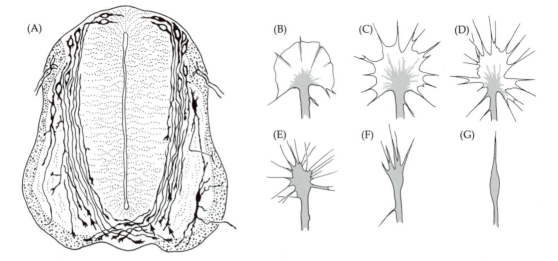

FIGURE 12. *Sketches of growth cone morphologies.* *(A) Original drawing by Cajal of growth cones (arrows) in the embryonic chick spinal cord. (B–E) Appearance of growth cones on highly adhesive surfaces in vitro. (F) Appearance of growth cone on a surface of limited* *adhesiveness. (G) Appearance of a growth cone in vivo when the axon is growing along a preexisting nerve bundle. (A after Ramón y Cajal, 1890; B–G after Bray, 1982a.)*

these structures *cones d'accroissement* (Figure 12) (Ramón y Cajal, 1890, 1911, 1929). It was Harrison, however, who first described a living growth cone and made the fundamental observation that growth cones in tissue culture are constantly moving by local extension and retraction (Figure 13) (Harrison, 1910, 1935).

At the level of the light microscope, growth cones in tissue culture look like flattened clubs with numerous fine extensions (Figures 12 and 13) (Johnston and Wessells, 1980; Bunge et al., 1981; Letourneau, 1982; Bray, 1982b; Landis, 1983). The broader extensions are called lamellipodia and the finer ones microspikes or filopodia. The terminal expansion that is usually obvious in tissue culture is not always seen when axons are growing in situ (Figure 12); presumably the bulbous expansion in vitro is not necessary for axonal elongation. At the ultrastructural level, the growth cone appears quite different from the adjacent neurite (Figure 14). Unlike the trailing process, the growth cone is jammed with organelles (although growth cones in the central nervous system may have a sparser distribution of organelles than those in the periphery). Especially prominent are actin microfilaments in filopodia and lamellipodia. In addition, growth cones contain numerous cisternae, smooth endoplasmic reticulum, dense-core vesicles, and lysosomes (Yamada et al., 1971; Bray and Bunge, 1973; Bunge et al., 1981; Letourneau, 1982; Landis, 1983). These structures are presumably the basis for the membrane incorporation that must be occurring at the growing tips (see next section).

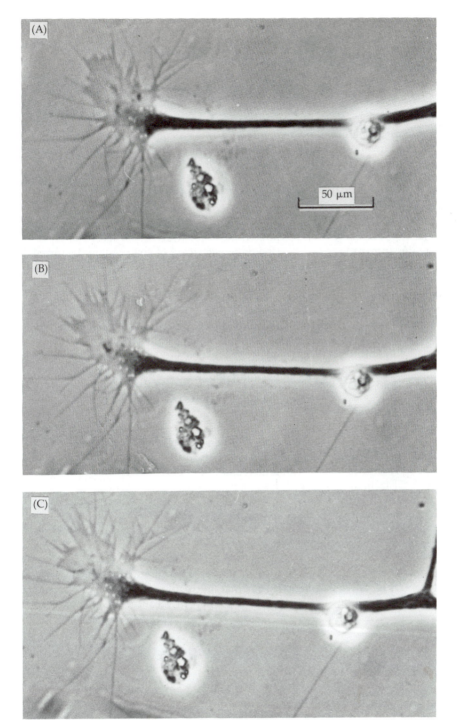

FIGURE 13.   *Rapid movements of growth cone filopodia in tissue culture. These three frames (A–C) show the changes in the filopodial pattern of a growth cone from a sensory neuron; the pictures were taken at 20-second intervals. (Courtesy of D. Bray.)*

Ross Granville Harrison (1870–1959)

Ross Harrison was born in the Philadelphia suburb called Germantown. He received his Ph.D. in 1894 from the department of zoology at Johns Hopkins University in a cohort that included T. H. Morgan and E. G. Conklin. After obtaining a medical degree in 1899 at Bonn, he became a member of the anatomy department at Johns Hopkins; in 1907 he moved to Yale where he was, for many years, the head of the zoology department.

Harrison's major contributions to neuroembryology concern axons, their mode of outgrowth, and the manner in which they find their way (Hamburger, 1980). Although the controversy is now nearly forgotten, in the early part of the twentieth century the issue of how axons formed was by no means settled. W. His and S. Ramón y Cajal supported the idea that axons grew from parent cell bodies; others, however, promoted the so-called "cell chain" or "plasmodesm" theories of axon formation. The adherents of this view maintained that axons were built by linking up individual segments that were independently created, perhaps by Schwann cells. In experiments that made use of the then novel technique of embryonic transplantation (one of Harrison's fortes), he dispatched the notion that axons arise from Schwann cells. Harrison did this by removing the dorsal part of the neural tube (i.e., the neural crest) in frog embryos, thus eliminating Schwann cells. In these experimental tadpoles he found ventral roots with nerve fibers of normal construction (Harrison, 1924).

This set to rest the idea of independent axonal segments and also confirmed the neural crest origin of Schwann cells. The ultimate solution to the problem of axon growth, however, required a more direct approach. In Harrison's words, "The really crucial experiment remained to be performed, and that was to test the power of nerve centers to form new fibers within some foreign medium, which could not by any possibility be suspected of contributing organized protoplasm to them" (Harrison, 1910, p. 790). In order to achieve this, he took pieces of embryonic frog neural tube and grew them in drops of lymph. The outgrowth of nerve fibers could then be followed directly under the microscope. Thus, Harrison not only settled the question of axonal origin, but also invented the technique of tissue culture (Harrison, 1907, 1910). Harrison also confirmed Cajal's inference that growth cones represent the elongating tips of axons. Ironically, the invention of the tissue culture technique was not exploited by Harrison (or others) for several decades.

In addition to these major contributions to understanding neuronal growth, Harrison made important discoveries in a number of other areas. In a variety of transplant experiments using pigmented and unpigmented embryos, he showed that cells destined to become lateral line sense organs migrate over long and stereotyped pathways (Harrison, 1903). He is also credited with putting the technique of experimental microsurgery on a solid footing, with developing the concept of the morpho-

Mechanisms of neurite growth

In principle, neuronal processes might grow by incorporating new membrane near the cell body, at the level of the growth cone, or along the entire length of the process. A variety of studies indicate that, prior to innervating a target, neurite extension occurs at the level of the growth cone. Support for this conclusion comes from experiments in which particles that adhere to neurites are observed over time. Particles of carmine stuck to a growing process do not move relative to the cell body, although the length of the process increases (Bray, 1970, 1973a).

genetic field (see Harrison, 1918, and Chapter 3), and with contributing importantly to understanding the origin of bilateral symmetry (Harrison, 1921). His idea that organ primordia are polarized along three main axes and that this polarization must have a detailed cellular basis remains a major issue in neuroembryology (Chapter 3).

V. Hamburger, who knew Harrison well, remembers his personal qualities in the following way:

Harrison was anything but cerebral. On the contrary, he was very close to the phenomena, and very down to earth. He had a knack for identifying basic problems (like the origin of symmetry) in a way that could be subjected to experimental analysis, and his experimental skill and analytical imagination succeeded in solving problems on the level on which they were conceived. He positively disliked too much speculation and theorizing; he would never have coined terms like "organizer." He was a pragmatist, a reductionist, and a skeptic. He was relaxed and much less tense than Spemann. Personally he was unassuming, low key. He never was a good speaker or an electrifying lecturer. But his quiet way of going about research, of doing it all himself, of restraint, of knowing the limits of his, and our, endeavors, made a deep impression on many, including myself. (Hamburger, personal communication)

Many expected that Harrison would receive the Nobel prize along with his friend and colleague H. Spemann in 1935 (see Box A in Chapter 3), but this was not to be. In fact, Harrison had been suggested for this honor in 1914, but the prizes were suspended at that point because of World War I. He was again suggested in 1933, but according to the Nobel committee, "Opinions diverged and in view of the rather limited value of the method [of tissue culture],

and the age of the discovery, an award could not be recommended" (Nobel Committee, 1962). The prize in physiology and medicine that year was given to Harrison's classmate T. H. Morgan for his work on chromosomes. The Nobel committee notwithstanding, Harrison's contributions to understanding the development of the nervous system, and to biology in general, certainly rank him as one of the great developmental biologists of the early twentieth century.

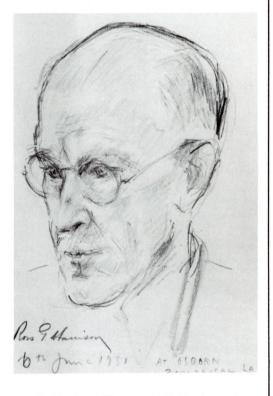

Ross G. Harrison. (Courtesy of V. Hamburger.)

Therefore, growth must be occurring distally (Figure 15). In corroboration of this, a lectin label applied to a growing neurite is, after a short time, no longer apparent at the growing tip (see Landis, 1983). Finally, when a neurite is cut, the amputated segment continues to elongate for several hours (Figure 16) (Hughes, 1953; Shaw and Bray, 1977; Wessells et al., 1978; see also Bray et al., 1978).

The mechanism of membrane addition at the growing tip is still debated. It seems likely that preformed membrane vesicles originating from the Golgi apparatus are transported to the distal neurite and fuse with the growth cone membrane (Landis, 1983). Whatever the mecha-

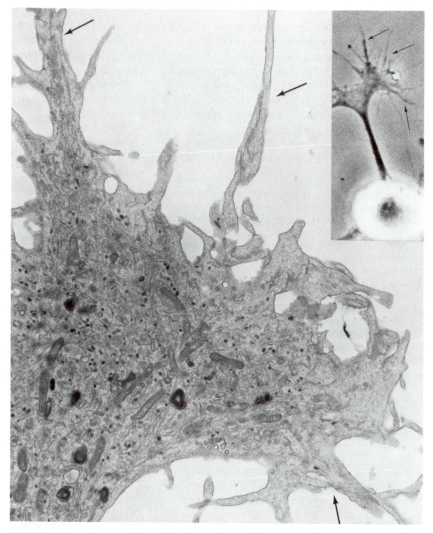

FIGURE 14.   *Electron microscopical appearance of growth cones. This low-power view shows a thin section of a mammalian sympathetic neuron in vitro. Inset is a light microscopical (phase-contrast) picture of the same growth cone. Arrows point to the same filopodia in the light and electron micrographs. Organelles typically found in abundance in growth cones in tissue culture include mitochondria, filaments, vesicles of all shapes and sizes, and smooth endoplasmic reticulum. The major organelles in filopodia are actin microfilaments; most other organelles are relatively sparse in the filopodia themselves. ×14,000. (Courtesy of M. Bunge and D. Bray.)*

nism of membrane addition, the driving force behind elongation of neurites is almost certainly the continual tug of the growth cone, presumably in a manner similar to lamellipodial movement in fibroblasts and other nonneural cells (Bray and Bunge, 1973; Bray, 1973b, 1979, 1982a). Most growth cone filopodia extend, stick briefly to the substrate,

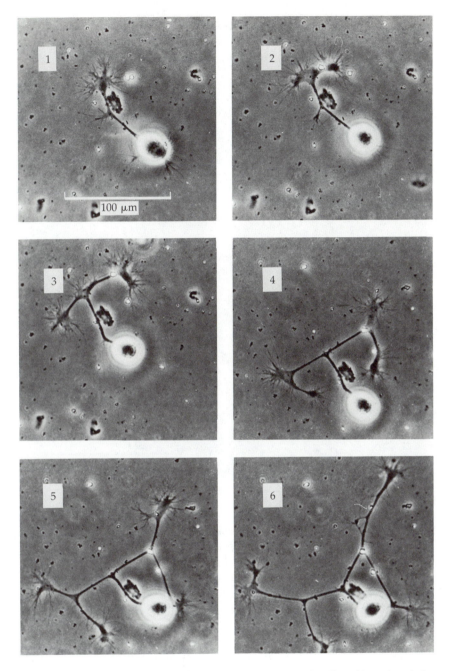

FIGURE 15. *Growing axons incorporate new membrane distally. This series of pho-tomicrographs shows growing neurites from a rat sympathetic neuron in tissue culture. The culture surface has been seeded with carmine particles. Examination of neuritic growth with reference to particular particles reveals that the particles maintain their approximate position with respect to the cell body, whereas the distal neurites extend substantially. Successive frames (1–6) were taken at approximately 30-minute intervals. (From Bray, 1970.)*

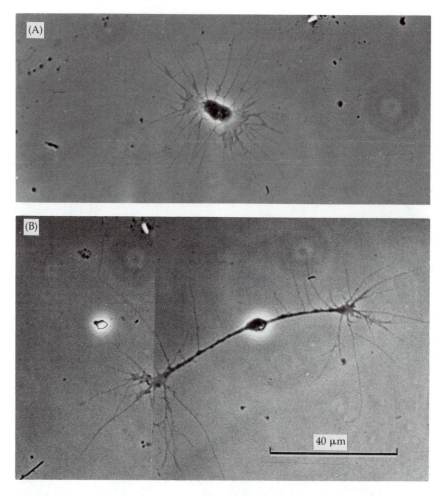

FIGURE 16. *Growth of an amputated distal neurite. (A) This bead was formed upon retraction of an amputated neurite about 15 minutes after being severed from its cell body. The neurite originated from a sympathetic neuron growing in vitro. (B) Eighty minutes later the bead has extended processes in two directions; each process is tipped by a growth cone. This experiment shows that growing neurites are, in the short run, independent of the metabolism of the cell body. Apparently there is no inherent polarity in growing axons as growth cones form at both ends of the amputated neurite. (Courtesy of D. Bray.)*

and then withdraw (Bray, 1973b; Wessells et al., 1974; Bunge, 1977). Adhesion of a filopodial process to the substrate apparently prevents its resorption; thus, when force is generated, the trailing growth cone moves forward. As in the ruffling membranes of fibroblasts, actin and myosin are major components of growth cones: indeed, actin microfilaments are the major organelles in filopodia (Letourneau, 1979; Kuczmarski and Rosenbaum, 1979; Letourneau, 1981; Bray and Gilbert, 1981). The interaction of actin filaments and myosin is probably the basis of growth cone traction. In confirmation of this, agents that interfere with actin (such as cytochalasin B) stop neurite extension (Yamada et al., 1971). The mechanism of filopodial extension is not known, but Ca^{2+} appears to be involved (Anglister et al., 1982).

In summary, the growth cone is the driving force behind neurite extension. The mechanism of elongation is not known in detail, but membrane components synthesized in the cell body are probably transported distally and inserted at the growth cone, which moves forward by extension, substrate attachment, and subsequent traction. Of course, even after attachment to a target, axons elongate as the animal grows; this process does not involve growth cones, but apparently depends on continued axonal tension (Bray, 1984).

CONCLUSIONS

Accurate location of neurons and their processes is fundamental to the establishment of correct patterns of neuronal connections.

In vertebrates, an important step in this process is the migration of neuronal precursors from their site of origin to definitive locations. Developing cells from the two major sources of neurons—the neural crest and the ventricular zone of the neural tube—migrate substantial distances. Some cortical neurons appear to make this journey by crawling along a particular class of glial cell (radial glia). Many other sorts of neurons, however, migrate without benefit of such preexisting guides. A reasonable view might be that preexisting glial scaffolds are not a prerequisite for accurate migration but organize this phenomenon in particular ways in the cortex. More generally, neuronal precursors are guided by cellular and extracellular cues in the matrix through which they move; the nature of the map they must read during this process is not yet understood. The mechanism of migratory movement is probably similar to the movement of fibroblasts and other cells that advance by making adhesive contacts at their leading edges and then pulling themselves forward. Therefore, differential adhesiveness is probably the key element in the determination of migratory pathways.

A unique feature of developing neurons is the extension of processes. This special form of cell movement occurs at growth cones, which advance in a manner similar to the advance of entire cells. It is attractive to suppose that the same cues that determine the migratory path of neuronal precursors direct the subsequent outgrowth of neuronal processes (see Chapter 5).

Axon Outgrowth and the Generation of Stereotyped Nerve Patterns

INTRODUCTION

Whereas previous chapters dealt with general developmental issues that are also relevant to the nervous system, the outgrowth of axons is a peculiarly neural phenomenon. Axonal signaling has a number of advantages over other means of cell communication. First, information received by one cell can be rapidly transmitted to another. Second, by branching, axons can convey the state of one nerve cell to many target cells. Third, the state of many cells can be communicated to a single neuron by convergent innervation. Finally, axons usually innervate specific sets of cells (or even parts of cells); thus neuronal communication is remarkably precise. The purpose of this chapter is to consider how growing axons find appropriate targets.

STUDIES OF AXON OUTGROWTH
IN RELATIVELY SIMPLE SYSTEMS

The most direct way to study how an axon traverses the distance to its target is to observe outgrowth during development. This approach was first taken in the 1930s by C. C. Speidel, who followed the course of axon outgrowth in the nearly transparent tadpole tail (Speidel, 1933, 1941). More recently, this strategy has been applied to the appendages (legs and antennae) of some insects (Bentley and Keshishian, 1982; Ho and Goodman, 1982; Goodman et al., 1982a,b). When they first develop, insect appendages comprise a single epithelial layer surrounding a loose mesoderm. Sensory neurons differentiate from the epithelium throughout the course of embryonic development and send processes toward the corresponding central ganglia (Figure 1) (Wigglesworth, 1953, 1959; Lawrence, 1969; Sanes and Hildebrand, 1976). The morphology and trajectory of particular axons can be studied in fixed appendages after intracellular injection of the cell bodies with dyes such as Lucifer Yellow or after staining with antibodies (Taghert et al., 1982). These approaches are also being used to study axon trajectories in the insect central nervous system (Raper et al., 1983a,b).

The processes of sensory neurons in insect appendages must navi-

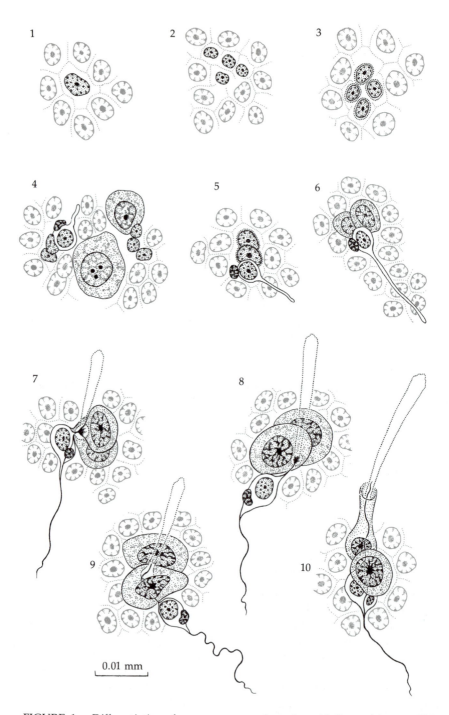

FIGURE 1. *Differentiation of sensory neurons from the epithelium of insects. This diagram shows the stages in the differentiation of a sensory hair in the fourth-stage larva of the bug* Rhodnius prolixus *(silver stain). As the nerve cell differentiates, it elaborates a process that innervates the base of the hair and an axon that grows toward the corresponding central ganglion. (From Wigglesworth, 1959.)*

gate to a central ganglion (Sanes and Hildebrand, 1975; Bate, 1976). In the developing locust, for example, two solitary pairs of axons emerge from sensory neurons in the antennae and run to the ganglia of the central nervous system (Bate, 1976). The axons from antennal sensory receptors that differentiate later grow toward the central ganglion in close association with the initial pair of pioneers. Thus, the adult nerve bundle from an antenna represents an agglomeration of axons around these initial fibers. A similar sequence occurs in the growth of other sensory axons in invertebrates (Meinertzhagen, 1973; Lopresti et al., 1974; Edwards, 1977).

The behavior of these fibers can be interpreted in two ways. The view that prevailed until recently was that the initial axons were capable of navigational feats that later axons could not perform. From this perspective, the axons that differentiated later simply followed the pioneers and had little or no ability to navigate in their own right. If this were the case, then destroying the pioneers ought to cause disruption of subsequent axon growth; in particular, it ought to abolish the stereotyped nerve bundles that characterize insect appendages as well as most other neuronal pathways (Figure 2). Using a laser microbeam, J. S. Edwards and his collaborators could, in fact, destroy pioneer fibers arising from the cricket cercus (Edwards et al., 1981). The result of this

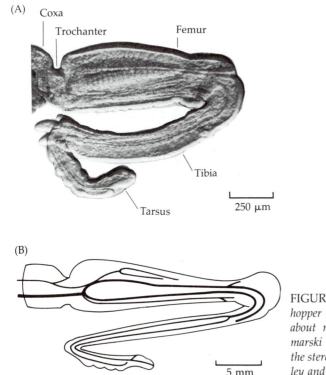

(A) Coxa
Trochanter   Femur
Tibia
Tarsus
250 μm

(B)
5 mm

FIGURE 2.   *The growth of sensory axons in the grasshopper leg. (A) Photomicrograph of a grasshopper leg about midway through embryonic development (Nomarski optics). (B) Diagram of the adult leg, showing the stereotyped nerve pathways in the limb. (After Bentley and Keshishian, 1982.)*

experiment was equivocal. When the pioneer fibers were destroyed, the subsequent outgrowth of sensory axons toward the cricket central nervous system formed a number of small bundles rather than a normal nerve; they did, however, reach the central nervous system.

Subsequent experiments have suggested that *all* neurons in the insect appendage are capable of the same navigational feats and that the pioneers are simply first to do the job. The complicated and yet stereotyped outgrowth of axons from sensory neurons in the grasshopper leg has now been studied in some detail (Bentley and Keshishian, 1982; Ho and Goodman, 1982; see also Goodman et al., 1982a,b). A differentiating neuron first sends out extensive filopodia, which traverse distances equivalent to several cell diameters (Figure 3). C. M. Bate (1976) first noted that other cells along the way seem particularly important in determining the route of growth, and he suggested that each cell encountered might act as a sort of "stepping-stone." Indeed, when the growth cones of sensory axons contact other differentiating neurons along the pathway, they form junctions capable of passing dye from one cell to the other; filopodia extending in other directions disappear and the extensions in the direction of the contacted neuron are stabilized (Figure 3). This process is repeated until the next neuron is contacted, and so on (see Figures 2 and 3). Each stepping-stone cell eventually extends its own axon; these axons apparently go through the same routine as the so-called pioneers, fasciculating with the axons that preceded them.

Unlike the experiments of Edwards in the cricket, deletion of the earliest differentiating neurons in the locust leg does not lead to abnormal trajectories of later developing axons (Bentley and Keshishian, 1982; see also Nardi, 1983). Evidently, any axon is capable of defining the normal pathway in the absence of the earlier pioneers. On the other hand, removing the intermediate stepping-stone cells alters the normal pathway (Bentley and Caudy, 1983). These observations suggest that the growing tips of all the sensory axons in the insect limb recognize appropriate signals along the route.

In summary, invertebrate axons appear to be capable of independent navigation to their targets. The stereotyped pathway of these nerve fibers apparently reflects the obedience of all axons in insect appendages to the same rules of outgrowth. The fact that sensory axons grow in the same general direction (i.e., proximally) argues for some inherent polarity in the appendage, a phenomenon reminiscent of the more general encoding of positional information discussed in Chapter 2.

STUDIES OF AXON OUTGROWTH
IN MORE COMPLEX SYSTEMS

Axon outgrowth is more difficult to observe in vertebrates. At this level, most work has focused on the extension of motor neurons to muscles rather than the ingrowth of sensory axons. The most instructive ex-

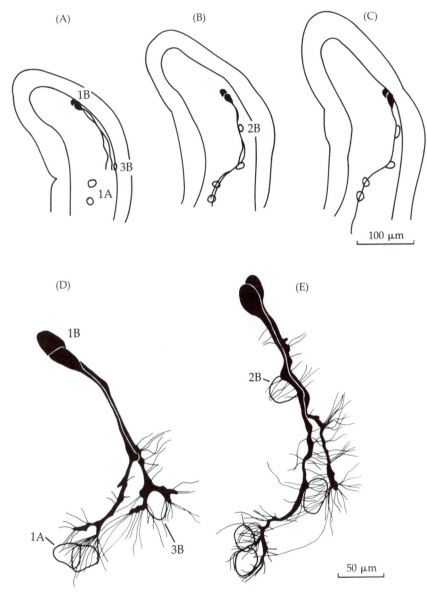

FIGURE 3.   *Direct observation of the development of nerve pathways in the grasshopper limb. (A–C) Camera lucida drawings of developing sensory neurons and their axons in whole-mounted grasshopper legs from successive embryonic stages (somewhat earlier than the leg shown in Figure 2A). Sensory axons (filled) take stereotyped routes as they navigate centrally; the course is similar to the adult pattern of nerves (cf. Figure 2). (D,E) Growth cones send out extensive filopodia in the direction of the future pathway. Filopodia that contact another differentiating neuron ("guidepost" cell; open) adhere to it preferentially, thus consolidating the axonal route. These more detailed camera lucida drawings were made from two different whole mounts after intracellular marking of the 1B cells with Lucifer Yellow. Stage corresponds approximately to B. (After Taghert et al., 1982.)*

ample has been the outgrowth of spinal motor neurons to muscles in the chick limb. As in studies of morphogenesis (Chapter 3), the chick limb is particularly attractive because of its accessibility in ovo.

Establishment of stereotyped projection patterns in vertebrates

The result of limb innervation in vertebrate development is well-defined groups of neurons (motor neuron pools) that follow stereotyped pathways to particular muscles (Figure 4). The way in which this adult pattern of nerves comes about is not well understood. As soon as motor

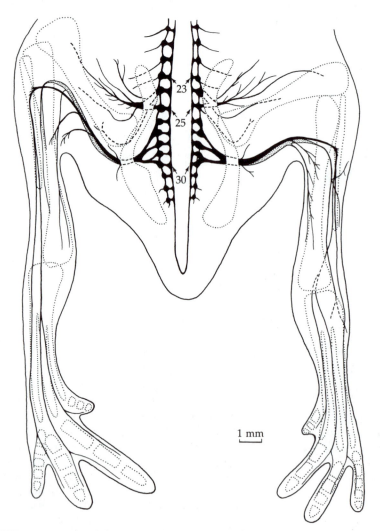

FIGURE 4. *Drawing of the pattern of innervation in the chick hind limbs. The drawing was made from a silver-stained embryo at 10 days of incubation (stage 36). Stipple indicates skeletal elements; numbers indicate segments. Note the minor differences in branching between the right and left sides. (After Fouvet, 1973.)*

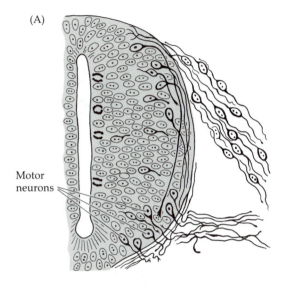

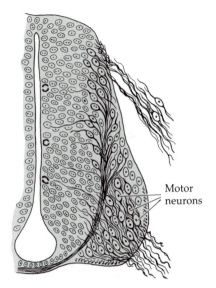

FIGURE 5. *The appearance of motor neurons in chick spinal cord at the time of motor axon outgrowth. (A) Drawing of the lumbar cord of a 3-day-old chick embryo (cross section of half the cord and the surrounding tissue). At the time that motor axons first grow out of the spinal cord, the cells lack dendrites and sometimes retain a basal process that extends toward the ventricular epithelium. Some motor neurons are still being born at* *this stage (note mitotic figures). (B) A day later, most motor neurons have migrated to their definitive position in the lateral motor column. As in the genesis of cortical structures (Chapter 4), the cells born last migrate through regions occupied by older cells to reach a more superficial (in this case, lateral) position. (After Ramón y Cajal, 1929.)*

neurons are generated, they migrate away from the ventricular epithelium and become part of a morphologically homogeneous motor column (Figure 5) (Hollyday and Hamburger, 1977). Axon outgrowth and functional innervation of muscle occurs very early: almost as soon as motor neurons arise, they send axons to the periphery (Figure 5) (Ramón y Cajal, 1929; see also Heaton et al., 1978). Thus, motor neuron pools are still in the process of segregating when axon outgrowth begins. When motor axons first enter the chick limb, they bear no obvious relation to one another (Hollyday, 1980a). Subsequently, the axons distribute themselves within the limb in patterns that gradually become recognizable as those of the adult nerves (Figure 6; cf. Figure 4). During this process the limb bud contains a central core of precartilage that separates two mesenchymal condensations called the dorsal and ventral premuscle masses (Figure 7). Thus, axons do not actually grow to particular muscles but to regions of what appears to be homogeneous mesenchyme. Taken together, these several observations make plain that neither motor neuron pools, their targets, nor the nerve pathways are well defined at the time innervation of the limb occurs.

Extracellular recordings made from embryonic nerves suggest that the adult projection pattern of peripheral axons is established from early stages (Landmesser and Morris, 1975; Landmesser, 1978; Scott, 1982).

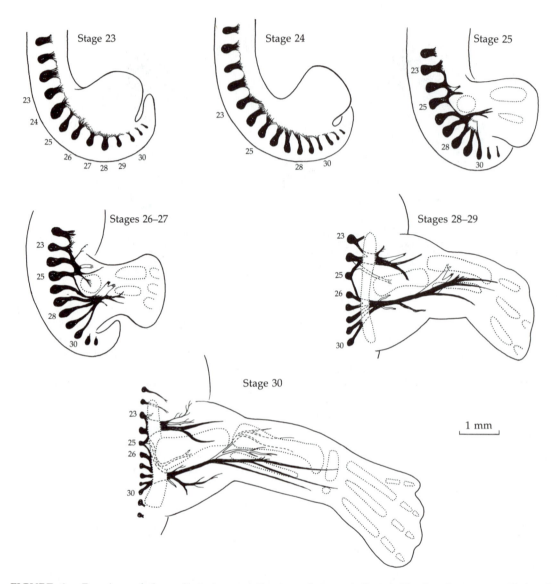

FIGURE 6. *Drawings of the earliest stages of the formation of nerves in the hind limb of the chick. The sections are parasagittal, so the origins of the spinal nerves are shown in cross section; stages and somite numbers are indicated. The dorsal nerves are filled and the ventral nerves open. Stipple indicates skeletal elements. (After Fouvet, 1973.)*

This impression has been confirmed by retrograde labeling with horseradish peroxidase (see Box A). When small amounts of peroxidase are injected into the embryonic muscle masses or skin in the chick hind limb at 4–5 days incubation, the neurons take up the enzyme and transport it retrogradely. The embryonic neurons identified in this way occupy the same relative position in the embryonic spinal cord and

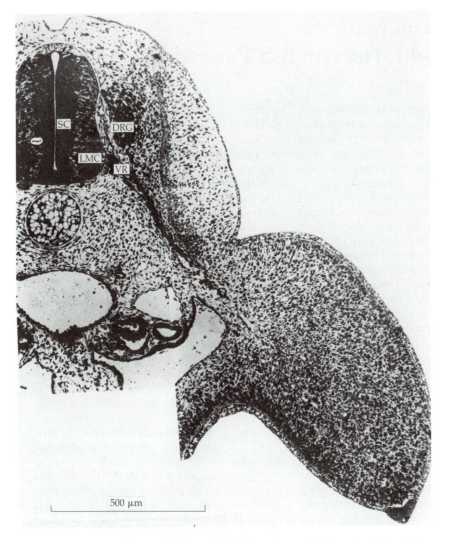

FIGURE 7.   *Transverse section through a chick embryo at 3½ days incubation (stage 23) at the level of the anterior limb bud. The spinal cord (SC) and the lateral motor column (LMC) are indicated. The motor axons leave the spinal cord in the ventral root (VR) to reach the base of the limb. At this stage, individual muscles are not identifiable; only ventral and dorsal premuscle masses are present. DRG, Dorsal root ganglion. (From Bennett, 1981.)*

dorsal root ganglia as the adult complement of neurons (Figure 8) (Landmesser, 1978; Hollyday, 1980b; Scott, 1982; Honig, 1982). Similar labeling in mammalian embryos shows that the adult pattern of nerve projections is also established at very early stages (Smith and Hollyday, 1984; see also Smith and Hollyday, 1983; Rubin, 1985b).

The early presence of adult projection patterns suggests little error

Cell Marking
with Horseradish Peroxidase

In recent years the technique of marking neurons with the enzyme horseradish peroxidase (HRP) has become a major tool. In its brief history, this method has probably been used by more neurobiologists than have used the Golgi stain since its discovery in 1870.

Although the Golgi technique was unequivocally the invention of a single person, the widespread use of peroxidase is difficult to attach to the efforts of any individual. Perhaps this is because several different advances led to its current applications. First was the observation by P. Weiss and H. B. Hiscoe in 1948 that materials are continually transported along axons. This observation led to work on the now well-established, but incompletely understood, phenomenon of axonal transport. Second was the idea that transported macromolecules might act as markers. The notion of using horseradish peroxidase for this purpose probably arose from the use of this molecule in extracellular marking studies pioneered by W. Straus, M. Karnovsky, and R. C. Graham, who showed that a reaction product catalyzed by this enzyme forms a dense precipitate that can be seen in both light and electron microscopes (Mesulam, 1982). In 1971 K. Kristensson and Y. Olsson first used HRP to label neurons retrogradely in the peripheral nervous system (Kristensson and Olsson, 1971). J. H. and M. M. LaVail then demonstrated the efficacy of HRP in the central nervous system and worked out much of the cell biology of its transport (LaVail and LaVail, 1972).

Horseradish peroxidase is a heme protein found in the roots of the horseradish and has a molecular weight of about 40,000 daltons. The advantages of this particular agent are striking. It is readily taken up by nerve cells; because of its size, HRP tends to remain inside the cells and their axons and dendrites. Most important

is the amplification that occurs because this protein is an enzyme. It is not the transported molecule itself that is seen in the microscope but rather a reaction product produced by incubation with an appropriate substrate and hydrogen peroxide. In consequence, a relatively small number of enzyme molecules can create an easily visualized precipitate. Interestingly, the sequence of reactions involved is similar to the reactions that produce melanins, a large family of plant and animal pigments.

Numerous variations in HRP methodology have now been described (see, for example, reviews in Heimer and Robards, 1981; Mesulam, 1982). In general, the enzyme is used in three ways by neurobiologists. The most common use is as a retrograde label. In this approach, HRP (as crystals or solution) is placed on or near injured axons. Retrograde axonal transport then carries the enzyme molecules to the cell bodies, which are made visible by catalysis of an appropriate substrate such as diaminobenzidine, tetramethylbenzidine, or pyrocatechol. This simple, yet powerful approach shows the location of nerve cells that project to a given region and has radically changed the ease with which one can obtain information about neuronal projections. A variant of this approach is uptake of the enzyme by intact axon terminals; for example, intraocular injections retrogradely label cells in the superior cervical ganglion. Terminal uptake can be augmented by electrical stimulation and can also be used to distinguish active from inactive terminals (Holtzman et al., 1971; Heuser and Reese, 1973; Ceccarelli et al., 1973).

A second way of using the enzyme is to introduce it near injured nerve cell bodies. The enzyme is then taken up by cell somata (presumably by endocytosis) and transported distally by anterograde axonal transport. This ap-

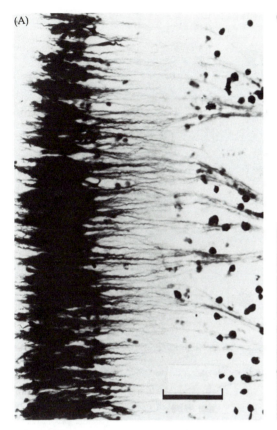

(A)

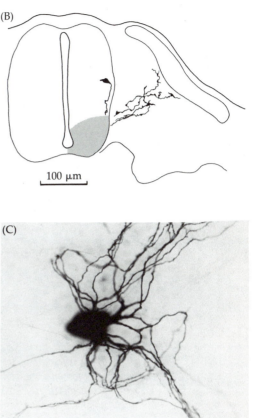

(B)

100 μm

(C)

(A) Preganglionic neurons in the embryonic rat spinal cord (E14) retrogradely labeled after HRP injection into the stellate ganglion (T1–T3 indicate thoracic segments). (B) Anterograde transport of HRP into motor neuron axons after injection into the spinal cord of an embryonic chick. (C) Mammalian sympathetic neuron after intracellular injection of HRP through a micropipette. (A from Rubin, 1985b; B after Hollyday, 1983; C from D. Purves, unpublished.)

proach can demonstrate the projection site and the anatomy of terminal arborizations and thus provides information complementary to the retrograde transport approach (see figure). Finally, HRP can be introduced into the electrolyte solution filling a micropipette, a technique that permits intracellular marking of individual cells after electrophysiological studies. This approach was first used to mark crustacean neurons with the fluorescent dye Procion Yellow by A. O. Stretton and E. A. Kravitz (1968); in the mid-1970s a number of workers adapted HRP to this intracellular method (see Mesulam, 1982). Intracellular injection has remarkable power because it provides a Golgi-like picture of cells whose properties and connections can be studied in detail prior to staining.

It is hard to overestimate the importance of this technique in neurobiology generally and developmental studies in particular.

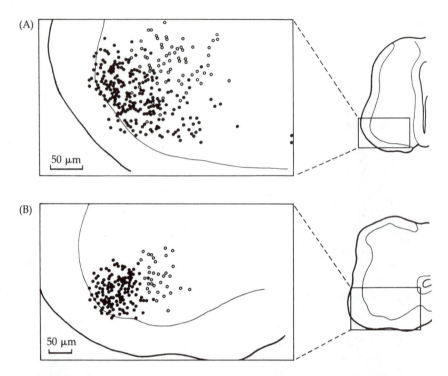

FIGURE 8. *Location of motor neuron pools at early stages in the chick spinal cord. Horseradish peroxidase injection into ventral (open circles) and dorsal (filled circles) muscle masses on day 6 of incubation (A: stage 28) shows approximately the same mediolateral distribution as injection of particular muscles in the ventral and dorsal thigh at later stages (B: day 11; stage 37). Apparently the motor neurons that send axons to different muscles are distinct from early stages. (After Landmesser, 1978.)*

in the establishment of peripheral innervation. On the other hand, M. R. Bennett and his collaborators have found some initial mistakes in the development of wing bud innervation in the chick (Pettigrew et al., 1979; see also McGrath and Bennett, 1979; Bennett et al., 1980; Hollyday, 1983). A. H. Lamb has also reported some evidence of initial error in the innervation of the frog limb. Motor neurons that ultimately innervate distal limb musculature are transiently associated with developing muscles in the proximal part of the frog hind limb at early developmental stages (Lamb, 1976). The degree of error, however, is not very substantial (no more than 10 percent). Moreover, diffusion of peroxidase away from the injection site (or uptake by nearby fibers of passage) is difficult to control in young embryos. Thus, the degree of apparent error observed at early stages is, if anything, an overestimate. The dominant theme of initial innervation in the peripheral nervous system seems to be appropriate connectivity from the outset.

Significance of stereotyped nerve branching

Although the adult pattern of nerve branching is generally taken to indicate that particular motor axons follow well-defined routes to their targets, the significance of nerve pattern vis-à-vis the innervation of specific targets is not at all clear. One puzzling fact is that the limb appears to dictate a normal pattern of nerve branching regardless of the axons that enter it. Thus, changing the segmental source of limb innervation by limb transplantation in the rostrocaudal axis does not change the final pattern of limb nerves (Harrison, 1907; Detwiler, 1936; Hamburger, 1939; Piatt, 1956; Hollyday et al., 1977). A similar conclusion derives from limb duplication experiments. In the chick wing, the posterior division of the brachial nerve splits into three branches at the elbow: a muscle branch, a purely cutaneous branch, and the median nerve (which innervates both distal muscles and skin). When a tandem limb is created by grafting one wing bud onto another, the median nerve from the first elbow reaches the second elbow and is confronted there by the same choice of pathways that faced the brachial nerve at the proximal joint. If nerve routes were simply determined by preexisting paths that appealed to axons arising from different motor neuron pools, then the axons that chose the median nerve path at the proximal joint should prefer that path at the second opportunity. However, the median nerve also trifurcates to project to the very muscles that were avoided in the proximal limb segment (Lewis, 1978; see also Stirling and Summerbell, 1979; Summerbell and Stirling, 1981; Stirling, 1983; Whitelaw and Hollyday, 1983b).

These experiments argue that the stereotyped pattern of nerves in the limb does not arise through a simple matching of neurons with particular targets, but involves a more complicated interaction of axons and the matrix they traverse.

Evidence for axonal pathfinding

Although branching nerve patterns are probably not a consequence of axons seeking specific targets, axons do seem to be biased to grow in particular directions. For example, A. Stefanelli (1951) and E. Hibbard (1965) showed that rotation or transposition of Mauthner cells in fish or in amphibians fails to prevent the Mauthner cell axons from eventually finding their way (Figure 9). A related observation is that the few pyramidal cells in the mammalian cortex that by chance are improperly oriented still seek out their normal targets (Van der Loos, 1965). Similarly, the axons of some autonomic ganglion cells initially grow in the wrong direction before making a hairpin turn to reach an appropriate destination (Lichtman, 1977; Purves and Hume, 1981). Other examples of axonal pathfinding in abnormal circumstances occur in invertebrates (see, for example, Ghysen, 1978), in the cortical connections of mutant

(A) NORMAL ORIENTATION

(B) REVERSED ORIENTATION

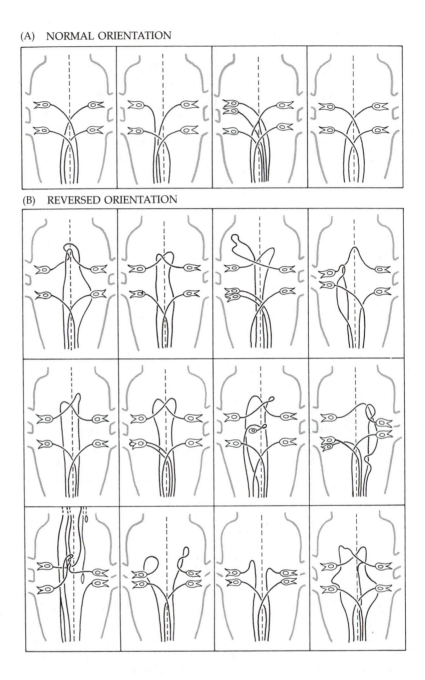

mice (Caviness, 1976; Caviness and Rakic, 1978), and in the retinotectal system of lower vertebrates (Chapter 11). Thus many classes of axons find their way even when they are misdirected or are forced to start from an ectopic location.

The ability of misrouted axons to find their way has been further tested by deletion or reversal of short segments of spinal cord in chick

FIGURE 9. *The ability of axons to find their way after misrouting. This series of drawings shows the results of transplantation experiments carried out on Mauthner cells in the brain stem of an amphibian (Pleurodeles waltlii). A partial duplication of the medulla was induced by grafting a medullary segment from a donor animal; thus, the upper pair of Mauthner cells in each panel is supernumerary. In (A), the grafted segment was placed in the normal rostrocaudal orientation (each of the panels represents a separate experiment). In these cases the axons follow what would be considered a more or less normal route (i.e., the same route as the lower pair of host cells). The panels in (B) show the results when the graft was placed in reversed anterior–posterior orientation. In most experiments, the supernumerary pair of Mauthner cell axons first grew rostrally with respect to the host, that is, in the wrong direction. In every case, however, the misguided axons eventually corrected themselves and grew down the cord, decussating in the process. Misdirected Mauthner axons evidently sense their error when they emerge from the graft into rostral tissues of the host, which they would not normally encounter. These results imply that cues in the tissues through which vertebrate axons grow are instrumental in guiding them. (After Hibbard, 1965.)*

embryos (Lance-Jones and Landmesser, 1980a,b, 1981a,b). In these experiments, axons from spinal cord segments adjacent to a deletion found their usual targets but largely ignored nearby targets that remained denervated because of the missing segments (Lance-Jones and Landmesser, 1980a; see also Landmesser, 1980; Whitelaw and Hollyday, 1983a). Axons growing out of spinal cord pieces that had been shifted by two or three segments as a result of cord reversal were also able to find their normal targets with little error (Figure 10) (Lance-Jones and Landmesser, 1980b, 1981b). When, however, larger segments of spinal cord were reversed, axons grew to abnormal locations (see also Hollyday et al., 1977). These results suggest that axons are only capable of compensating for relatively minor dislocations.

Finally, V. Whitelaw and M. Hollyday (1983b,c) have examined whether motor axons in the chick hind limb can find targets in novel positions. They found that in serially duplicated limbs (e.g., thigh-thigh-calf-foot), the second thigh segment was innervated by axons that normally innervate calf; similarly, in thigh-calf-calf-foot limbs, the second calf was innervated by the motor neurons that normally innervate the foot. This result, like the tandem elbow experiment (see earlier), shows that motor axon pathfinding is not predicated on innervation of specific targets (see also Summerbell and Stirling, 1981).

Taken together, these experiments present a paradox: particular axons are biased to grow to specific places, yet axons from different motor neuron pools can substitute for one another in the establishment of normal nerve patterns.

MECHANISMS OF DIRECTED AXON OUTGROWTH

Unraveling the mystery of stereotyped projection patterns will ultimately depend on a detailed understanding of the mechanisms that

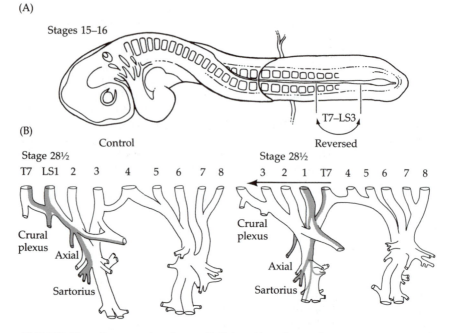

(A)

Stages 15–16

T7–LS3

(B)

Control

Stage 28½

T7 LS1 2   3   4   5   6   7   8

Crural
plexus

Axial

Sartorius

Reversed

Stage 28½

3   2   1   T7   4   5   6   7   8

Crural
plexus

Axial

Sartorius

FIGURE 10. *Compensation for small dislocations of axonal starting position in the chick embryo. (A) Lengths of spinal cord comprising several segments (T7–LS3, in this case) can be reversed at early embryonic stages (2½ days of incubation; stage 15–16). (B) The pattern of axon projection at later stages (about 6 days incubation; stage 28½) can be determined by anterograde transport of horseradish peroxidase injected into one or two spinal cord segments. The normal projection pattern of segments T7 and LS1 is shown on the left; on the right is the projection after the reversal operation shown in A (arrow). The ectopic motor neurons eventually find correct peripheral nerves and innervate appropriate muscles. (From Lance-Jones and Landmesser, 1980b.)*

bias axons to grow in a particular direction. A number of different factors influence axonal trajectories (see also Box B).

Stereotropism

Perhaps the simplest explanation of directed growth is mechanical routing of axons to the right place, a process called stereotropism. Early evidence taken to support this idea was the finding that explanted nerve cells send out neurites along scratches in the surface of a culture dish or along lines of tension in a plasma clot (Weiss, 1934, 1941). It seems likely that mechanical factors such as paths of least resistance, interfaces, aligned tracts of cells, and surface contours all influence axons in different circumstances (Horder, 1978; Horder and Martin, 1978; Bray, 1982). A case in point is the behavior of axons in the cuticle of the bug *Rhodnius* (Wigglesworth, 1953). When the contour of the cuticle is altered by a small lesion, axons that find their way into the resulting trough are unable to escape and circle aimlessly. Some workers, T. J. Horder, for example, have gone so far as to suggest that mechanical and temporal factors are a sufficient explanation of patterned innervation (Horder, 1978; Horder and Martin, 1979).

A more specific notion of mechanical routing is the so-called blueprint hypothesis, which postulates that a pattern of holes or spaces is generated in the neuroepithelial matrix before axon outgrowth (Singer et al., 1979). Axons in the spinal cord of the embryonic newt, for example, appear to grow into such spaces, which are regarded as guiding them to appropriate destinations. Similarly, axons growing out from the mouse retina enter open spaces in the region of the optic nerve head (Figure 11) (see also Krayanek and Goldberg, 1981). In a mutant mouse in which these spaces are obliterated, axon outgrowth is impeded (Silver and Robb, 1979; Silver and Sidman, 1980); thus, such neuroepithelial spaces appear to be a prerequisite for normal axon outgrowth in some circumstances. A further example in an invertebrate is

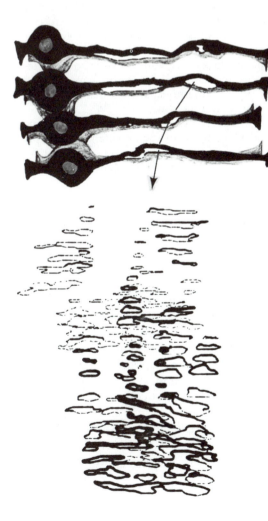

FIGURE 11. *Diagram of the disposition of neuroepithelial cells in the mouse optic cup. Intercellular openings in the region of the optic disk are thought to form sets of interconnected tunnels (arrow) through which retinal axons grow. The series of 1-μm sections shown below suggests that adjacent cells cooperate to keep the spaces in register. (After Silver and Sidman, 1980.)*

Axon Outgrowth during Regeneration

Studies of axon outgrowth during regeneration provide additional information about the behavior of growing axons and raise important clinical issues.

Most classes of peripheral axons regenerate readily after they are severed and often regain their normal targets (muscles or sensory receptors in the skin, for example). In general, regenerating axons have a strong predilection for the normal sites of termination within target tissues. Thus, motor axons reoccupy the endplate zone of muscle fibers (Gutmann and Young, 1944; Bennett et al., 1973; Letinsky et al., 1976; Sanes et al., 1980), and at least some sensory axons return quite precisely to specialized sensory receptors in the skin (Burgess and Horch, 1973; Burgess et al., 1974) or to muscle spindles (Thulin, 1960; Bessou et al., 1965; Brown and Butler, 1976). Although regenerating axons are often able to find appropriate postsynaptic elements within a target, in most vertebrates, especially in mammals, they have little luck finding their original targets within the larger context of the limb or some other body part (Bernstein and Guth, 1961; Brushart and Mesulam, 1980; see also Chapter 10). Thus, when motor axons regenerate, they appear to innervate deprived muscles or skin on a first-come, first-served basis.

In the light of this inability of regenerating mammalian axons to navigate normally, it is surprising that peripheral nerve regeneration is topographically accurate in some other vertebrates. Appropriate reinnervation of various muscles has been demonstrated in experiments on salamander limbs and the extraocular muscles (Grimm, 1971; Cass et al., 1973; Fangboner and Vanable, 1975). The stimulus for this effort was the claim by R. W. Sperry and H. L. Arora (1965) that regenerating axons of the third cranial nerve of a fish partition themselves correctly between the several extraocular muscles. The upshot of this work is that in some vertebrates, the tissues of the mature limb continue to provide interpretable cues that enable the axons to find their way.

In the central nervous system of mammals (including man), an additional phenomenon is apparent: severed central axons are loath to grow at all, extending only short distances beyond a lesion. In a series of simple, yet powerful experiments, A. J. Aguayo and his colleagues have explored the basis of this deficiency by transplanting a segment of pe-

the tendency of sensory axons to grow into the tubular spaces that become the wing veins in *Drosophila* (Palka et al., 1983).

In spite of these observations, the notion of preexisting mechanical pathways does not provide an adequate explanation of axonal navigation. First, such preexisting pathways are not apparent along the route of most axons that have been studied. Second, it is difficult to imagine how preformed spaces could serve to tell particular axons how to get onto or off of major pathways. Third, even if such mechanical guides were general, one would still have to explain how such guides were themselves established. Although mechanical factors may help to guide the outgrowth of axons, this class of ideas cannot explain many features of axonal behavior.

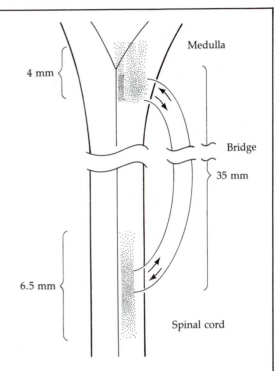

Diagram of a peripheral nerve bridge experiment demonstrating that central axons can grow long distances when presented with the environment of a peripheral nerve. Here a peripheral nerve bridge in the rat links the medulla and the thoracic spinal cord. After a suitable interval, application of horseradish peroxidase to the bridge retrogradely labels neurons in both the medulla and thoracic cord, thereby indicating that some central axons can extend 3 cm or more after transection. (After Aguayo et al., 1982b.)

ripheral nerve to a central site, and vice versa (Aguayo et al., 1979; Bray et al., 1981; Aguayo et al., 1982; Benfey and Aguayo, 1982). They showed that central axons can actually extend many millimeters after an injury but are prevented from doing so by some aspect of the central environment. Thus, when central axons are confronted with the distal stump of a *peripheral* nerve, they perform about as well as severed peripheral axons. The most likely villain in this piece is the central glial cell. This idea has become more attractive with the discovery of various trophic interactions between nerve and glial cells (see Bray et al., 1981). The fact that central axons *can* extend long distances offers some promise, in principle, of addressing spinal and other lesions where injured axons have to go a long way to reestablish their normal connections. Aguayo has shown that bridges of peripheral nerve can serve as bypass conduits to route at least some axons across spinal lesions in rats (see figure) (Aguayo et al., 1982).

Taken together, these findings add a further element of complexity to the already difficult question of how axons find their way. In many animals it appears that some aspect of maturation obliterates or makes uninterpretable the road signs that served so well during development.

Tropism based on differential adhesiveness

The observation that growth cone filopodia seem to explore the local environment (Chapter 4) suggests another, more subtle way that surfaces can direct axonal growth. That surface properties are capable of influencing the direction of neurite growth has been shown by P. Letourneau in tissue culture (Letourneau, 1975a,b; see also Collins and Garrett, 1980). When neurons are seeded onto a culture plate with a surface bearing geometrical patterns of artificial materials to which neurites adhere differentially, axons follow the pattern described by the substance to which they adhere best (Figure 12; see also Figure 5 in Chapter 4). Detachment of individual filopodia by micromanipulation

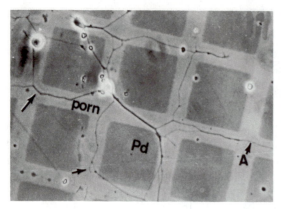

FIGURE 12. *Demonstration that neurite growth can be guided by differential adhesivity to the substrate. The surface of a culture dish was coated in a gridlike pattern with avenues of polyornithine (porn) amidst squares coated with palladium (Pd). The growth cones adhere preferentially to the polyornithine. When sensory neurons from chick embryos are seeded onto such a surface, the growing neurites follow the avenues of the more adhesive substrate. A, Neurite. ×180 (From Letourneau, 1975b.)*

confirms the importance of filopodial attachment in the direction of neurite extension (Wessells and Nuttall, 1978). D. Bray (1979, 1982) has further shown that the vector of the force generated by growth cone adhesiveness is an important determinant of direction: when a growing neurite is pulled to one side with a fine glass needle, the direction of advance is immediately changed by this stress (Figure 13) (Bray, 1979; see also Bray, 1984).

The ability of growing axons to follow an adhesive pathway in a selective manner probably operates in life as well as in the culture dish. For example, growth cones frequently advance preferentially across epithelial layers covered by basal lamina. Thus, in the moth wing, sensory axons grow on the basal lamina between two epithelial layers (Nardi and Kafatos, 1976). By transplanting portions of epithelium, a gradient of adhesivity that increases in the direction of axon growth can be demonstrated (Nardi, 1983; see also Berlot and Goodman, 1984). The behavior of growth cones at limb segment boundaries in the grasshopper leg also suggests gradients of adhesivity in epithelia (Bentley and Caudy, 1983). Finally, axons growing in situ (or in vitro) often fasciculate in a highly selective manner. For example, axons of sibling neurons in the grasshopper embryo can grow in different directions at a point of choice based on which preexisting axon they prefer to extend along (Raper et al., 1983). The molecular basis of selective adhesion is considered in Chapter 11.

Galvanotropism

Early accounts of axon guidance routinely included a discussion of electrical influences (see, for example, Ariëns Kappers et al., 1936; Weiss, 1941). Electrical guidance fell from fashion over the years but has been revived recently by the experiments of L. Jaffe and his collaborators. These experiments indicate that voltage gradients are commonplace in developing embryos and can indeed influence axonal growth (Jaffe, 1979, 1981).

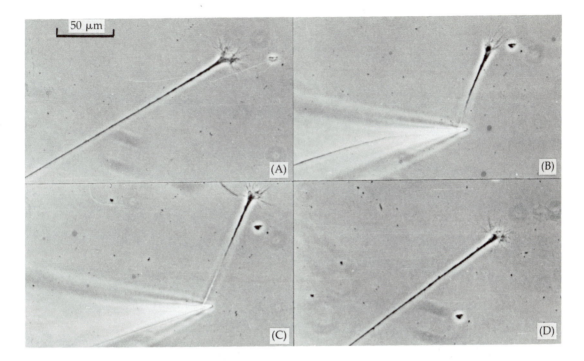

FIGURE 13. *Redirection of a growing neurite by mechanical displacement of the trailing process. (A) Distal neurite and growth cone of a cultured sympathetic ganglion cell, growing diagonally from left to right. (B) Within a minute of displacing the neurite with a micro-* *needle, the direction of growth is changed. (C) Twelve minutes later the neurite continues to extend in the new direction. (D) Fifteen minutes after the removal of the microneedle the neurite has resumed its original direction of growth. (From Bray, 1979.)*

The renaissance of this line of research depended on the invention by Jaffe and R. Nuccitelli (1974) of a vibrating probe that can measure very small voltage differences in the fluid surrounding living tissues (Figure 14). Using this probe, they found that steady currents on the order of 1–100 $\mu A/cm^2$ are generated by developing systems such as germinating plants, fucoid eggs, vertebrate embryos, and regenerating limbs (Jaffe, 1981). Endogenous electrical fields have also been measured in the vicinity of muscle fibers (Betz et al., 1980; Betz and Caldwell, 1984; Caldwell and Betz, 1984; Betz et al., 1984). In general, such fields are generated by local electrogenic membrane pumps; the circuit is completed by adjacent regions which are leaky to the particular ion involved (Jaffe, 1979, 1981). Associated voltage gradients of a few millivolts to 0.1 V or more have been measured.

Such fields can influence both the rate and the direction of neurite extension from cultured cells (Figure 15); neurites grow more rapidly toward the negative pole than toward the anode, and gradually turn in the direction of the cathode (Jaffe and Poo, 1979; Hinkle et al., 1981; Patel and Poo, 1982, 1984; see also Borgens et al., 1981). This cathodal influence can be observed in electrical gradients as small as 7 mV/mm!

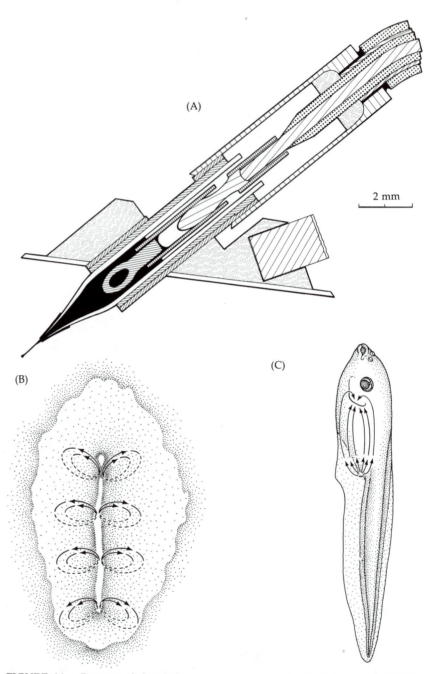

(A)

2 mm

(B)

(C)

FIGURE 14.   *Patterns of electrical current measured in developing embryos. (A) Vibrating probe used to measure tiny electrical fields in the vicinity of developing organisms or cells. The probe is shaped more or less like a ball point pen; the ball at the tip (20–30 μm in diameter) vibrates laterally at 200 Hz over a distance that is typically 30 μm. The vibration converts any potential difference between the extremes of this excursion into a sinusoidal output, the amplitude of which is a measure of the potential difference. (B) Pattern of current determined from such measurements around an early chick embryo (cf. Figure 6 in Chapter 1). (C) Pattern measured in a* Xenopus *tadpole (stage 49). (A,B after Jaffe, 1981; C after Jaffe and Poo, 1979.)*

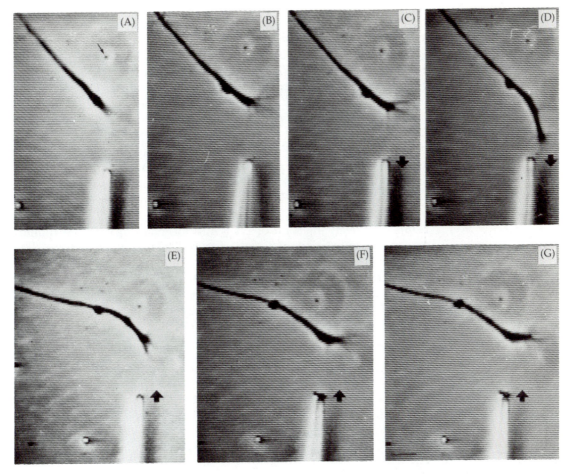

FIGURE 15. *Influence of an electrical field on the direction of neurite growth. This series of micrographs shows the attraction of a neurite from a cultured amphibian neuron toward the tip of an electrode when it is the cathode (C–D), and subsequent growth away from the electrode when the polarity is reversed and it becomes the anode (E–G). No current is being passed in A and B. The interval between frames is 15–20 minutes; the current passed was 200 nA. Arrows show direction of current. (From Patel et al., 1984.)*

M.-M. Poo and his colleagues have shown that membrane proteins such as acetylcholine receptors can move rather dramatically under the influence of fields similar in magnitude to those that can be measured in some living systems with the vibrating probe (Jaffe and Poo, 1979; Poo, 1981). This finding is important because it implies that the electrophoresis of particular molecules at the growing tip of an axon might affect the direction of growth.

The idea that embryonic currents influence axon outgrowth (or other aspects of embryonic pattern) is often given rather short shrift. Although evidence for physiological effects on axon outgrowth is still lacking, axon growth is clearly responsive to field strengths that are probably present at the relevant embryonic stages.

Chemotropism

Another possible mechanism of axon guidance that has been widely considered is navigation along gradients of a diffusible signal emanating from an axon's target. Recent experiments on the tropic influence of the protein nerve growth factor (NGF) have given advocates of this view a specific example that appears to support this means of axon guidance (the discovery and significance of NGF are treated in detail in Chapter 7).

A tropic effect of NGF has been shown in tissue culture experiments in which local application of this molecule to growing neurites of dorsal root ganglion cells causes them to change their direction of growth over a remarkably brief time (Figure 16) (Gundersen and Barrett, 1979, 1980; see also Campenot, 1977; Ebendal and Jacobson, 1977; Letourneau, 1978). Moreover, injection of NGF into the brain of neonatal rodents causes sympathetic axons to take a completely aberrant pathway into the spinal cord and to ascend toward the site of NGF injection (Menesini-Chen et al., 1978; see Figure 6 in Chapter 7).

It seems unlikely, however, that nerve growth factor or a similar agent could serve as a comprehensive explanation of axon guidance. In the first place, normal concentrations of NGF in target tissues are ex-

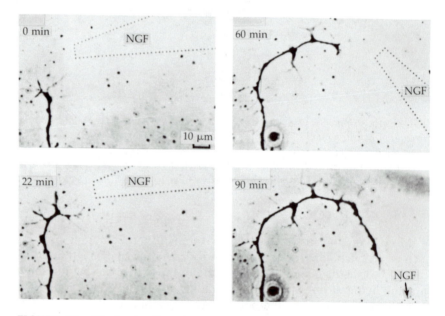

FIGURE 16. *The tropic effect of nerve growth factor. These sequential photomicrographs show the response of the distal tip of a dorsal root ganglion cell neurite exposed to NGF diffusing from the tip of a micropipette (dotted line; numbers in the upper left indicate elapsed minutes). Ninety minutes after the start of the experiment, the neurite had extended 108 μm and had turned almost 160° from its original direction of growth, presumably in response to movements of the NGF pipette. (Courtesy of J. Barrett.)*

tremely low (see Chapter 7): there is a difference of many orders of magnitude between the concentrations used to demonstrate tropism and the NGF levels that exist in vivo. Second, the targets of sensory and sympathetic ganglion cells (the major classes of neurons known to be sensitive to nerve growth factor) are ubiquitous. It is therefore difficult to imagine how gradients of diffusible molecules could, by themselves, cause the highly stereotyped patterns of outgrowth apparent in normal development. Third, sympathetic and sensory axons follow the same initial pathways as motor axons, although they innervate different targets. Finally, nerve patterns tend to be normal when developing muscles are killed by X irradiation of the somitic mesoderm prior to its migration (Lewis et al., 1981; see also Christ et al., 1977). Nerves that grow into such limb buds show the usual branching pattern, with one important exception: whereas the main nerve trunks and their cutaneous sensory branches are fully developed, the nerve branches which in a normal limb would innervate muscles are almost completely absent (Lewis et al., 1981; see also Whitelaw and Hollyday, 1983a). Thus, the proximal nerve routes appear to be independent of the target tissues; on the other hand, the formation of distal branches to individual muscles may require a signal from the target.

In summary, it seems more likely that NGF and other similar agents that arise from axonal targets serve as local attractants to axons that have reached the vicinity of those targets by other means.

CONCLUSIONS

Growing axons often cross substantial distances enroute to their targets. The manner in which this occurs in invertebrates suggests that axons respond continually to directional cues in their local environment. Less direct observations in vertebrate limbs are consistent with this idea. Studies of axon outgrowth in the vertebrate limb also show that the initial projection of axons to muscle (or skin) occurs with relatively little projection error (and that axons can compensate for minor dislocations). On the other hand, axons are in some ways interchangeable during the establishment of nerve patterns. Thus, axons that do not normally innervate the limb form a normal pattern of limb nerves when given the opportunity; moreover, the same axons may make different choices at homologous points in serially duplicated limbs. Although it is widely assumed that active seeking of appropriate pathways is a major contributor to stereotyped nerve patterns in vertebrates, this idea still has very little experimental support and should be regarded with caution. The paradox presented by the evidence for the selective guidance of axons and the evidence that axons can substitute for one another in generating stereotyped branching patterns will only be resolved when a great deal more is known about the mechanisms that direct axons.

A number of such mechanisms have been considered, including mechanical guides, pathways of differential adhesiveness, electrical fields, and tropic gradients emanating from targets. Although each has some merit, none of these mechanisms by itself provides a satisfactory explanation of the full range of behavior shown by growing axons. The most plausible general explanation of axon outgrowth is that a number of influences act together to assure accurate navigation and that the mechanisms that lead axons to their targets (e.g., gradients of differential adhesiveness) may be quite different from the mechanisms that signal the arrival at an appropriate target (e.g., local signals of diffusible agents arising from the target cells).

Neuronal Death During Development

INTRODUCTION

The death of cells is a normal event throughout the life of animals. In many organ systems, cells turn over continuously, sometimes at an impressive rate. Human red blood cells, for example, have an average lifetime of about 120 days; the cells of many epithelial linings turn over even more rapidly. From this perspective, the nervous system is exceptional: most neurons do not turn over at all. Given the stability of neurons in maturity, the death of many nerve cells during embryonic development comes as something of a surprise.

That cell death is a prominent feature of normal development has long been recognized (Glücksmann, 1951; Saunders and Fallon, 1966). The phenomenon is traditionally divided into three categories. Phylogenetic cell death refers to the elimination of entire structures during the course of development. An example is the loss of the tail from developing vertebrate embryos (frogs and humans, for instance). A second category is morphogenetic death; this refers to the loss of cells during the shaping of tissues. The loss of the digital webs between fingers and toes in the limb buds of mammalian embryos is an example in this category. Finally, histogenetic cell death refers to a diffuse loss of cells from an organ during the course of normal development. Although these distinctions are not very rigorous, histogenetic cell death is the category most relevant to the development of the nervous system.

Acceptance of the notion that some neurons die in the course of normal development came relatively late in the history of neuroembryology. A number of neuroembryologists in the early 1900s alluded to the likelihood of neuronal death during development (see, for example, Collin, 1906), but it was not until the middle of the century that the prevalence (and significance) of this phenomenon was generally appreciated (Oppenheimer, 1981a; Cunningham, 1982). There are several reasons for this. Although as many as half or more of the neuronal precursors originally present in various parts of the nervous system degenerate during early development, the signs of degeneration are transient. Thus, casual observation of any particular neural structure does not necessarily convey the magnitude of this developmental pro-

Counting Cells

It might seem a straightforward matter to assess by accurate cell counts the degree of neuronal degeneration during the development of a particular region of the nervous system. However, this information is actually quite hard to come by, and a number of acrimonious disputes about neuronal death have revolved around methodology. B. Q. Banker, for example, has argued that little or no death of neurons occurs in the embryonic spinal cord of mammals (Banker, 1982). She attributes the discrepancy between her results and numerous other studies supporting motor neuron loss in the lateral motor column to inadequate attention to cell count correction methods (see below). Although her analysis is controversial, her article and the ensuing discussion point up the difficulties of accurately counting developing nerve cells.

There are at least four problems faced by neurobiologists carrying out this kind of work. First, young neurons are often difficult to distinguish from glial cells during early development. Although this problem may ultimately

be solved by the use of glial-specific markers, at present one runs the risk of overestimating neuronal populations by including glial cells. A second problem is that cell counts must be related to a well-defined area or volume. Counting cells in a central nucleus is relatively simple as long as the nucleus remains discrete throughout the developmental period of interest. In many regions, however, boundaries are not easily recognized and the size and shape of neuronal groups changes dramatically. This problem has been overcome to a degree by retrograde labeling of cells with horseradish peroxidase (see Box A in Chapter 5), but this method suffers from the assumption that developing cells take up the marker equally well at different developmental stages and that diffusion of the marker is equally restricted in small and large targets. A third problem concerns counts made in histological sections. Counting neurons in sections requires correction for "double counting," that is for counts of the same cell in two or more adjacent sections (see figure). A number of formulas have

cess. It is only when cells are systematically counted at the beginning and at the end of the period of cell death that this phenomenon is apparent (see Box A); even then the magnitude of cell death may be difficult to estimate because of concurrent proliferation and degeneration.

The normally occurring death of many neuronal precursors appears to arise from one of two developmental strategies. Some neurons are programmed to die by virtue of intrinsic instruction; in many cases, however, the death of particular neurons is not preordained but depends on interactions with other cells.

PROGRAMMED CELL DEATH

The small number of cells in some invertebrates, such as the nematode *C. elegans,* has allowed embryologists to follow the development of individual cells and their progeny from the earliest stages of develop-

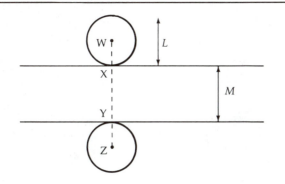

$$P = A \frac{M}{L + M}$$

M. Abercrombie (1946) pointed out that cell counts made from microtome sections must be corrected for split-cell counts. This need is made clear by the diagram on the left: any cell (circles) whose center lies between points W and Z will be represented in section X-Y. Therefore, simple counts of cells, cell nuclei, or any other organelle will overestimate the number of cells present. The correction formula suggested by Abercrombie is shown on the right. P is the corrected number of cells (or nuclei) per section, A the raw count, M the section thickness, and L the average diameter of the cells.

been developed to make such corrections: the most widely used of these was described by M. Abercrombie in 1946. All these formulas, however, depend on estimates of the smallest fragments counted as neurons, or on the size of a subcellular element (e.g., the nucleolus) that is small relative to the section thickness. A fourth problem is that in some (perhaps most) parts of the nervous system, proliferation and cell death are overlapping events. Thus, the number of cells counted in a particular region may not accurately reflect the degree of cell death; if cell proliferation and neuronal death occur at the same rate in a given region, the vast majority of neurons could die without an appreciable change in the number of cells counted. Finally, cell counting is a decidedly tedious business that only the most conscientious investigators are likely to carry out with care and accuracy.

ment (Chapter 2). As described earlier, individual cells follow a highly stereotyped sequence of divisions that largely determines the number and type of the progeny. An integral part of this process is the invariable degeneration of particular cells in the lineage (Figure 1). There are certain fixed rules in this process in *C. elegans*: the posterior daughter of an anterior–posterior cell division is more likely to die; and one daughter cell of a division nearly always survives (Sulston and Horvitz, 1977). What evidence there is suggests that cell death in these circumstances is largely autogenous and under genetic control (Horvitz et al., 1982; Hedgecock et al., 1983).

Because all the cells in a lineage may not be needed in a given part of the animal, the programmed death of some progeny seems an expeditious way of achieving regional diversity in both the numbers and types of neurons present in the adult. In grasshoppers, for example, programmed cell death allows differences to emerge between segmental ganglia. Thus, cell degeneration is more pronounced in abdominal seg-

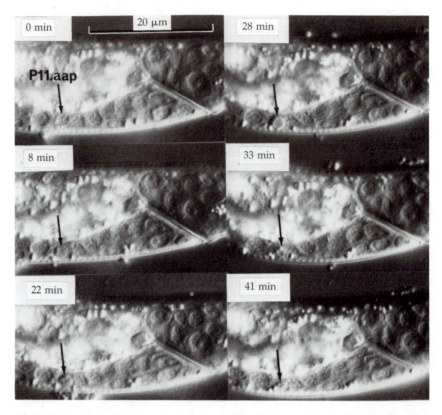

FIGURE 1. *Programmed cell death in the developing nematode* C. elegans. *This sequence of photomicrographs shows the death of a particular cell in the lineage that contributes to the ventral nerve cord (see Chapter 2). Degeneration occurs over a period of about 30 minutes. The dying cell is indicated by the arrow in each frame. (From Sulston and Horovitz, 1977.)*

ments than in thoracic segments, thereby leading to a disparity in ganglionic size (there are about 3000 neurons in mature thoracic ganglia, compared with 500 in abdominal ganglia) (Goodman and Bate, 1981; Bate and Grunewald, 1981). By the same token, programmed death in a lineage can alter the types of cells that result. For instance, some cells that survive in the region of the nematode vulva die in other regions (Figure 2) (Horvitz, 1981; see also Bate et al., 1981). Presumably the cells that degenerate in the nonsexual regions (i.e., homologues of the surviving cells in the vulval region) are generated because they are a necessary part of the lineage strategy: the sister of a cell that degenerates produces progeny that are essential in all regions.

Analogous studies have not been carried out in vertebrates; therefore it is not really known whether programmed degeneration occurs at very early stages. By the same token, not all cell death in invertebrates is programmed (see, for example, Shankland, 1984). Because a single cell in invertebrates often carries out a function that is subserved by hundreds or thousands of cells in the vertebrate nervous system, it

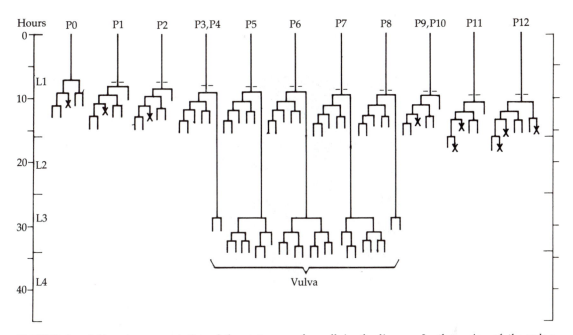

FIGURE 2. *Schematic representation of the postembryonic development of the ventral nerve cord and vulva in a* C. elegans *hermaphrodite. P0–P12 are precursors that generate the ventral nerve cord and its associated ganglia; each* **X** *represents the programmed degeneration of a cell in the lineage. In the region of the vulva, precursors that die elsewhere survive. Thus, altering the program of degeneration leads to regional differences in both numbers and types of cells. L1–L4 indicate larval stages. (After Sulston and Horvitz, 1977.)*

seems unlikely that exactly the same strategy for achieving the right types and numbers of components would be used at all phylogenetic levels. Relatively simple animals evidently rely on strict lineage programs to generate small and precise numbers of nerve cells in appropriate distributions. Although more complex nervous systems may employ programmed cell death as well, they also appear to use a more flexible strategy based on neuronal redundancy.

TARGET-DEPENDENT NEURONAL DEATH

Death of neurons is a prominent feature of embryonic development in vertebrates. For many of these cells, death is not a result of lineage but occurs because of competition between nerve cells at the level of the target they innervate.

Relation between the number of cells in nerve centers and the size of their targets

Experiments early in this century showed that the final number of neurons in various vertebrate nerve centers is determined by the presence and relative size of the neuronal target (Figure 3). In 1909, M. L.

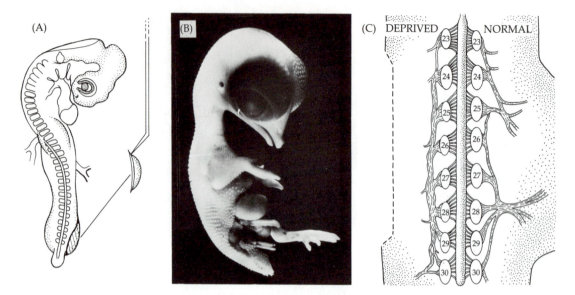

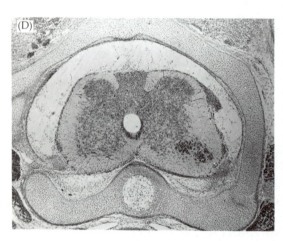

FIGURE 3. *The effects of limb bud ablation in chick embryos. (A) At approximately 2½ days of incubation, a leg primordium can be excised with a fine glass needle. (B) A 10-day chick embryo whose right leg primordium was extirpated as in A. (C) Reconstruction of the lumbosacral spinal cord, spinal ganglia, and peripheral nerves in a 6½-day embryo, one of whose legs was extirpated at 2½ days. Note the smaller size of the relevant spinal ganglia on the operated side. (D) Cross section of the lumbar spinal cord from a 9-day chick embryo, showing the appearance of the lateral motor column on the normal side and the contralateral side on which the leg primordium was extirpated at 2½ days of incubation. The lateral motor column on the deprived side is virtually absent. (A after Hamburger, 1977; B from Hamburger, 1977; C after Hamburger, 1958; D from Hamburger, 1958.)*

Shorey found that removal of limb buds from chick embryos or amphibian larvae depleted limb motor neurons and neurons in the related sensory ganglia. This relationship was confirmed by S. Detwiler (1920, 1936), who found that implantation of an extra limb bud in early amphibian embryos induced a corresponding increase in the population of neurons in the related sensory ganglia. A final contribution to these early observations was the demonstration by V. Hamburger (1934) (see Box B) of a proportional relationship between the amount of the target removed and the number of neurons in the innervating population (see also Piatt, 1946; Prestige, 1967a,b).

Each of these experiments indicated that the target is somehow instrumental in defining the final population of innervating cells. What was unclear, however, was the mechanism by which this regulation was achieved. In general, the interpretation of such results until the 1950s was that the missing target failed to recruit or induce differentiation of a population of precursor cells whose numbers were consequently altered. Although S. Ramón y Cajal and others considered the possibility that neuronal death occurs normally, the prevailing view was that "the immense majority of the neuroblasts survive to term and succeed in collaborating with the normal structures of the adult nervous system" (Ramón y Cajal, 1929; see also Collin, 1906; Oppenheim, 1981a).

Experiments carried out on sensory ganglia in chick embryos by Hamburger and R. Levi-Montalcini in the late 1940s were crucial in changing this dogma (Hamburger and Levi-Montalcini, 1949). They first confirmed that target ablation (limb bud removal) caused marked atrophy of the corresponding sensory ganglia. Hamburger and Levi-Montalcini then went on to show that this hypoplasia occurs at least in part because many neurons that are initially present in sensory ganglia degenerate after limb bud ablation (see also Hamburger et al., 1981). More important, they showed that this phenomenon is also characteristic of sensory ganglia in *normal* chick embryos. That is, cell death occurs not only after ablation of the target but as an ordinary feature of embryonic development.

Not surprisingly, the misconceptions of several decades were not resolved at one fell swoop. In interpreting their work in 1949, Hamburger and Levi-Montalcini continued to support the idea that the influence of the target on developing nerve centers is explained by an effect on the proliferation of neuronal precursors as well as by an effect on the degree of cell death. Whether the target has any influence on precursor proliferation is not completely settled to this day, but studies using modern techniques such as thymidine autoradiography indicate that the ablation of a neuronal target probably has little or no effect on nerve cell proliferation (Currie and Cowan, 1974; Carr and Simpson, 1978a,b; see also Hamburger, 1958).

Subsequent to this initial description, normally occurring neuronal death has been found in a variety of systems including spinal motor neuron pools (Hamburger, 1958, 1975), spinal preganglionic neurons (Levi-Montalcini, 1950; Oppenheim et al., 1982), autonomic ganglia (Aguayo et al., 1973, Landmesser and Pilar, 1974b; Hendry and Campbell, 1976; Wright et al., 1983), brain stem nuclei (Dunnebacke, 1953; Cowan and Wenger, 1967, 1968; Rogers and Cowan, 1973; Alley, 1974; Sohal, 1976a), and cells projecting entirely within the central nervous system (Sohal and Narayanan, 1974; Cowan and Clarke, 1976; Rager, 1980; O'Leary and Cowan, 1982, 1984; Rakic and Riley, 1983). In all of these systems, the extent of cell death is considerable (30–75 percent; Figure 4).

Whether all developing systems of neurons are subject to degeneration is unclear. The cerebral cortex, which for a long time was thought to display only minimal cell death, has been shown to undergo at least a modest degree of neuronal degeneration during development (Lewis,

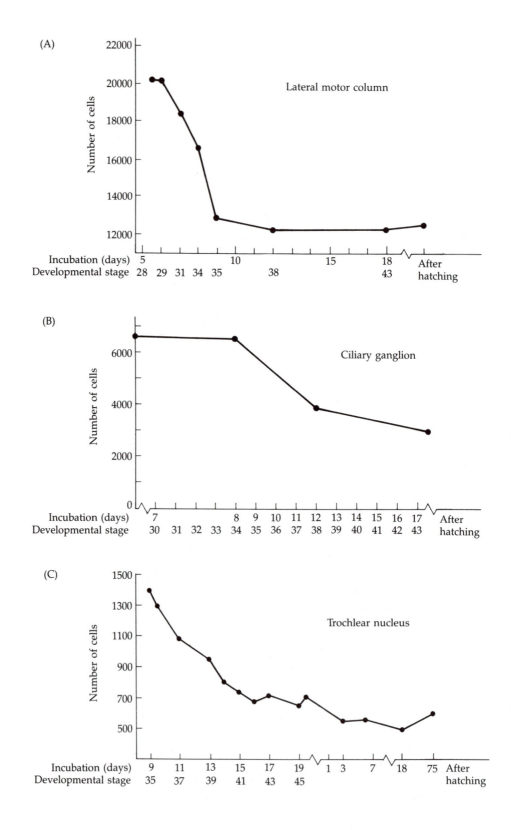

◄ FIGURE 4. *Normally occurring neuronal death in different parts of the embryonic nervous system in the chick. (A) Lateral motor column of the spinal cord; (B) ciliary ganglion; (C) trochlear nucleus in the brain stem. Hamilton–Hamburger stages and days of incubation are indicated below each graph. In each system a massive loss of neurons occurs in early embryonic life. (A after Hamburger, 1975; B after Landmesser and Pilar, 1974b; C after Cowan and Wenger, 1967.)*

1975; Finlay and Slattery, 1983; Pearlman, 1985; see also Oppenheim, 1981a). Nonetheless, some systems, such as pontine nuclei in birds, are evidently not subject to this phenomenon (Armstrong and Clarke, 1979). Moreover, target-dependent death may not be characteristic of invertebrate development (Figure 5) (Sanes et al., 1976; Whitington et al., 1982; see also Whitington and Seifert, 1982).

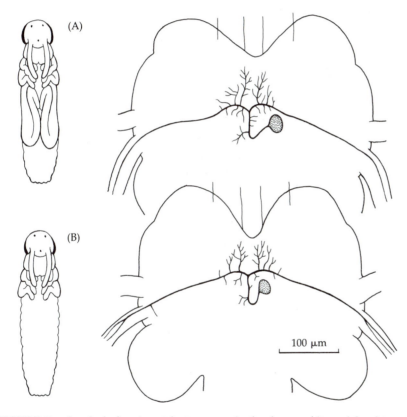

100 μm

FIGURE 5. *Survival of an invertebrate neuron in the absence of its peripheral target. (A) Camera lucida drawing of a grasshopper metathoracic ganglion in which an identified motor neuron that projects to the leg has been injected with the fluorescent dye Lucifer Yellow. (B) Ganglion from another embryo at a comparable stage in which the same cell has been injected; as indicated in the accompanying cartoon, the metathoracic legs were removed at an earlier embryonic stage. Extirpation of the target has no apparent effect on the survival or even the detailed morphology of the motor neuron, a result very different from that observed in vertebrate embryogenesis (cf. Figure 3). Whether the axon succeeds in innervating other targets is not known. (After Whitington et al., 1982.)*

Viktor Hamburger (b. 1900)

Viktor Hamburger was born in Landeshut, Silesia (now a part of Poland, but then a province of Germany). Although his father was a businessman, much of Hamburger's youth was spent in a rural setting where his interest in biology was encouraged by teachers and a friend who was later a leading taxonomist at the Berlin Museum of Natural History. He attended the Universities of Breslau, Heidelberg, Munich, and Freiburg and received his Ph.D. in zoology under the supervision of H. Spemann in 1925 (see Box A in Chapter 3). He then took a post as a research associate at the Kaiser Wilhelm Institute for Biology in Berlin in the laboratory of O. Mangold and, after two years, became a privatdozent and instructor at the Zoological Institute of the University of Freiburg (see Holtfreter, 1965, for a marvelous account of academic life in Germany during that period).

In 1932 Hamburger received a yearlong Rockefeller fellowship to work in F. R. Lillie's laboratory at the University of Chicago, at that time one of the few laboratories in the world studying the embryology of the chick; his purpose was to apply Spemann's microsurgical methods to the chick embryo. When he arrived in Chicago in 1932 his intention was to stay only a year. However, the rise of the Nazi party in early 1933 resulted in a letter from the dean of the faculty at the University of Freiburg informing Hamburger that, due to "the cleansing of the professions," he had been dismissed from his position in Germany. Thus, he stayed on as a Rockefeller fellow at the University of Chicago until 1935 when he was appointed to the zoology faculty at Washington University in St. Louis, where he has remained.

Hamburger's research proceeded along four different but related lines. The first of these, fundamental to the other three, was his classic study of the normal development of the chick embryo. "Our real teacher," Hamburger said, "has been and still is the embryo—who is, incidentally, the only teacher who is always right" (Holtfreter, 1965). Because of Hamburger's work, this preparation now provides the standard for much vertebrate neuroembryology; the staged series published with H. Hamilton (Hamburger and Hamilton, 1951), which summarizes the major developmental landmarks of the chick, is one of the most cited papers in the biological literature.

The second avenue of Hamburger's work

Proximate cause of target-dependent neuronal death

When considering the possible mechanisms of target-related neuronal death, it is obviously important to know as much as possible about the details of degeneration. What is the timing of this process? What is the appearance of cells undergoing degeneration? What do timing and appearance suggest about the cellular mechanisms that bring about neuronal demise?

The timing of cell death is usually quite sharp and often occurs at approximately the same time that axons reach their targets. In the chick embryo spinal cord, dorsal root ganglia, and ciliary ganglion, the period of cell death spans just a few days in early development (approximately days 5 through 12 of incubation; see Figure 4). There are, however, some exceptions to this acuteness (see Box D). In mammalian sympa-

and perhaps the most important, concerned the discovery and elucidation of neuronal death in normal embryonic development (see text). A number of earlier investigators had noted that removal of a peripheral target—for example, the limb bud in a tadpole or a chick embryo—resulted in developmental failure of the related nerve centers. Hamburger, with his colleague R. Levi-Montalcini, showed that *normal* nerve cell death is also dictated by the peripheral target. These studies on normally occurring neuronal death in the chick embryo form the basis for present thinking about competitive processes in the nervous system.

The third line of Hamburger's research was his discovery with Levi-Montalcini in the late 1940s and early 1950s of the protein nerve growth factor (see Chapter 7). Since the 1950s, work in numerous laboratories has characterized the nerve growth factor molecule and established a good understanding of its biological significance (Chapter 7).

The final line of Hamburger's research concerned the development of behavior. Using his knowledge of the normal development of the chick embryo, Hamburger explored the earliest stages of embryonic motor activity in a series of experiments carried out in the 1960s. Contrary to the view widely held by behavioral psychologists, he showed that the earliest movements of embryos are independent of sensory stimulation (Hamburger et al., 1966).

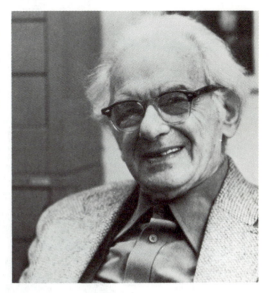

Viktor Hamburger in his office at Washington University in 1982. (Courtesy of Outlook magazine.)

The importance of these observations is discussed in Chapter 14.

To a remarkable degree, Hamburger's work has set the course of developmental neuroembryology in this century. However, only in the last decade or so have neurobiologists (as distinguished from embryologists) recognized the fundamental significance of his contributions.

thetic ganglia, for example, a substantial amount of cell death has been reported to occur postnatally (Hendry and Campbell, 1976; Wright et al., 1983; see, however, Davies, 1978).

Morphological observations on degenerating neurons have been made at both the light and electron microscopical levels (Figure 6). A perplexing finding is that the ultrastructural appearance of cells undergoing normal degeneration is not always identical to the appearance of neurons that degenerate following target ablation (Pilar and Landmesser, 1976). Cells that die a natural death in the chick ciliary ganglion develop a normal complement of rough endoplasmic reticulum and polyribosomes, which then become dilated and otherwise abnormal during degeneration. Target-deprived ciliary ganglion cells fail to develop these cytoplasmic changes. In this case, degeneration is characterized primarily by changes in the nucleus, changes that appear only

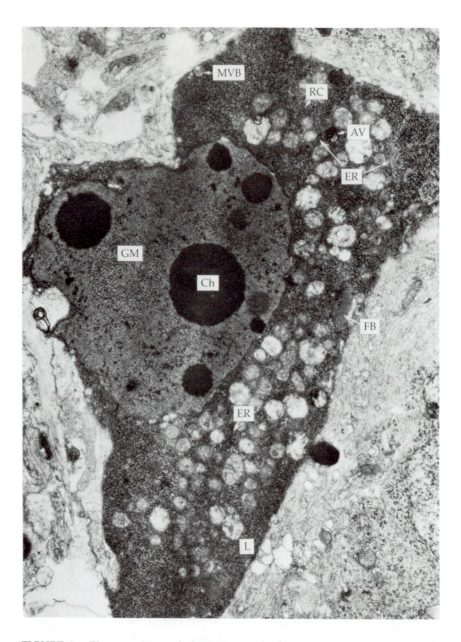

FIGURE 6. *Electron microscopical appearance of a degenerating neuron in the lateral motor column of a normal 6-day chick embryo. The neuron stains much more darkly than normal, as is typical of degenerating cells; the mitochondria are swollen and the nucleus is pyknotic with several masses of condensed chromatin (Ch). The small number of such profiles relative to the magnitude of neuronal loss (see Figure 4A) suggests that degeneration and phagocytosis occur quite quickly. AV, Autophagic vacuole; L, primary lysosomes; MVB, multivesicular bodies; GM, granular masses; ER, endoplasmic reticulum; RC, ribosome crystals; FB, filament bundles. ×10,800. (From Chu-Wang and Oppenheim, 1978.)*

during the end stage of normally occurring neuronal death. On the other hand, similar observations in other parts of the nervous system have not shown any particular difference in the appearance of cells degenerating normally and those degenerating after peripheral ablation (Chu-Wang and Oppenheim, 1978; Sohal and Weidman, 1978; Hughes and McLoon, 1979).

Evidently neurons develop and differentiate more or less normally before death. For example, appropriate levels of the enzymes choline acetyltransferase and acetylcholinesterase are found in spinal motor neurons destined to die because of peripheral ablation (Oppenheim et al., 1978). In the chick ciliary ganglion, neurons differentiate, send out dendrites, and become innervated before the phase of cell death (Landmesser and Pilar, 1974a). All this suggests that the early biology of neurons is much the same whether they eventually die or survive.

BOX
C

Cell Death Induced by Hormones

Cell death can be triggered in the nervous system and elsewhere by the action of hormones. An extreme example is the tobacco hornworm moth (*Manduca sexta*) in which about half of the neurons in abdominal ganglia degenerate in association with the emergence of the adult moth from its pupal case (Truman and Schwartz, 1982; Truman, 1983). This massive degeneration is under the control of ecdysone and related hormones and is quite stereotyped in its distribution. Cell death can occur by direct action of hormones on developing nerve cells or secondarily by the induction of metamorphosis (see Box B in Chapter 1). In anurans, metamorphosis is triggered by an increase in circulating levels of thyroxin (Kollros, 1968). The resorption of the tail, for example, is related to the level of this hormone, and isolated tails can be induced to undergo metamorphosis (histolysis) in a bath to which thyroxin has been added (Weber, 1962). Because neurons depend on targets for survival, the resorption of a structure like the tail also leads to degeneration of the related nerve cells (Brown, 1946).

Thyroxin can also trigger neuronal death directly. For example, Mauthner cells in the brain stem of larval anurans gradually increase in size but atrophy and die about the time the animal matures (Stefanelli, 1950). The targets of the Mauthner cells degenerate during metamorphosis, but this is probably not the cause of neuronal death because interrupting connections to the target has no effect on the Mauthner cells (Weiss and Rossetti, 1951). However, when larvae are treated with exogenous thyroxin, the Mauthner cells atrophy prematurely; conversely, when metamorphosis is blocked with thiourea, the Mauthner cells survive indefinitely (Fox and Moulton, 1968; Kollros, 1968, 1981). Similar effects of thyroxin on cell survival have been reported for the lateral motor column and the mesencephalic nucleus of frogs (Beaudoin, 1956; Kollros and McMurray, 1956; Decker, 1976).

The effects of hormones on neuron survival are not limited to animals that undergo metamorphosis. In the rat cerebellum, for example, low levels of thyroxin increase the degree of granule cell death (Lewis et al., 1976). The dependence of neurons in the developing cerebellum and elsewhere on thyroid hormones probably contributes to the mental retardation (cretinism) that accompanies congenital hypothyroidism.

Evidence for competition in neuronal death

These findings, together with the observation that death is accentuated by the extirpation of neuronal targets, imply that nerve cell survival involves acquisition of a target-derived agent that is in limited supply.

In several systems it is possible to inject horseradish peroxidase into the target prior to the time of cell death to determine what percentage of the initial population has already reached their destination. In the developing visual system of the chick, virtually all of the neurons that supply efferent innervation to the retina are retrogradely labeled by peroxidase injection into the eye before the onset of cell death (Cowan and Clarke, 1976). Similarly, nearly all the cells in the ciliary ganglion are labeled by ocular injection at the beginning of the cell death period (Pilar et al., 1980). Finally, retrograde labeling of motor neurons in the chick spinal cord shows that these cells also reach their target prior to the phase of cell death (Chu-Wang and Oppenheim, 1978; see also Prestige and Wilson, 1974). Therefore, failure of axons to reach the target is probably not a cause of normally occurring neuronal death.

Several additional experiments make a direct case for competition at the level of the target. Increasing the bulk of the target by implantation of a supernumerary limb salvages neurons that otherwise would have died (Hollyday and Hamburger, 1976; Hollyday et al., 1977; see also Hamburger, 1939; Bueker, 1945). That target augmentation increases the ultimate size of mature neural centers was already known from the experiments of Detwiler (1920); the contribution of modern experiments has been to show that this occurs because normal cell death is forestalled (Figures 7 and 8). Experiments in which a smaller number of neurons innervate a target of normal size point to the same conclusion. In the ciliary ganglion of the chick, neurons reach their target (the eye) by way of three postganglionic nerves. By cutting some of the postganglionic nerves, G. Pilar, L. Landmesser, and L. Burstein (1980) reduced the number of ciliary ganglion cells before the normal cell death period (Figure 8). The result of this mismatch was that an appreciably larger fraction of the remaining ciliary ganglion cell population survived to maturity. This outcome implies that when the number of competing

FIGURE 7. *Increased survival of motor neurons following augmentation of the periphery. (A) A 6-day chick embryo with a right supernumerary leg, which had been grafted at 2½ days of incubation. (B) A 12-day chick embryo with a right supernumerary leg (normal left leg is not visible). The corresponding motor columns of animals with an extra leg showed increased numbers of motor neurons on the side related to the graft (on the order of 10 to 30 percent). (C) Cross section through the lumbar cord of a 12-day embryo with a right supernumerary leg. The number of motor neurons on the right side (as well as the number of dorsal root ganglion cells) is increased. (D) A highly unusual frog, which in nature had four hind limbs—three on the right and one on the left. Inset: A cross section of the lumbosacral cord of this animal showed hypertrophy of both the ventral horn and the dorsal columns on the side with the extra limbs. (A,B,C, from Hollyday and Hamburger, 1976; D from Bueker, 1945.)*

neurons is reduced a greater proportion of the competitors survive (see, however, Lamb, 1984). A third approach is to produce a mismatch by augmenting the number of neurons that innervate a target before the period of cell death. D. O'Leary and M. Cowan have done this in the chick visual system; they found that when both isthmo-optic nuclei are induced to innervate one eye by early enucleation, fewer neurons in these centers survive (O'Leary and Cowan, 1984).

Based on this evidence, the conventional view is that the neurons innervating a target compete with one another and that the losers die. The major purpose of this competitive phenomenon is presumed to be

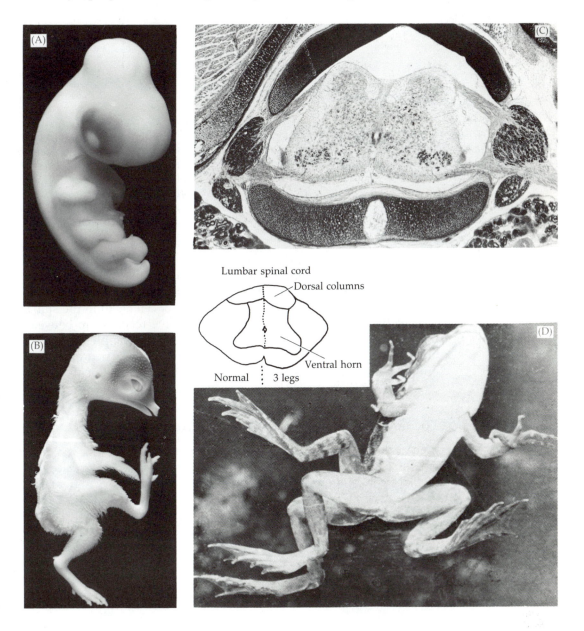

Lumbar spinal cord
Dorsal columns
Ventral horn
Normal : 3 legs

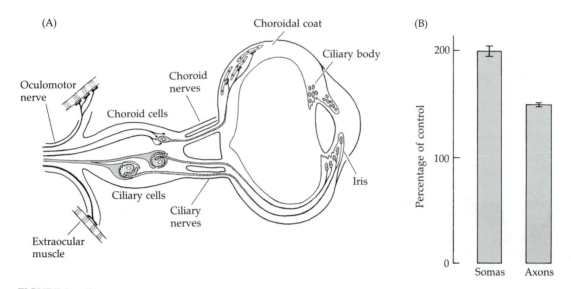

FIGURE 8. *Competition between neurons for survival during normal vertebrate development. (A) Diagram of the innervation of the chick iris by the ciliary ganglion at hatching. Because axons from the ganglion reach the eye by way of several branches, it is possible to reduce the number of cells in the ganglion substantially by cutting all but one of these nerves. Interrupting most of the postganglionic branches at the onset of the cell* *death period resulted in a loss of about two-thirds of the neurons in the ganglion. (B) Subsequent examination of the number of axons at stages 39–40 in the remaining nerve branch (or of the number of nerve cells filled by retrograde transport of horseradish peroxidase) indicates that reducing competition in this way salvages many nerve cells that ordinarily degenerate. (A after Landmesser and Pilar, 1974b; B after Pilar et al., 1980.)*

matching the size of innervating populations to the capacity of their targets (see Hamburger and Oppenheim, 1982). As Hamburger put the matter at the end of his paper on the nature of cell death in the spinal cord of the developing chick, "The quantitative relationship between the number of motor neurons and the size of the peripheral field of innervation is established by a selective survival of those neurons which find an adequate peripheral milieu, and the degeneration of all others" (Hamburger, 1958, p. 399).

The object of competition during neuronal death

Much present work on cell death is aimed at understanding what constitutes "an adequate peripheral milieu." If normally occurring cell death involves competition, what is it that neurons compete for? A great deal of circumstantial evidence suggests that nerve cells compete for factors produced by the target cells. Many of the arguments for this point of view are discussed in the following chapter, which considers the trophic effects of target cells on the neurons that innervate them. To summarize, some classes of neurons (mammalian and avian sensory and sympathetic ganglion cells) depend for survival on the protein nerve growth factor (NGF). A variety of studies show (1) that NGF is produced by the relevant targets; (2) that innervating axons have specific receptors for the protein; (3) that axon terminals are able to take up the molecule at the level of the target; (4) that axons transport NGF to the parent cell bodies; (5) that in the absence of peripherally derived NGF the innervating neurons die, and (6) that exogenous NGF can spare neurons that would otherwise die. The dependence of particular classes of nerve cells on a target-derived agent suggests that all neurons compete for factors produced by their targets. In accord with this idea, experiments both in vivo and in vitro show that the survival of other classes of neurons can be enhanced by target-derived factors different from NGF (see Chapter 7).

Although the idea of neuronal competition for target cell factors is attractive, some observations on neuronal death in vertebrate embryogenesis are not easily explained in this way. A. Lamb (1980, 1981a) has presented several results on cell death that challenge this view. For example, when both sides of the caudal spinal cord are made to innervate a single leg in the developing frog, the number of motor neurons that survive to maturity is larger than would be expected if the two sides of the spinal cord had simply competed with one another for the single limb (Figure 9). In this instance, the degree of motor neuron

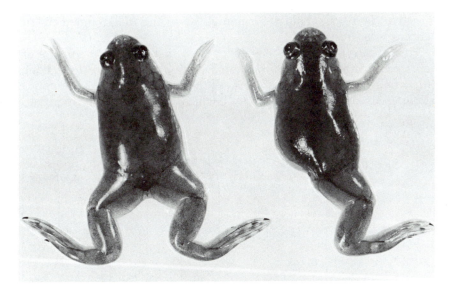

FIGURE 9. *A normal juvenile frog (left) and a "monopodal frog" created by an earlier operation in which one limb bud was extirpated and the contralateral nerves deflected into the remaining limb. Retrograde labeling with horseradish peroxidase shows that in many cases such limbs are innervated by appropriate motor neuron pools on both sides of the spinal cord. The degree of cell death in these pools, however, is not commensurate with the reduction of the target tissue by about half—considerably more motor neurons survive than would be expected. On the basis of this result, A. Lamb has argued that neuronal death in the lateral motor column of* Xenopus *must have some basis other than peripheral competition. (From Lamb, 1981a.)*

death in the spinal cord was reported to be roughly normal even though twice as many neurons projected to the remaining leg. On the other hand, a similar experiment in the chick visual system (see earlier) showed that cell death was much increased when neurons from both isthmo-optic nuclei were made to innervate a single eye (O'Leary and Cowan, 1984).

Another line of evidence that argues for some caution in the interpretation of normally occurring neuron death in vertebrate embryos concerns the timing of axon outgrowth. Within 2 hours after injection of tritiated-thymidine into 5½-day-old chick embryos, about 15 percent of the dorsal root ganglion cells that have incorporated thymidine show typical signs of degeneration (Carr and Simpson, 1982). Because this is too little time for a cell to be produced, differentiate, and send an axon to the periphery, these results suggest that competition (if that is the appropriate explanation here) may not always occur at the level of the target (see also Hamburger et al., 1981).

A third fly in the ointment is that a paradigm similar to the ciliary ganglion experiment of Pilar and his collaborators (Figure 8) has given opposite results when carried out in the frog spinal cord (Lamb, 1979). When Lamb removed a portion of frog spinal motor neurons before the cell death period, he found that death among the residual population went on apace (see also Lamb, 1981a,b). The proportion of motor neurons that died was about the same as when the full complement of neurons was present.

Finally, several workers have suggested that the major purpose of nerve cell death is sharpening the specificity of neuronal projections rather than simply matching the sizes of pre- and postsynaptic populations (see, for example, Hughes, 1968). In the developing frog limb,

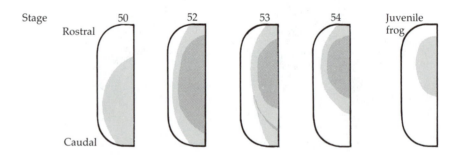

FIGURE 10. *Erroneous projection as a possible cause of cell death. Diagram shows the location of neurons in the lateral motor column that project to the knee flexors in* Xenopus *tadpoles at different stages of development (stage 50 to juvenile). Dorsal view; rostral is up and lateral to the left. Patterns were determined by retrograde axonal transport of horseradish peroxidase injected into the designated limb region (the intensity of shading corresponds to the density of retrogradely labeled cells). The change in the area occupied by retrogradely labeled cells during development suggests that some motor neurons initially project to inappropriate targets and that mismatched cells are eliminated during the cell death period. (After Lamb, 1976.)*

a wide range of spinal cord levels initially project to the knee flexors; later, however, only the more rostral innervation persists (Figure 10) (Lamb, 1976, 1977; Bennett and Lavidis, 1981; see also Bennett and Lai, 1981a,b). Lamb has argued that this changing pattern is the result of selective cell death, a phenomenon that he invokes to explain the apparent absence of much competition in some of his results (see earlier). Similar evidence (and interpretation) has come from studies of developing limbs in chicks (Pettigrew et al., 1979; Laing, 1982) and axolotls (McGrath and Bennett, 1979). Although some of these results are controversial, neuronal survival may well be influenced by qualitative as well as quantitative aspects of neuronal targets.

Taken together, these several findings suggest that competition may be a complex affair in which neurons do not simply battle with one another for a target-derived elixir. Nonetheless, in many situations acquisition of adequate amounts of target-derived factors appears to be crucial for neuronal survival.

Role of synaptic connections in neuronal death or survival

Because most neurons appear to die after reaching their targets, a natural question is whether survival depends on the formation of connections with target cells. This issue is complicated because in some cases (dorsal root ganglia, for instance) the innervation of the peripheral targets occurs without benefit of synapses. Nevertheless, the role of specialized connections with target cells in neuronal death is of considerable interest.

In the musculature of the chick iris, the bulk of synapse formation coincides with the major wave of neuronal death in the ciliary ganglion (Landmesser and Pilar, 1974b; Narayanan and Narayanan, 1981). This finding suggests that synapse formation per se might indeed be involved in determining the death or survival of the innervating neurons. The formation of just a few synapses with target cells does not protect a neuron against eventual death because some degenerating synapses are found in target tissues during the normal cell death period (Landmesser and Pilar, 1976); nor does innervation make cells immune to cell death because all the ganglion cells can be activated by preganglionic stimulation before their demise (Landmesser and Pilar, 1974a,b). On the other hand, death or survival might depend on the formation of an adequate number of synapses with target cells or on the quality of their function. A relationship between synaptic function and a neuron's ability to survive is further supported by the observation that blockade of neuromuscular transmission prevents the death of many motor neurons in the chick spinal cord (Figure 11) (Laing and Prestige, 1978; Pittman and Oppenheim, 1979; Creazzo and Sohal, 1979; Sohal et al., 1979; Olek, 1980; Oppenheim, 1981b; Ding et al., 1983; see also Hamburger et al., 1981). These experiments were carried out by applying a neuromuscular blocking agent such as curare or α-bungarotoxin to a chick embryo just before the normal period of cell death. The ensuing muscle

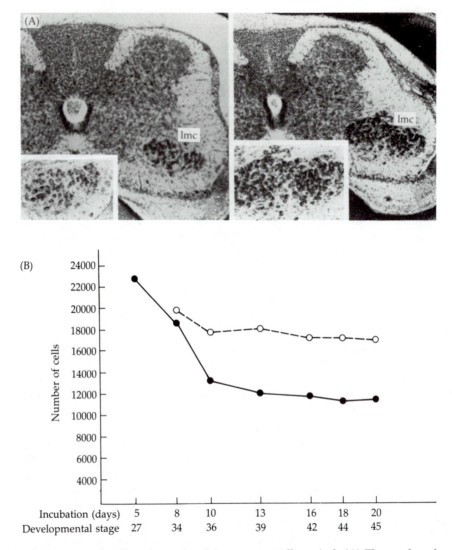

FIGURE 11. *The effect of neural activity on nerve cell survival. (A) The number of motor neurons persisting in the lateral motor column of the developing chick spinal cord can be influenced by neuromuscular blocking agents. A cross section of the lumbar cord of a normal 10-day chick embryo (left) is compared to a similar section from a curare-treated embryo at the same age. Insets are enlargements of the lateral motor column (lmc; ×110). (B) Graphic summary of the effects of curare treatment. The solid line shows the normal course of motor neuron death in control animals (cf. Figure 4A). Neuromuscular blockade with curare for about 3 days during this period (days 6 through 9 of incubation) reduces the degree of nerve cell degeneration. When motility returns, the surplus motor neurons die (not shown). Each point represents the average of 2 to 10 embryos. (A from Pittmann and Oppenheim, 1979; B after Pittmann and Oppenheim, 1979.)*

paralysis was associated with a dramatic survival of motor neurons well beyond the time when they would ordinarily have died (Figure 11). When the blocking agent was removed, the surplus motor neurons belatedly succumbed (Pittman and Oppenheim, 1979; see, however, Oppenheim, 1984). Conversely, excessive stimulation of developing muscles may enhance the death of motor neurons (Oppenheim and Núñez, 1982).

A possible explanation of these results is that functional innervation regulates target production (or secretion) of the agent or agents on which cell survival is predicated (see earlier). Thus, as a muscle is innervated and becomes active, its overall production of a trophic factor may be lowered to a level that can support only some of the neurons originally projecting to it. In this view, blockade of synaptic transmission maintains muscle fibers in a state resembling their condition prior to nerve contact, a condition in which the production and/or secretion of target factors is relatively high (see Chapter 8). Support for this general idea comes from the observation that nerve growth factor production by smooth muscle in the iris increases markedly after denervation (Ebendal et al., 1980). An important point is that if innervation modulates production of target factors, then competition will depend on the state of the postsynaptic cell as well as on interactions between axons (Purves, 1980).

INNERVATION-DEPENDENT NEURONAL DEATH

A final determinant of neuronal survival is the innervation that neurons receive (see also Chapter 8). For example, the removal of peripheral sense organs causes degeneration of neurons in the central nuclei to which the sensory axons project. Thus, removal of the eye (Levi-Montalcini, 1949) or the otocyst (Filogamo, 1950; Parks, 1979) from an early avian embryo induces degeneration of neurons in the corresponding sites of central projection (see also Sohal, 1976b; Okado and Oppenheim, 1984). Similarly, removal of the eye in newborn mice is followed within a week by a massive degeneration of the superior colliculus (DeLong and Sidman, 1962) and lateral geniculate (Heumann and Rabinowicz, 1980). Conversely, abnormally large axonal projections can rescue target cells that would otherwise die (Cunningham et al., 1979). All this suggests that the number of neurons in some parts of the nervous system is regulated by afferent connections in addition to (or perhaps instead of) retrograde regulation from targets. The mechanism of these anterograde effects on survival is not known. However, it is quite possible that retrograde and anterograde regulation of neuronal survival work in concert in motor and sensory systems. For instance, there is normally a substantial loss of cells from the retinal ganglion cell layer during the first two postnatal weeks in hamsters. When one eye is removed at birth, the frequency of degenerating retinal cell profiles in the contralateral eye is reduced (Sengelaub and Finlay, 1981; see also

Cell Death and Neuronal Proliferation in Maturity

In most regions of the vertebrate nervous system, neuronal proliferation and cell death are restricted to early development. In a few situations, however, these phenomena are ongoing. One such case is the olfactory epithelium, in which neurons undergo continual degeneration and replacement (Graziadei and Monti-Graziadei, 1978, 1979a,b). Neurons are generated from stem cells in the base of the epithelium and mature in about a week (see figure). These cells establish synaptic connections centrally but degenerate after about a month. The reason for such turnover is not entirely clear. One possibility is that neurons in such exposed epithelia die because of "wear and tear." Careful morphological observations by P. P. C. Graziadei and G. A. Monti-Graziadei, however, show little evidence of injury, and these workers suggest that neuronal turnover in the olfactory epithelium simply represents the normal life span of these cells (Graziadei and Monti Graziadei, 1978). In some animals (and perhaps in parts of the nervous system of all animals), the growth of targets may also require modification of neuronal number throughout life. Examples are the fish retina and the skate spinal cord, which continue to add neurons as the animals grow (Leonard et al., 1978; Birse et al., 1980; Johns, 1981). Some evidence for neuronal turnover has also been described in the brain of songbirds (see Chapter 14). Even in some parts of the mammalian brain, the numbers of neurons may increase (or decrease) substantially for long periods after birth (Kaplan and Hinds, 1977; Rootman et al., 1981; Bayer et al., 1982).

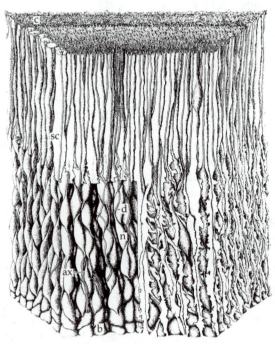

Diagram of the olfactory epithelium in the rat. The mature nerve cells (n) that die are continually replaced by proliferation of precursors (b) at the base of the epithelium. d, Dendrites; ax, axons; sc, supporting cells; c, cilia at the epithelial surface. (From Graziadei and Monti-Graziadei, 1978.)

Lund, 1973). Taken together with the fact that early eye removal induces degeneration of target neurons, these results suggest that retinal afferents control the number of cells in retinal targets and that the amount of available target regulates the number of retinal ganglion cells that survive. Such loops of interdependence in neuronal death or survival are probably ubiquitous.

CONCLUSIONS

Cell death is commonplace in development, and the nervous system is no exception. In invertebrates, the descendants of particular precursors degenerate in what appears to be a predetermined and highly stereotyped fashion. This strategy is presumably well suited to regulating cell numbers and establishing regional diversity in relatively simple systems. In vertebrates, however, the death of neurons is not preordained but seems to involve competitive interactions between nerve cells at the level of their targets. One obvious aim that is served by this phenomenon is matching the size of an innervating population of cells to the capacity of its target. Because relatively large populations of neurons in vertebrates carry out particular functions, some mechanism for regulating the size of synaptically connected populations is essential. In contrast, invertebrates may achieve this matching in a much more programmatic way because one or a few neurons are often the sole executors of a given function. Present evidence supports the idea that vertebrate neurons commonly die because of failure in competition for a factor or factors produced by the target: the protein nerve growth factor serves as a paradigm for this idea (Chapter 7).

The phenomenon of cell death in vertebrates underscores the importance of competitive strategies in neural development. Neuronal number in various populations is not prespecified, at least in any detailed sense; rather this property is determined by feedback (and feedforward) from other cells. The usefulness of such flexibility is also apparent during the subsequent formation of neural circuits. Indeed, the competitive acquisition of trophic factors appears to be a common denominator of early neuron survival and later modulation of neuronal connections (see Chapters 12 and 13).

Trophic Effects of Targets on Neurons

CHAPTER

7

INTRODUCTION

Conventional synaptic effects are usually measured on a time scale of milliseconds or seconds; there are other interactions between nerve cells, however, that transpire over days, months, or indeed the lifetime of the animal. Such long-term effects are called "trophic," from the Greek, meaning to nourish. Of course, trophic interactions between nerve cells and their targets do not represent nourishment in any literal sense. What is acquired by the nerve cells is not some ordinary metabolite but a specific agent to which some neurons are sensitive and others are not. Thus, these interactions are restricted in roughly the same way that hormone or neurotransmitter effects are restricted. Indeed, hormones, neurotransmitters, and trophic agents probably represent a continuum of extracellular messengers: they are distinguished primarily by the strategy of their action.

NERVE GROWTH FACTOR:
THE PREEMINENT EXAMPLE OF A TROPHIC AGENT

The devastating effects of early target removal make plain that many kinds of neurons must find suitable targets in order to survive (Chapter 6). The interpretation of normally occurring neuronal death in vertebrates is that individual neurons within an innervating pool require a target-derived factor that is available in limited supply. Whereas this proposition is speculative for most populations of nerve cells, for two neuronal classes there is good evidence that a specific agent is indeed required for neuronal survival. The agent is nerve growth factor (NGF).

Discovery of nerve growth factor

Although the history of trophic agents could perhaps be traced from the turn of the century when S. Ramón y Cajal expressed enthusiasm for trophic interactions as important mechanisms in neural development (see Ramón y Cajal, 1929, p. 400), the discovery of nerve growth factor proper begins with experiments carried out by E. Bueker (1948), a student of V. Hamburger in the late 1940s. The role of target tissues in the development and survival of neural centers was already an area of vigorous research (Chapter 6). Shortly after he left Hamburger's laboratory, Bueker undertook experiments in which mouse tumors were implanted into chick embryos to explore whether rapidly growing neoplastic tissues might provide an easier way of augmenting the periphery than implantation of a supernumerary limb. In addition, it was felt that an effect derived from tissue that could be grown in large quantities would be more amenable to chemical analysis (V. Hamburger, personal communication). Bueker transplanted three different tumors: mouse adenocarcinoma (which failed to grow in the chick embryo), Rous sarcoma (which caused extensive hemorrhage), and mouse sarcoma "180" (which grew quite well). Bueker characterized the growth of mouse sarcomas and the response of nearby nerves. He found that as the tumor grew it was invaded by nerve bundles. He also noted that the ipsilateral dorsal root ganglia at the level of the tumor were enlarged compared to the contralateral ganglia. In contrast, the spinal motor column was unaffected. From these observations Bueker surmised that the nerve fibers in the tumor were sensory and that the motor system was refractory to this effect. Because the nature of the interaction between targets and their innervating centers was only beginning to be understood in 1948, the significance of Bueker's observation was not immediately appreciated (Levi-Montalcini, 1975; Hamburger, 1980). However, Hamburger and R. Levi-Montalcini (see Box A) went on to explore this intriguing result. To his later regret, Bueker expressed little interest in further investigation of the sarcoma effect.

In their initial experiments, Levi-Montalcini and Hamburger confirmed and extended what Bueker had seen using Levi-Montalcini's improved methods of staining nerve fibers with silver. They found that sensory, and also sympathetic, ganglia in the vicinity of the sarcoma implants were obviously enlarged compared to more distant ganglia (Figure 1) (Levi-Montalcini and Hamburger, 1951, 1953). That this effect was due to an agent secreted by the implant was demonstrated by the persistence of the effect when the tumor was placed on the chorioallantoic membrane instead of in the embryo proper. Because in these circumstances the only link between the tumor and the nervous system was the circulation, the effect had to be mediated by a substance secreted by the tumor. Levi-Montalcini and Hamburger called this agent the nerve growth factor.

Some of the excitement and anticipation generated by this discovery can be appreciated from Levi-Montalcini's description of the effects of the tumor implant on the chick sympathetic system.

> We should like to emphasize the exceptional character of the response of the visceral nervous system to the tumor. The results reveal a morphogenetic effect for which there is no parallel. The selective susceptibility of some neurons to the effect of the tumor and the absence of species specificity may suggest an analogy between this and hormonal effects. One aspect of the effect of the tumor does not fit in this picture, however. The tumor promotes an

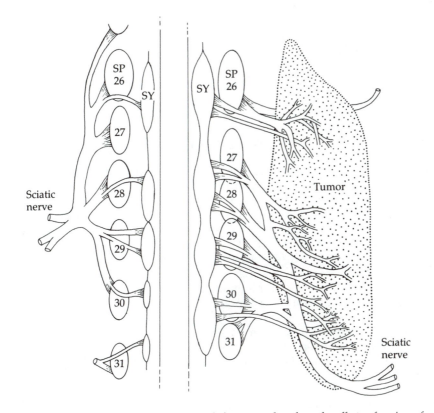

FIGURE 1. *The discovery of nerve growth factor was based on the effects of a piece of mouse sarcoma tumor on the developing nervous system of chick embryos. This drawing shows the lumbosacral region of a 15-day-old chick embryo into which a tumor (dotted line) was implanted a few days earlier. The sympathetic chain (SY) and spinal ganglia (SP) in the region of the tumor implant are obviously enlarged. In addition, the peripheral nerves are hypertrophied and appear to be directed toward the tumor. Numbers indicate spinal segments. (After Levi-Montalcini and Hamburger, 1951.)*

excessive growth of the sympathetic system with total disregard of the requirements of the whole organism. In fact, it upsets its harmonious development to such an extent that it causes profound changes in the sequence of developmental processes. Whereas, under normal conditions proliferation and differentiation of the sympathetic ganglia are held within limits and kept in pace with the development of other structures, we find that under the impact of the tumor the sympathetic system overtakes other systems. The increase in the size of the sympathetic chain ganglia, which in one particular case amounts to more than eight times the normal size, is even more impressive if one realizes that the embryos were considerably smaller than normal embryos, due to toxic tumor effects. The latest stages investigated are 16- and 17-day embryos, and there is no indication that the hyperplastic process has come to an end at that time.

The accommodation of an enormous number of nerve fibers in the viscera is equally intriguing. It indicates another severe infraction of the laws which govern the mechanics of development. Under

Rita Levi-Montalcini (b. 1909)

A native of Turin, Italy, Rita Levi-Montalcini entered medical school in that city in the early 1930s in a remarkable class that included S. Luria and R. Dulbecco. A major figure at the school was the professor of anatomy, Giuseppe Levi; Levi-Montalcini undertook her first research in the Anatomical Institute in Turin under his guidance, learning the rudiments of tissue culture, which was then a novel technique. When she graduated in 1936 her indecision about pursuing a clinical career in neurology and psychiatry (as opposed to throwing herself fully into research) was resolved by Mussolini's "Manifesto per la difensa della razza." This document, signed by a number of Italian scientists in 1938, barred both academic and professional careers to "non-Aryans." Thus, in 1939 she accepted an offer from a neurological institute in Brussels and moved there just before the declarations of war between Germany and France and England. However, when it appeared certain that Belgium would also be invaded, she returned to Italy. Faced with the alternative of moving to the United States or pursuing research in difficult circumstances and staying with her family, she chose the latter course. Levi-Montalcini built a small laboratory at her home and proceeded to carry out experiments with no more

than an incubator, a microscope, a microtome, and some access to the literature. G. Levi had also returned to Italy from Belgium, and together they began an investigation of the chick embryo, exploring the effect of the periphery on developing nerve centers with silver staining (Levi-Montalcini and Levi, 1942, 1944; see also Levi-Montalcini and Levi, 1943). Remarkably, Levi-Montalcini made a number of important observations under these conditions, including the degeneration of cells in peripherally deprived sensory ganglia and the discovery of migratory processes in the cephalic nerves and cerebellum (Levi-Montalcini and Levi, 1944; Levi-Montalcini, 1964). The impetus for many of these studies was V. Hamburger's earlier work, with which she was thoroughly acquainted

During this time, Levi-Montalcini's home in Turin became a meeting place for the friends and former students of G. Levi, as well as a laboratory. By 1942, however, the intense bombing of Turin forced Levi-Montalcini to move to the countryside. Here conditions for research were even more primitive, and her experimental eggs were often consumed after they had yielded up their results. In spite of these deprivations, she completed a study of the acoustical-vestibular centers of the chick, a

normal conditions nerve fibers are admitted to organs according to a rigid time schedule, and the quantity of the entering fibers is strictly limited; each organ has a characteristic density, and regulative mechanisms are in operation to prevent hyperneurotization. In the present instance, all barriers seem to have broken down, and the organs surrender to the invading fibers. It remains to be seen whether some properties of the nerve fibers are changed, such as their invasiveness or growth potential, or whether the organs themselves are directly affected by the tumor. An even more striking instance of the abnormal behavior of visceral nerve fibers is represented by their perforation of the intima of the veins, and the formation of nerve agglomerations in the lumen of these vessels. Nothing can be said concerning the nature of the agent and our research is now heading in this direction (Levi-Montalcini, 1953, p. 342–343).

study that was published in the United States some years later (Levi-Montalcini, 1949).

When the Nazis invaded Italy after Mussolini's fall in 1943, Levi-Montalcini and her family fled again to Florence, where they became refugees, surviving by anonymity. Finally, with the end of the war in 1945, she returned to Turin and became the assistant of Levi, who resumed his position as professor of anatomy at the University. In 1946 she received a letter from Hamburger, who had read her articles with Levi on the relation between the periphery and the developing nerve centers; because they disagreed on the interpretation of similar results (Hamburger, 1934), Hamburger invited her to work for a 1-year period in his laboratory in St. Louis. Thus, in 1947 Levi-Montalcini finally left Turin to spend "the next 26 years, the happiest and most productive of my life" at Washington University (Levi-Montalcini, 1975). In 1974 she returned to Rome, where she has carried out numerous additional studies on NGF at the Instituto di Biologia Cellulare.

The collaboration with Hamburger, which started in 1947, was certainly one of the most fruitful in developmental neurobiology, and the major results of their work are well known to everyone in this field. Their observations on tumor implants (see text) led eventually to the discovery of nerve growth factor by Levi-Montalcini, who committed her career entirely to NGF and carried their joint early work to its logical conclusion. The fact that she succeeded so brilliantly in unraveling the nature and bio-

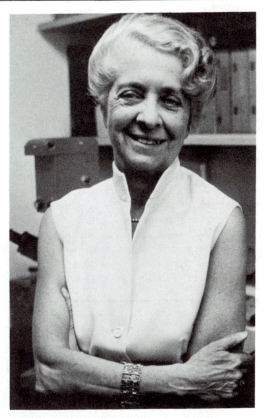

Rita Levi-Montalcini in 1977. (Courtesy of V. Hamburger)

logical importance of NGF over a period of 30 years is not only a tribute to her personally but also to the persistence of the scientific spirit against all odds.

Characterization of the nerve growth factor molecule

Perhaps the crux of any biochemical identification and purification is the quality of the assay for the substance in question. Levi-Montalcini recognized the necessity of such an assay if further progress were to be made with nerve growth factor, and in the early 1950s she traveled to Brazil where she solved this problem during a stay in H. Meyer's laboratory. During the months she spent in Rio de Janeiro, Levi-Montalcini devised a semiquantitative means of measuring the stimulating effects of the tumor using chick sensory or sympathetic ganglia incubated in a simple tissue culture medium. The result of incubating ganglia in proximity to a piece of tumor was a remarkable outgrowth of thousands of nerve cell processes (neurites) from the explanted ganglia

Why Does a Mouse Sarcoma Secrete NGF?

A great deal of interest has recently been focused on oncogenic genes, discrete segments of host DNA that are appropriated by certain viruses and are instrumental in viral replication. These same viruses (acute transforming retroviruses) can also change normal cells into malignant ones; the appropriated host genes are therefore suspect as the agents of transformation and have been called oncogenes (Bishop, 1982; see also Downward et al., 1984). The oncogene of the simian sarcoma virus is a host gene that codes for platelet-derived growth factor (PDGF) (Doolittle et al., 1982).

Because PDGF is a growth factor for human fibroblasts, smooth muscle cells, and glia, it is plausible that several important aspects of tumor behavior (unrestrained growth, invasion of other tissues) are a result of the excessive production of various growth factors. In this light, E. Bueker's discovery of growth factor activity in a mouse sarcoma has a certain logic. By the same token, amplification of growth factor production by viruses may aid in the discovery of as yet unrecognized trophic agents (Skene, 1983).

(Figure 2) (Cohen et al., 1954; Levi-Montalcini et al., 1954). Although a reliable radioimmunoassay for measuring NGF concentration is now available (Korsching and Thoenen, 1983), Levi-Montalcini's original bioassay is still commonly used; the halo effect is considered the ultimate criterion of the potency of NGF preparations.

Armed with this assay, Levi-Montalcini and a succession of colleagues set about identifying the NGF molecule and evaluating its biological role. The critical step in this work was made possible by a series of largely serendipitous events. S. Cohen and Levi-Montalcini had been attempting to define the active agent in the tumor extract and knew from chemical analyses that the active fractions contained both nucleic acid and protein. In order to distinguish the activity of the nucleic acid and protein moieties, they undertook experiments using snake venom, an excellent source of phosphodiesterase—the destruction of the nucleic acid by the esterase was expected to indicate whether the active agent was the protein. In what must have been a perplexing result, Cohen and Levi-Montalcini found that the control assays, which contained no tumor extract but only snake venom, showed an even greater degree of nerve-growth stimulation than the cultures containing the tumor extract. Amazingly, a further series of experiments showed that snake venom actually contained a protein (now known to be a form of NGF) that had exactly the same properties as the agent derived from the mouse tumor (Levi-Montalcini and Cohen, 1956; Cohen and Levi-Montalcini, 1956; Cohen, 1959). The fact that NGF was present in snake venom suggested to Cohen that it might be worthwhile looking at the mammalian analogue of the snake venom gland, the salivary gland. In

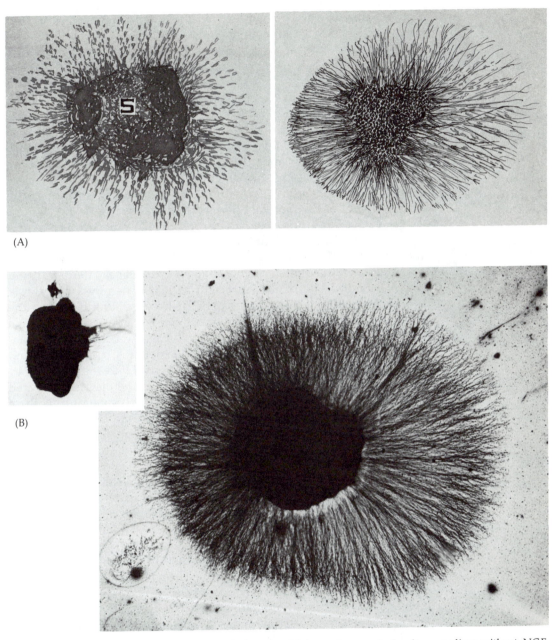

FIGURE 2. *Biological assay for nerve growth factor. (A) Drawing sent from Brazil by R. Levi-Montalcini to V. Hamburger in 1951, showing the first evidence of the effect of mouse sarcoma on neurite outgrowth in vitro. On the left is a small piece of mouse sarcoma (S); on the right is an explanted chick sensory ganglion showing a profusion of neurites after only a few hours of coculture. (B) Inset is a photomicrograph of a chick dorsal root ganglion from an 8-day embryo grown for 24 hours in a control culture medium without NGF. Addition of one biological unit of NGF to the medium stimulates a halo of neurites growing from another explanted ganglion within the same period of culture. By making serial dilutions of media containing an unknown amount of nerve growth factor the approximate concentration of this agent can be determined. Sympathetic ganglia can also be used in the assay. (Courtesy of R. Levi-Montalcini and V. Hamburger.)*

fact, a salivary gland of male mice—the submaxillary—does indeed contain very large amounts of nerve growth factor (Cohen, 1960). The crucial advantage of this discovery was that the salivary gland provided the large amount of starting material needed to isolate and characterize the NGF molecule.

The purification and detailed characterization of NGF took an additional decade. In 1969, V. Bocchini and P.U. Angeletti described a reliable method of preparing nerve growth factor from mouse salivary glands; this method yielded a highly purified preparation of the protein. This procedure is still standard and uses about 900 pairs of submaxillary glands from male mice for a single run. Two years later, R. H. Angeletti and R. A. Bradshaw (1971) reported the amino acid sequence of the active subunit of the molecule purified in this way (Figure 3).

Nerve growth factor isolated from homogenates of the male mouse submaxillary gland is a complex of three subunits—α, β, and γ—in the ratio $2\alpha{:}\beta{:}2\gamma$. The molecular weight of the complex is about 130,000, and it has a sedimentation coefficient of 7 S (Varon et al., 1967a,b, 1968). The α subunit has a molecular weight of 26,000; its physiological role is still obscure (Server and Shooter, 1977). The γ subunit has about the same molecular weight as the α subunit and is a peptidase with some homology to bovine trypsin (Varon et al., 1968; Bradshaw, 1978). Neither the α or γ moiety has obvious effects on neurons; it is the β subunit that promotes neurite outgrowth and cell survival (Greene et al., 1971). This moiety is also known as 2.5 S NGF and is the material prepared by the Bocchini and Angeletti method (1969). The β subunit consists of two identical monomers, each of which comprises 118 amino acids; these form a noncovalently bound dimer with a molecular weight of 26,518 (see Figure 3). Interestingly, the amino acid sequence of the β subunit monomers has considerable similarity to proinsulin, insulin, the insulinlike growth factors, and relaxin (Angeletti and Bradshaw, 1971; Frazier et al., 1972; Angeletti et al., 1973; Bradshaw, 1978).

Incorporation of labeled amino acids into submaxillary gland nerve growth factor indicates that NGF is synthesized in the gland (Levi-Montalcini and Angeletti, 1968; Berger and Shooter, 1978; Greene and Shooter, 1980). This work also showed that the β subunit monomer is formed by the cleavage of a pro-β molecule with a molecular weight of about 22,000. The cleavage can be catalyzed by the γ subunit (arginine provides the carboxyl terminal of the β subunit, and the γ subunit is an arginine-specific esteropeptidase); whether this is a normal prerequisite for NGF activation is unclear.

BIOLOGICAL ROLE OF NERVE GROWTH FACTOR

Once the NGF molecule had been isolated and characterized, a variety of detailed studies addressing its biological role were undertaken. Most information about the biology of NGF pertains to neural development in birds and mammals; the role of NGF in other animals is less clear, but this (or a similar) agent is probably important in fish and amphibians

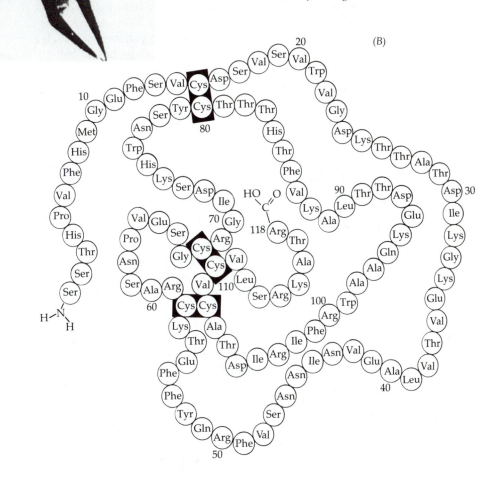

FIGURE 3. *The nerve growth factor molecule. (A) Crystals of NGF grown by hanging drop vapor diffusion. (B) The amino acid sequence of one of the monomers of β (2.5 S) NGF purified from the mouse submaxillary gland. Two such monomers make up the β subunit, the biologically active component of the NGF molecule. Each monomer comprises 118 amino acids and has a molecular weight of 13,259. (A from Server and Shooter, 1977; B after Angeletti and Bradshaw, 1971.)*

(Benowitz and Greene, 1979; Yip and Grafstein, 1982; Yip and Johnson, 1983; Levi-Montalcini, personal communication).

Specificity of nerve growth factor effects

It is now generally accepted that nerve growth factor does not affect all types of neurons (Levi-Montalcini and Angeletti, 1968; Mobley et al., 1977; Harper and Thoenen, 1980). Rather, its influence is largely limited to two parts of the nervous system: sympathetic chain ganglia and sensory ganglia of neural crest origin. Effects on other parts of the nervous system have been suggested but remain uncertain or controversial (Mobley et al., 1977). For example, the pelvic ganglia in mammals (which have properties of both sympathetic and parasympathetic ganglia) show some sensitivity to nerve growth factor but are not dependent upon it to the same degree as the ganglia of the sympathetic chain in the thorax and upper abdomen. Similarly, there is some uncertainty about whether NGF affects all the cells within dorsal root ganglia or whether there is a subpopulation of sensory neurons that are insensitive. Finally, evidence that some central neurons such as the adrenergic cells of the locus coeruleus respond to nerve growth factor has been presented (Björklund and Stenevi, 1972), but these observations are disputed (Menesini-Chen et al., 1978).

Nerve growth factor also has important effects on nonneural cells. Daily injections of NGF into perinatal rats transform chromaffin cells in the adrenal medulla into what appear to be ordinary sympathetic neurons (Figure 4) (Aloe and Levi-Montalcini, 1979). Thus, NGF causes induction of tyrosine hydroxylase and dopamine-β-hydroxylase in these cells (Otten et al., 1977) and even extension of neurites (Olson and Malmfors, 1970; Unsicker and Chamley, 1977). Conversely, reducing the availability of NGF may destroy chromaffin cell precursors and immature chromaffin cells in the adrenal medulla (Aloe and Levi-Montalcini, 1979). NGF-treated chromaffin cells isolated in culture also send out neurites and show catecholamine-specific fluorescence. Because these phenomena can be abolished by addition of glucocorticoids to the culture medium, NGF effects may normally be inhibited by the high

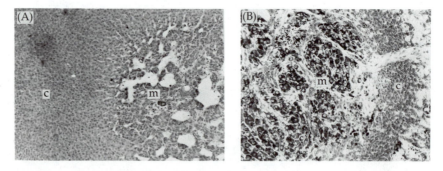

FIGURE 4. *The effect of nerve growth factor on developing adrenal medullary cells. (A) This photomicrograph shows a cross section of the adrenal gland of a normal 10-day-old rat pup. The normal gland consists of a dense cortical layer of cells (c) surrounding a central medullary area (m) made up largely of endocrine cells and blood vessels. (B) A similar section from a 10-day-old rat treated for several days both before and after birth with injections of nerve growth factor. After NGF treatment, the medulla is greatly increased in volume as a result of the apparent transformation of many adrenal cortical cells into neurons that sprout profusely branching fibers. Both micrographs are magnified 105 times. (From Aloe and Levi-Montalcini, 1979.)*

concentrations of glucocorticoids in the adrenal glands (Unsicker et al., 1978). Nerve growth factor treatment of neonatal rats also stimulates an increase in the number of mast cells (Aloe and Levi-Montalcini, 1977).

Clearly, NGF affects a variety of cell types; in the nervous system, however, its influence is restricted to a few classes of neurons.

Biological sources of nerve growth factor

One biological source of NGF is, or course, the submaxillary gland of the adult male mouse, where NGF is found in the convoluted tubules and saliva (but not the acini) (Levi-Montalcini and Cohen, 1960; Caramia et al., 1962; Wallace and Partlow, 1976; Schwab et al., 1976; Murphy et al., 1977). However, removal of the mouse submaxillary gland at birth has no obvious effect on the development of NGF-sensitive neurons (Levi-Montalcini and Angeletti, 1968). In fact, no one has a very good idea why NGF is found in such high concentrations in this gland. Although it is a sympathetic target, the submaxillary is not innervated more intensely than any other organ that receives postganglionic sympathetic fibers. Moreover, even though male mice have about 10 times as much NGF in their salivary glands as female mice (testosterone stimulates NGF production), the sympathetic ganglia that innervate the glands are about the same size in both sexes (Levi-Montalcini and Angeletti, 1964; see also Hendry and Iversen, 1973). Oddly enough, other closely related mammals such as rats and rabbits do not have high levels of NGF in their salivary glands (Levi-Montalcini and Angeletti, 1968). More recently, high concentrations of NGF have been found in another peculiar location, the guinea pig and bovine prostate gland (Harper et al., 1979, 1982, 1983). The reason for this is as mysterious as the high NGF levels in salivary glands.

The apparent role of nerve growth factor in the development of sympathetic and sensory ganglia suggests that this agent ought to be generally present in the targets of sensitive neurons. This logic has led a number of workers to assess NGF levels in a variety of sympathetic end organs. Evidence concerning target concentrations and synthesis has been difficult to obtain, and this aspect of the NGF story remains its weakest part. Early studies purported to demonstrate NGF in nearly all body tissues except kidney and brain. In retrospect, the concentrations of NGF present in most target tissues are simply too low to be measured with the methods initially used (Harper and Thoenen, 1980). Using a two-site enzyme immunoassay, S. Korsching and H. Thoenen have demonstrated that NGF is indeed found in the targets of sympathetic ganglion cells in amounts proportional to the density of innervation (Korsching and Thoenen, 1983). The levels of NGF measured are in the range of 1 ng/g of target tissue. Tissues not well innervated by sympathetic fibers, such as heart ventricle and skeletal muscle, have amounts of NGF below the level of detectability (about 0.3 ng/g).

Demonstration of synthesis by sympathetic targets has also proved difficult. Aside from its production in salivary gland tubules (which probably has nothing to do with sympathetic innervation), until recently the only evidence for NGF synthesis by a sympathetically innervated tissue was NGF production by the iris (Ebendal et al., 1980). Even in this case it is necessary to denervate the iris in order to measure NGF production. This apparent enhancement of NGF synthesis following denervation is an interesting fact in its own right, suggesting that the elaboration of trophic factors by targets is modulated by the innervation they receive. This work on the iris has now been confirmed and extended by the demonstration that sympathetically innervated targets contain messenger RNA for NGF, whereas a variety of other tissues do not (Shelton and Reichert, 1984). Nerve growth factor can also be synthesized by several tissues in vitro. Among the cells that produce NGF, or a molecule immunologically indistinguishable from it, are fibroblasts, 3T3 cells, and cultured muscle cells (Oger et al., 1974; Young et al., 1975; Murphy et al., 1977; Greene and Shooter, 1980).

Effects of nerve growth factor on neuron survival

Nerve growth factor appears to be a requirement for the maturation and survival of two types of mammalian and avian neurons: sympathetic chain and dorsal root ganglion cells. To reiterate, these cells (as well as many other types of neurons) normally die in substantial numbers during the course of development (Chapter 6). The most plausible explanation of cell death in these systems is failure in competition for a peripherally derived trophic factor.

In the late 1950s, the development of an antiserum to nerve growth factor (made by injecting a partially purified NGF preparation into a rabbit and harvesting the blood serum a few weeks later) gave Levi-Montalcini and her colleagues the opportunity to test directly the idea that NGF might be a survival factor for developing sympathetic neurons (Levi-Montalcini and Booker, 1960). Newborn mice and rats were injected over a period of several days with small doses of antiserum to determine whether this treatment had any effect on the development of sensory and sympathetic ganglia. The dramatic result was that sympathetic ganglia nearly disappeared after only a few days (Figure 5) (Levi-Montalcini, 1972). Surprisingly, the absence of sympathetic ganglia has relatively little effect on the maturation of rats or mice.

The drastic effects of antiserum on the developing sympathetic nervous system (referred to as immunosympathectomy) provided an important link in a chain of evidence that ultimately showed that the molecule first extracted from a mouse tumor plays an important role in the normal development of some parts of the mammalian nervous system. Another link in this argument is that systemic treatment of developing mammals with exogenous NGF causes marked hypertrophy of the peripheral sympathetic system (Angeletti et al., 1971; Aloe et al., 1975). In vitro studies using dissociated sympathetic ganglion cells confirmed that a major effect of NGF is promotion of cell survival (Levi-Montalcini and Angeletti, 1963; Varon et al., 1973; Greene, 1977a; Chun

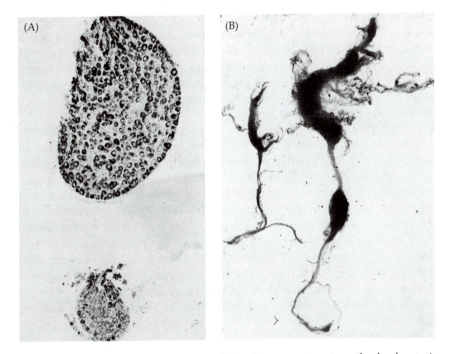

FIGURE 5. *The effects of a course of NGF antiserum treatment on the development of sympathetic ganglia in neonatal rodents. (A) Cross section of a superior cervical ganglion from a normal 9-day-old mouse (above) compared to a similar section from a 9-day-old mouse injected daily since birth with NGF antiserum (below). The superior cervical ganglion of the treated mouse shows marked atrophy, with obvious loss of nerve cells. (B) Whole mounts of the stellate and thoracic chain ganglia of control (right) and experimental (left) mice similarly treated and examined at 20 days of age. The sympathetic chain from the mouse injected since birth with NGF antiserum shows gross atrophy. (From Levi-Montalcini, 1972.)*

and Patterson, 1977a,b,c; Berg, 1982). Since NGF deprivation enhances the death of sympathetic ganglion cells (and since an excess promotes survival), it seems likely that the amount of NGF normally available regulates the number of neurons that survive to maturity in this system.

The effects of NGF antiserum on sensory neurons is more complicated. In spite of the decimation of sympathetic ganglia, antiserum given to perinatal animals has little or no effect on the maturation of the dorsal root ganglia. Embryonic dorsal root ganglion cells do, however, depend on NGF for survival in culture (Levi-Montalcini and Angeletti, 1963; Greene, 1977b); moreover, these neurons send out a profusion of neurites in response to NGF treatment in vitro (recall that this is the basis of the NGF bioassay), and they hypertrophy when NGF is administered to chick embryos (see Figure 1). Thus, the lack of an appreciable effect from antiserum treatment was perplexing. It is now clear that the reason for this difference between sympathetic and sensory ganglia is the developmental period during which the two classes of cells are sensitive. If mammalian sensory ganglia are deprived of NGF at earlier embryonic stages of development, a severe depletion of sensory ganglion cells is apparent (Gorin and Johnson, 1979; Johnson et al., 1980). Early exposure to antiserum was achieved by immunizing a pregnant mother (the guinea pig is the animal in which this procedure works best): because NGF antibodies cross the placenta, the developing embryo is exposed during gestation.

A general concern with NGF antiserum experiments is that the antibodies might have a nonspecific but nonetheless lethal effect on sensitive cells. For example, the antiserum might kill sympathetic and sensory cells by binding to them and activating a cytotoxic reaction mediated by the complement system rather than by deprivation of physiological amounts of endogenous NGF. A number of studies have examined this point, and although one can argue that the experimenters had a vested interest in showing that the effect of anti-NGF is physiological, the outcome has consistently been that anti-NGF appears to act by depriving the sensitive cells of their normal source of nerve growth factor (Levi-Montalcini and Angeletti, 1966; Goedert et al., 1980). Indeed, antibodies to NGF are equally effective in complement-deficient mice (Ennis et al., 1979).

Tropic effect of nerve growth factor

Another major effect of NGF is its tropic influence; a tropic effect (as distinguished from a trophic effect) refers to the direction of neuritic growth (Chapter 5). In the case of NGF, tropism has been assessed by asking whether neurites growing from the cell bodies of NGF-sensitive neurons are responsive to concentration gradients of nerve growth factor.

Two sorts of experiments have been undertaken to explore this issue. In one approach, a gradient of NGF is created by allowing diffusion from the tip of a micropipette filled with an NGF solution (see Figure 16 in Chapter 5) (Gundersen and Barrett, 1979, 1980; see also Letourneau, 1978). These experiments show that NGF gradients can cause the neurites of an NGF-sensitive cell to change direction over just a few minutes. Another approach has been to inject large amounts of NGF into the brain stem of newborn rodents (Figure 6) (Menesini-Chen et al., 1978). Such injections cause postganglionic axons from sympathetic ganglia to grow into the spinal cord and up the dorsal funiculus, apparently seeking out ever higher concentrations of NGF. The developmental significance of this tropic effect is discussed in Chapter 5.

Local maintenance of terminal arborizations by nerve growth factor

Still another general effect of NGF on sensitive neurons concerns the maintenance of terminal arborizations. R. Campenot (1977, 1981, 1982a,b) showed that NGF can modulate the arborizations of sympa-

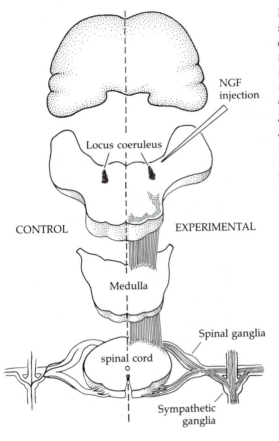

FIGURE 6. *Diagram of the highly abnormal entry of sympathetic fiber bundles into the spinal cord and medulla of neonatal rats after intracerebral injection of nerve growth factor. On the experimental side (right), nerve growth factor has been injected into the floor of the fourth ventricle near the locus coeruleus. Several days after this treatment, fibers from sympathetic ganglia have entered the spinal cord through the spinal ganglia and have ascended in the dorsal cord toward the region of the NGF injection. This bizarre rerouting of sympathetic fibers offers in vivo evidence for a tropic effect of nerve growth factor. (After Levi-Montalcini, 1976.)*

thetic ganglion cells grown in culture without affecting cell survival and, indeed, without involving the cell soma at all. In this work, dissociated sympathetic ganglion cells were placed in the central well of a chamber with three compartments (Figure 7). Each compartment was isolated from the others by a grease seal on the bottom of the culture dish; thus, NGF concentrations could be varied independently in the central and peripheral chambers. When all three chambers were filled with adequate concentrations of NGF, neurites of ganglion cells explanted into the central well sent processes into the two peripheral compartments. When NGF was removed from one of the peripheral wells, however, the neurites that had grown into that compartment gradually withered and retracted (Campenot, 1982b). Conversely, when NGF was removed from the central compartment but allowed to remain in the peripheral wells, the neurites and cells in the central compartment remained intact.

These results indicate that peripheral neurites can support the parent cell body by uptake of NGF. They also show that NGF has a maintenance effect on neurites, causing them to grow or recede as a function of local concentration. This local effect of trophic factors is a central

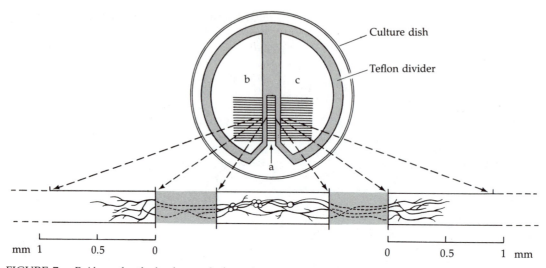

FIGURE 7. *Evidence for the local control of neurites by nerve growth factor. Diagram shows a culture dish with three sections (a,b,c) separated from one another by a Teflon divider sealed to the bottom of the dish with grease (top view). The central compartment (a) is open to the bulk of the culture medium; the medium in compartments (b) and (c) can be changed independently. Isolated rat sympathetic ganglion cells plated in compartment (a) will grow along avenues of collagen on the surface of the dish under the grease seal and into compartments (b) and (c). (An expanded view of neurites* *growing along such an avenue from the central compartment to the side chambers is shown below.) Neurite growth into the lateral chambers will occur as long as the chambers contain adequate concentrations of nerve growth factor. Removal of NGF from one or the other of the side chambers causes a local regression of neurites without affecting the survival of the cells in the central well. (NGF must, in these circumstances, be present in the central chamber.) This provides a direct demonstration of the local control of neuronal arborizations by a trophic agent. (After Campenot, 1981.)*

theme in later chapters which consider the maintenance and rearrangement of synaptic connections.

In summary, NGF has three major effects on sensitive neurons: it promotes cell survival, influences the direction of neuritic growth, and controls the extent of terminal arbors.

HOW DOES NERVE GROWTH FACTOR ACHIEVE ITS EFFECTS?

If nerve growth factor is produced by the targets of sympathetic and sensory ganglion cells, there must be a means by which axonal endings take up and transport this molecule (or a second messenger) back to the cell body. Indeed, there is good evidence that NGF is normally taken up peripherally and retrogradely transported (Figure 8) (Angeletti et al., 1972; Hendry et al., 1974a,b; Stöckel et al., 1974, 1975, 1976; Stöckel and Thoenen, 1975). When NGF labeled with radioactive iodine is injected into the eye, it interacts with sympathetic nerve endings; other proteins of similar size and physicochemical properties are not taken up to nearly the same degree (Hendry et al., 1974a,b; Iversen et al., 1975; Johnson et al., 1978; Dumas et al., 1979). Specific (saturable)

NGF receptors are present on the membranes of NGF-sensitive cells but are generally absent on cells that are unresponsive to NGF (Greene and Shooter, 1980; see, however, Max et al., 1978; Ebbott and Hendry, 1978). There appear to be several classes of receptors, but the significance of these varieties is not yet clear (Herrup and Shooter, 1975; Andres et al., 1977; Yankner and Shooter, 1982). Following interaction with receptors, NGF is internalized and transported back to the cell body, where it arrives in native form (Bradshaw, 1978; Greene and Shooter, 1980; Schwab and Thoenen, 1983).

The time course of accumulation in the superior cervical ganglion of labeled NGF injected into the anterior chamber of the eye (recall that the superior cervical ganglion supplies the sympathetic innervation of the iris) also indicates retrograde transport. The accumulation is negligible at first but peaks in about 16 hours (Johnson et al., 1978); this delay between the introduction of the agent at nerve endings and its arrival in cell bodies is consistent with retrograde transport along sympathetic axons (Figure 8). Moreover, there is very little label in the contralateral ganglion; this result indicates that accumulation depends on terminal exposure to NGF rather than on uptake via the circulation. The demonstration that endogenous NGF is also retrogradely transported confirms the view that this is the way NGF normally reaches sensitive neurons (Figure 9) (Palmatier et al., 1984).

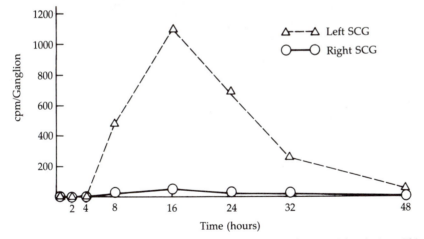

FIGURE 8. *Retrograde transport of nerve growth factor from peripheral sites. This graph shows the accumulation of radioactivity (measured as counts per minute, cpm) in rat superior cervical ganglia after injection of radiolabeled NGF into the anterior chamber of the left eye of an adult rat (10 ng of ^{125}I-labeled NGF). Counts in the ganglion on the same side as the injected eye (left SCG) accumulate gradually, reaching a peak in about 16 hours. This is consistent with uptake from the anterior chamber by postganglionic superior cervical ganglion axons and subsequent transport to the ganglion. The fact that little or no accumulation occurs in the contralateral ganglion (right SCG) indicates that very little labeled NGF is taken up via the circulation. (After Johnson et al., 1978.)*

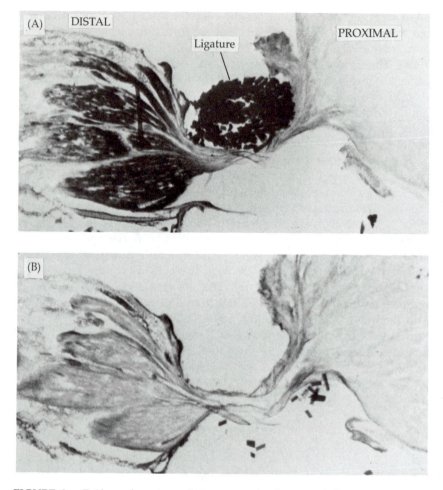

FIGURE 9. *Evidence for retrograde transport of endogenous NGF. (A) Ligated peripheral nerve of a guinea pig superior cervical ganglion treated with rabbit antiserum against guinea pig NGF (the NGF is made visible by a goat anti-rabbit antibody conjugated to horseradish peroxidase). Endogenous NGF accumulates in the nerve just distal to the ligation within 20 hours. (B) Ligated nerve stained with nonimmune rabbit serum serves as a control. ×60. (After Palmitier et al., 1984.)*

A number of observations underscore the importance of the retrograde access of NGF to sensitive cells during development. If the axons of sympathetic ganglion cells are cut early in development (or destroyed pharmacologically by 6-hydroxydopamine), then sympathetic ganglion cells show a variety of morphological and physiological reactions that can be partially or completely reversed by the administration of exogenous NGF (Levi-Montalcini et al., 1975; Hendry, 1975; Hendry and Campbell, 1976; Hamburger and Yip, 1984). Conversely, normally occurring neuronal death in spinal ganglia can be forestalled by peripherally applied NGF (Figure 10) (Brunso-Bechtold and Hamburger, 1979; Hamburger et al., 1981).

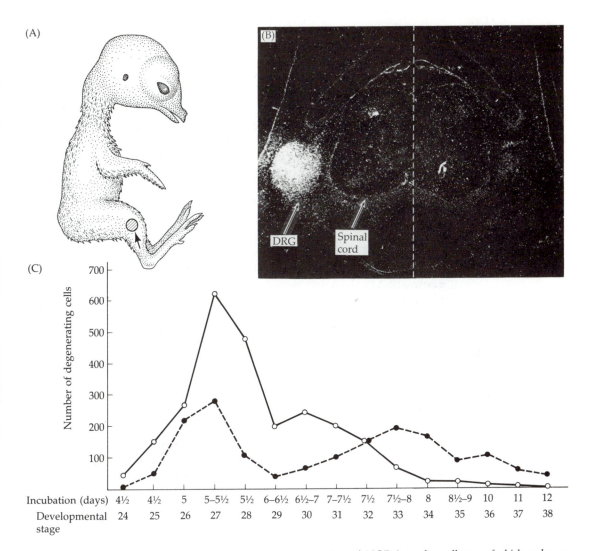

Incubation (days)	4½	4½	5	5–5½	5½	6–6½	6½–7	7–7½	7½	7½–8	8	8½–9	10	11	12
Developmental stage	24	25	26	27	28	29	30	31	32	33	34	35	36	37	38

FIGURE 10. *Reduction of normal neuronal death in chick spinal ganglia by exogenous NGF. (A) An NGF pellet can be implanted subcutaneously (arrow) in the leg of a chick embryo at about 10 days of incubation. (B) The radioactively labeled NGF is picked up peripherally and transported to the ipsilateral dorsal root ganglia. This dark-field photomicrograph shows intense labeling of a spinal ganglion (DRG) on the same side as the pellet but little labeling of the contralateral ganglion or spinal motor neurons. Dashed line indicates the midline. (C) In related experiments, daily subcutaneous injection of NGF into the yolk sac of chick embryos sharply reduces the number of degenerating cells seen in spinal ganglia during the normal cell death period. The mechanism of protection from cell death is presumably uptake and retrograde transport of NGF. The solid line shows the usual increase in the number of degenerating profiles in thoracic spinal ganglion 18 between about the fourth and eighth days of incubation. The broken line shows the reduction of degeneration caused by exogenous NGF. (A,B after Brunso-Bechtold and Hamburger, 1979; C after Hamburger et al., 1981.)*

The locus and mechanism of NGF action remains controversial (Greene et al., 1979; Thoenen and Barde, 1980; Yankner and Shooter, 1982; Schwab et al., 1982). Because NGF can maintain neurites locally, the machinery responsible for at least this effect must be located peripherally. However, the way that NGF regulates neurites is not known. The mechanism of action at the cell body is equally unclear. After binding to plasma membrane receptors, NGF is evidently internalized and transferred to membrane-enclosed cytoplasmic compartments but not to the nucleus (Figure 11) (Levi et al., 1980; Rohrer et al., 1982; Schwab et al., 1982; see, however, Yankner and Shooter, 1979). Whether NGF binding activates a second messenger system is not known, although some evidence supports this view (Herrmann et al., 1981). Evidently, NGF does not produce its effects by subsequent release from cytoplasmic compartments because direct intracellular introduction of NGF fails to produce neurite outgrowth from a class of neurons (pheochromocytoma cells) that normally respond to external NGF (Heumann et al., 1981; Seeley et al., 1983).

Numerous studies show that NGF affects many aspects of neuronal metabolism (Greene and Shooter, 1980; Yankner and Shooter, 1982). Among the more prominent effects that have been discerned are a stimulation of RNA synthesis, a selective stimulation of protein synthesis, effects on ion fluxes, and effects on the uptake of small molecules. The central question, of course, is which (if any) of these influences is a prerequisite to the major biological actions of NGF.

EVIDENCE FOR AGENTS ANALOGOUS IN FUNCTION TO NERVE GROWTH FACTOR IN OTHER PARTS OF THE NERVOUS SYSTEM

Because cell death, local maintenance of neurites, and the retrograde effects of interrupting connections between axons and their targets are common to many, if not all, nerve cells (see Chapters 6 and 13), it is attractive to suppose that neurons in other parts of the nervous system, which show little or no sensitivity to NGF, depend on trophic factors that serve the same general purpose. Although the pursuit of other trophic factors is at an early stage, evidence for analogous agents in a number of systems has accumulated rapidly.

The system that might be expected to operate in closest analogy with NGF-dependent sympathetic ganglion cells is the system of parasympathetic ganglia in vertebrates. One approach to demonstrating a similar trophic agent in the parasympathetic system has been to explore neuronal death and survival in the avian ciliary ganglion during the course of normal development. The upshot of such experiments is that isolated ciliary ganglion cells, like sympathetic ganglion cells, die in culture unless they are supported by their normal targets, or extracts of target tissues (Nishi and Berg, 1977, 1979, 1981; Adler et al., 1979; Manthorpe et al., 1980; Bonyhady et al., 1980; Barde et al., 1983). This result is expected if parasympathetic ganglion cells also depend on a target-derived trophic factor.

Several laboratories have characterized components in conditioned media or tissue extracts that may ultimately qualify as trophic factors for ciliary ganglion cells (Ebendal et al., 1979; Manthorpe et al., 1980;

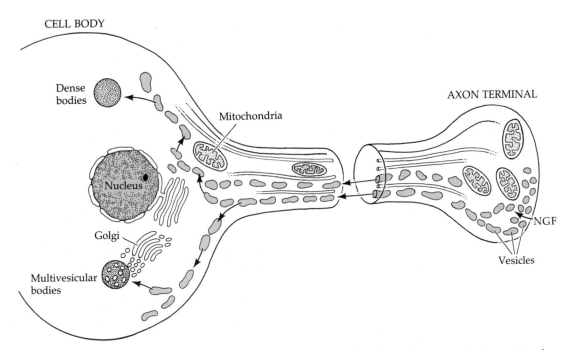

FIGURE 11. *Diagram of the current view of NGF uptake and subcellular distribution in sensitive neurons. NGF binds selectively to membrane receptors at the axon terminals of peripheral sympathetic and sensory neurons, where it is then internalized by endocytosis (arrow). Within the axon, NGF is localized in smooth cisternae and vesicles; after retrograde transort to the cell body, these membrane-bounded sacs apparently fuse with dense bodies and multivesicular bodies. There is no clear evidence for transfer of NGF to the cytosol itself or to the nucleus. (After Thoenen et al., 1979.)*

Bonyhady et al., 1980; Nishi and Berg, 1981; see also Coughlin et al., 1981). Two distinct components from eye tissues appear to have different effects on ciliary ganglion cells (Nishi and Berg, 1981). One component with a molecular weight of about 20,000 stimulates neuronal growth (assayed by cell size and protein synthesis), whereas a second, larger component (about 50,000) specifically stimulates the cholinergic development of these neurons (as measured by choline acetyltransferase) but has no effect on neuronal growth. The search for trophic molecules from other neural targets such as optic tectum, spinal cord, and skeletal muscle has only just begun but also appears promising (Dribin and Barrett, 1980, 1982; Bennett et al., 1980; Nurcombe and Bennett, 1981; Henderson et al., 1981; Hill et al., 1981; Kaufman and Barrett, 1983; Barde et al., 1983; Berg, 1984; Gurney, 1984).

The variety of trophic agents that apparently exists in the nervous system may also contribute to the apportionment of innervation to different targets. For example, the iris is innervated by two sets of autonomic nerves. The sphincter (constrictor) muscle is driven by parasympathetic ciliary ganglion cells, whereas the dilator is innervated largely by sympathetic ganglion cells. Evidently each of these neuronal

BOX

C

Familial Dysautonomia:
A Disorder of Trophic Function?

In 1949 C. M. Riley, R. L. Day, and their colleagues (Riley et al., 1949) described a peculiar syndrome that occurs in children and is characterized by low blood pressure (particularly upon standing), excessive sweating, diminished secretion of tears, vomiting, and a dramatic insensitivity to pain. In addition, these children tended to show weak tendon reflexes, poor coordination, and emotional and intellectual disorders. Since Riley and Day's initial description of 5 cases, approximately 200 additional instances of this bizarre disorder have been uncovered (Brunt and McKusick, 1970; Pearson, 1979). The disease is now recognized as an autosomal recessive disorder that occurs nearly exclusively in Jews whose ancestry can be traced to an area of eastern Europe including central and southern Poland, Galicia, the western Ukraine, northeastern Romania, and Lithuania.

The clinical picture suggests abnormalities of autonomic and sensory function, and pathological studies show that this is indeed the case.

The superior cervical ganglion, for example, has an average volume of only 34 percent of normal in cases that have been studied postmortem, and neuronal counts that are only 12 percent of normal (Pearson, 1979). As expected, peripheral sympathetic arborizations—which can normally be demonstrated by the freeze dry-aldehyde fluorescence technique—are markedly reduced or absent. Some parasympathetic ganglia are also affected; for instance, the sphenopalatine ganglion is the most drastically depleted of all the ganglia that have been examined. On the other hand, the ciliary ganglion is generally normal in these patients. Spinal ganglia are also depleted, but no consistent changes have been observed in the central nervous system. Finally, the fungiform papillae on the tongue are diminished or absent. These various neuropathological findings explain most of the clinical manifestations of this disease, which is now called familial dysautonomia.

For the most part, the cell classes affected populations is selectively maintained by a different trophic factor (or family of factors): the sympathetic axons by NGF, and the parasympathetic axons by a factor (or factors) derived from the sphincter muscle. It seems likely that the apportionment of sympathetic and parasympathetic terminals in these two different but contiguous muscles owes much to the specific and differential action of the trophic factors produced by the targets.

It might seem a simple matter to extract other trophic agents from target tissues, but this is unlikely to be straightforward. It was only good fortune that NGF is present in extremely high concentration in mouse salivary glands (for reasons that remain mysterious). This windfall enabled biochemists to isolate and eventually characterize the NGF molecule, and so far, no such source has materialized in the parasympathetic system or elsewhere. Nonetheless, rapid advances in biochemical and immunological techniques now make the identification of minute amounts of target-secreted trophic factors at least feasible. Using such methods, H. Thoenen and his collaborators have recently isolated in familial dysautonomia are the same cell classes that are sensitive to nerve growth factor in developing mammals. In consequence, a number of investigators have sought for abnormalities of nerve growth factor or nerve growth factor receptors in these patients (Siggers et al., 1976; Mobley et al., 1977; Schwartz and Breakefield, 1980). Although it is by no means certain that nerve growth factor is involved in familial dysautonomia, some abnormality of the NGF molecule, its receptors, or its synthetic pathway seems likely. In support of this, NGF antibody treatment of developing rats produces a syndrome reminiscent of this disease (Gorin and Johnson, 1979; Johnson et al., 1980; Aloe et al., 1981; see, however, Pearson et al., 1983).

A substantial advance in the effort to understand this disease is the isolation of the gene for human NGF using mouse DNA complementary to β-NGF (Ullrich et al., 1983; Scott et al., 1983). This provides a powerful tool for investigating neurological disorders in man that may involve NGF and, of course, may also provide large amounts of human NGF for possible therapeutic approaches. Taking advantage of this methodology, X. O. Breakefield and her colleagues have found that the gene for β-NGF is normal in patients with dysautonomia. The genes for the α and γ subunits have not yet been studied.

Whereas familial dysautonomia is by any standard a rare disease, many other neurological disorders of greater prevalence could well have a similar basis (i.e., arise from disordered trophic interactions between neurons and their targets). Examples that come to mind are some forms of muscular dystrophy, amyotrophic lateral sclerosis, other congenital sensory neuropathies, and some forms of mental retardation (see, for example, Pearson, 1979; Gurney, 1984). Another disease of trophic interaction may be the so-called Shy-Drager syndrome, a degenerative disorder of unknown cause that occurs in middle age and leads to progressive autonomic dysfunction (Shy and Drager, 1960). The major symptoms are severe orthostatic hypotension with progressive debility, which may lead to death in 5 to 15 years. The neuropathology of this disease shows degenerative changes in preganglionic neurons in the spinal cord and severe depletion of virtually all cranial nerve nuclei, as well as changes in the hypothalamus and elsewhere in the brain stem (Black, 1978). A detailed understanding of familial dysautonomia would provide considerable encouragement to neurologists struggling to understand these puzzling disorders.

and purified a molecule that is distinct from NGF and that has some trophic effects on sensory neurons (Thoenen and Barde, 1980; Barde et al., 1980; Edgar et al., 1981; Thoenen et al., 1981; Barde et al., 1982; see also Ebendal et al., 1979, 1983). The purified factor has a molecular weight of about 12,000 (1 μg was isolated from 1.5 kg of pig brain). Cultured chick sensory neurons can survive and grow in the absence of NGF when this agent is present (Turner et al., 1983). Thus it may be that a family of factors mediates the full spectrum of trophic interactions between particular neurons and their targets, even among some populations of NGF-sensitive neurons.

CONCLUSIONS

Cell death during normal vertebrate development indicates a profound dependence of neurons on the targets they innervate. In two specific parts of the nervous system, there is good evidence that this trophic interaction between neurons and targets is mediated by the protein nerve growth factor. Nerve growth factor, which is demonstrably produced by at least some of the relevant targets, binds to specific receptors on axon terminals and is taken up and retrogradely transported to nerve cell bodies. In addition to its influence on survival, NGF has local effects on growing neurites mediated by mechanisms that must be largely or entirely peripheral. These include both an influence on the direction of neurite growth and local maintenance of terminal arbors.

The overriding importance of NGF at present is that it provides a paradigm for trophic interactions common to many parts of the nervous system. It seems fair to suggest that NGF will ultimately be regarded as the first clear example of a class of trophic molecules that, although chemically different, all serve more or less the same physiological purpose. A comparison that makes this point is the importance of acetylcholine in the early decades of the century to unraveling the nature of chemical synaptic transmission.

Of course, there are still a number of serious problems concerning nerve growth factor, and one should not leap too quickly onto the trophic bandwagon. One problem is continuing uncertainty about exactly where NGF is made and in what quantities. This presumably arises largely from the fact that NGF is normally present in target tissues in concentrations that are at the limit of currently available detection techniques. A second problem is the phenomenally high concentration of NGF in a few peculiar places; why huge quantities of NGF are present in the salivary and prostate glands of some mammals remains a mystery. A third problem is evidence that NGF may not be the sole trophic agent for NGF-sensitive neurons such as dorsal root ganglion cells. Finally, NGF has additional actions that are not trophic, at least on the face of it. For example, NGF can influence the differentiation of adrenal medullary cells in vitro.

In spite of these and other problems, the current conception of the function of NGF provides one of the central themes in contemporary developmental neurobiology; the idea of trophic interactions based on the demonstrated role of NGF recurs in nearly all of the subsequent chapters of this book. Understanding the mechanisms of action of such agents and the rules that govern the competition for them seems likely to be one of the major tasks of neurobiologists in the next few decades.

Long-Term Effects of Neurons on Their Targets

INTRODUCTION

The influence of nerve growth factor on sensitive neurons is often considered a paradigm for trophic interactions exercised by targets on the nerve cells that innervate them (Chapter 7). There is another class of long-term interactions, however, that works in the opposite direction: anterograde trophic actions arising from neurons influence the survival and maintenance of target cells. Thus, neurons affect the properties of their targets, and targets affect the properties of neurons.

In general, these anterograde effects are less well understood than retrograde trophic effects. One reason for this is that no molecule has yet been identified that mediates long-term anterograde actions. Moreover, whereas retrograde trophic effects are evidently produced in an entirely chemical fashion, in many instances anterograde effects depend on synaptic activation of the postsynaptic cell.

LONG-TERM EFFECTS OF NEURONS ON MUSCLE

Perhaps the most thoroughly studied anterograde influence is the control of skeletal muscle properties by the motor neurons that innervate them (Harris, 1974; Purves, 1976; Grinnell and Herrera, 1981). Although much of this work has been carried out in adult animals in the context of reinnervation, the observations are equally relevant to development. An underlying theme of work on the long-term influence of nerve on muscle is the controversy between proponents of neural activity as a basis for anterograde effects and those who have favored chemical factors released from nerves as an explanation.

Effects of denervation on muscle fibers

Denervation of skeletal muscle in adult vertebrates results in a series of dramatic changes in the structure, biochemistry, and function of the postsynaptic muscle cells. The most obvious of these is muscle atrophy in which the mass of a denervated muscle is greatly reduced (Figure 1). The change in mass reflects a decrease in the diameter of each muscle

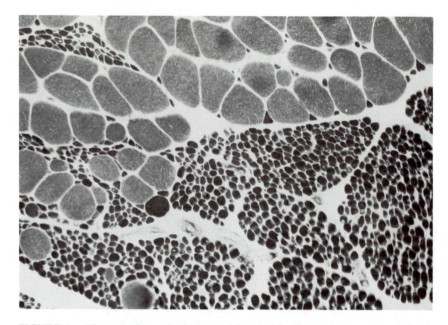

FIGURE 1. *The most dramatic evidence of the trophic effect of nerve on muscle is the atrophy of muscle fibers that follows denervation. This cross section is a biopsy of muscle from a patient with spinal muscular atrophy. In this fatal disorder, some spinal motor neurons die and others survive, thereby producing a picture of partial denervation. The large fibers are innervated, the smaller ones are denervated. The diameter of the large fibers is 70–80 μm. ATPase stain. (Courtesy of J. Carroll.)*

fiber, a decrease that in turn stems from a reduction of the major muscle proteins, actin and myosin (Tower, 1939; Close, 1972; Harris, 1974).

There are equally dramatic changes in the properties of the muscle fiber membrane following denervation. Thus, denervated fibers show a decreased sensitivity of voltage-sensitive Na^+ channels to the blocking action of tetrodotoxin (Harris and Thesleff, 1971), a tendency to generate spontaneous action potentials (visible as spontaneously occurring twitches of individual muscle fibers called fibrillations) (Tower, 1939; Purves and Sakmann, 1974), partial loss of the resting potential (Albuquerque and McIsaac, 1970), and increased membrane resistance (Albuquerque et al., 1971). Denervated fibers also show a renewed interest in receiving innervation. However, the most informative effect of denervation is a striking increase in the membrane response to acetylcholine (ACh), the transmitter agent at the vertebrate neuromuscular junction (Brown, 1937; Cannon, 1949; Kuffler, 1943; Axelsson and Thesleff, 1959; Miledi, 1960a,b; see also Hartzell and Fambrough, 1972).

The changes in muscles that have been denervated suggest that innervation somehow maintains muscle fibers in their normal state. Much of the early evidence appeared to favor the idea that motor nerve effects on muscle could be explained by the continuous release of a chemical (trophic) factor.

Evidence for a trophic factor
in the regulation of muscle properties

Experiments carried out in the early 1940s and 1950s showed that mammalian muscle fibers are more responsive to ACh following denervation (Ginetsinskii and Shamarina, 1942; Axelsson and Thesleff, 1959). Denervation supersensitivity is equally apparent in amphibian muscles (Miledi, 1960a,b) and in denervated insect muscles (Usherwood, 1969; Cull-Candy, 1978). In invertebrates and lower vertebrates, however, supersensitivity develops more slowly, and in some instances not at all (Frank, 1974).

Whereas the ACh sensitivity of innervated muscles is sharply limited to the subsynaptic region (see Figures 2 and 3A), within 2 or 3 days of denervation the entire length of a mammalian muscle fiber becomes responsive to ACh application. Extrajunctional ACh sensitivity after denervation reflects the incorporation of newly synthesized receptor molecules (Figure 2) (Brockes and Hall, 1975; see also Fambrough, 1970; Grampp et al., 1972; Sakmann, 1975); ACh receptors away from the endplate have a short lifetime (<24 hours), and steady state levels are maintained by continual synthesis (Devreotes and Fambrough, 1976). Such rapid extrajunctional turnover contrasts with receptor metabolism

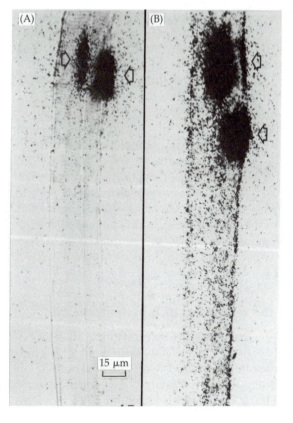

FIGURE 2. *Muscle supersensitivity after denervation is due to the appearance of extrajunctional acetylcholine receptors in the plasma membrane of denervated muscle fibers. (A) Autoradiograph of two isolated control fibers from an adult rat diaphragm that had been incubated with radioactively labeled α-bungarotoxin; the toxin binds specifically to acetylcholine receptors. The region of intense binding is the endplate (arrows)—very few silver grains are present over the extrajunctional portion of the fibers. (B) An autoradiograph of two fibers taken from a similarly treated diaphragm denervated several days previously. The marked increase in the density of silver grains over the fibers indicates a commensurate increase in ACh receptors (toxin binding sites). Note that the endplate region (arrows) retains its high concentration of receptors. (From Fambrough, 1981.)*

at the endplate, where the half-life of the receptors is about 8 days (Brockes and Hall, 1975).

That this influence of nerve on muscle is mediated by a chemical agent was suggested by the relation between the time of onset of denervation sensitivity (and of fibrillation) and the length of the distal nerve stump (Luco and Eyzaguirre, 1955; Emmelin and Malm, 1965). The longer the length of nerve left connected to the muscle, the more time it takes denervation changes to appear. The initial interpretation of this fact was that longer stumps contained a greater amount of residual trophic substance and would therefore maintain normal muscle properties for a longer period after denervation.

A second experiment that supported the idea of a neurotrophic signal involved cutting some of the inputs to frog sartorius muscle fibers (Miledi, 1960a). Because many of these fibers normally receive innervation at two different sites, this procedure leaves some fibers partially denervated but does not interfere with contraction because the synaptic effect of the remaining axon is sufficient to elicit an action potential. Within a few days of such partial denervation, R. Miledi found that the region around the denervated endplate showed local supersensitivity (and other changes) consistent with denervation. Because the activity of these fibers was presumably normal, this result also indicated that nerves supply a chemical agent to muscle cells that maintains their usual properties (Miledi, 1960a).

A third observation, also made by Miledi (1960b), was that ACh supersensitivity subsides in a denervated muscle well before regenerating motor nerve endings are sufficiently mature to cause contractions of the reinnervated fibers. Because supersensitivity began to subside during this inactive period, Miledi again concluded that a neurotrophic factor supplied to muscle by nerve was the most economical explanation (see also Miledi and Spitzer, 1974).

A final result that supported the idea of chemical mediation of denervation changes was the effect of blocking axonal transport by local application of drugs such as colchicine (Hofmann and Thesleff, 1972; Albuquerque et al., 1972). Colchicine blocks axoplasmic transport (by disrupting microtubules) and elicits denervation changes in muscle when applied to motor nerves. Because the nerve fibers conducted action potentials normally in these experiments, the effects of colchicine block were not caused by paralysis. Again, the simplest explanation seemed to be regulation of supersensitivity by a chemical signal derived from nerve.

Evidence for activity in the regulation of muscle properties

The evidence for neurotrophic chemical factors notwithstanding, it became evident by the mid-1970s that muscle activity is capable of influencing muscle fiber properties in a profound way. The key experiment that led to second thoughts about the inevitability of the trophic factor hypothesis was carried out by T. Lømo and J. Rosenthal (1972; see also

"Sciatin": Demonstration of a Neurotrophic Factor or a Cautionary Tale?

In 1978, T. H. Oh and G. J. Markelonis published a brief paper reporting that a protein extracted from chicken sciatic nerves is important in regulating acetylcholinesterase on the surface of cultured chick muscle fibers. In succeeding years these investigators and their colleagues explored the nature of this molecule and its biological effects and in 1982 described the amino acid composition of what they called "sciatin" (Markelonis et al., 1982). Their studies of the physicochemical properties of the molecule, its amino acid composition, and a partial amino acid sequence showed it to be strikingly similar to transferrin, a molecule that is widespread in vertebrates and is of fundamental importance in regulating the distribution and concentration of iron in cells. Indeed, purified chicken transferrin mimics the biological effect of sciatin in all particulars (Oh and Markelonis, 1982). The issue raised by this interesting series of papers is whether the transferrin-like molecule is an example of a "neurotrophic" factor.

That nerve extracts increase the general health of cultured muscle cells has been established by numerous observations. This, of course, presents a problem: Is an effect induced by a putative trophic agent specific and physiologically significant? Many conditions of culture are prerequisites for the good health of cultured cells; examples are the effects of collagen, insulin, pH, O_2 tension, and the availability of metabolic substrates. The initial assay used by Oh and Markelonis (1978) to isolate sciatin was the induction of muscle acetylcholinesterase by nerve extracts. In a subsequent paper, the assay for sciatin was "the degree of morphological maturation and the level of protein synthesis in embryonic muscle cells" (Markelonis and Oh, 1979). Later, the assay was a measurement of myoblast differentiation (Oh and Markelonis, 1980). Given these rather general indices of the effect of nerve extract on muscle, it is perhaps not surprising that sciatin is a molecule broadly involved in cell metabolism. Indeed, critics have suggested that sciatin is not a neurotrophic factor at all but simply an important molecule for muscle cell function that happens to be in nerve cells as well as elsewhere.

However, it may be premature to dismiss the sciatin story as irrelevant to neurotrophic interactions. Using an antiserum to sciatin, Markelonis and Oh have investigated the distribution of this molecule in embryonic and adult chicken tissues (Oh et al., 1981). Nonneural tissues such as skeletal muscle, smooth muscle, kidney, and liver were unstained by the antiserum. Cultured spinal cord neurons, cortical neurons, and sensory neurons, however, were well stained. The apparent localization of this molecule in neuronal perikarya suggests that it may still turn out to be a relatively specific neural agent that normally has a significant trophic influence on muscle cells.

Whatever the outcome, the story of sciatin makes the point that general assays of trophic effects (e.g., protein synthesis, differentiation) are likely to turn up molecules of broad metabolic importance. Deciding whether such molecules have special trophic significance in neural development may be difficult.

Jones and Vrbová, 1970), who, working in Miledi's laboratory, blocked nerve activity by the chronic application of local anesthetics (or diphtheria toxin). The idea of these experiments was to stop neural activity but to allow the nerve to remain intact with respect to the transport and release of a possible trophic factor. The locally blocked nerves continued to release ACh spontaneously (as evidenced by miniature endplate potentials); the related muscles, however, remained paralyzed for several days. At the end of such a period of nerve blockade, there was little or no evidence of nerve degeneration; nevertheless, the muscle fibers showed indisputable signs of ACh supersensitivity and other denervation changes (Figure 3). Lømo and Rosenthal also showed that direct electrical stimulation of muscles could prevent the onset of denervation changes, or reverse them once they had appeared.

A puzzle at this stage was how these findings could be reconciled with the fact that, by virtue of fibrillation (see earlier), denervated muscles are spontaneously active at rates similar to the levels of activity that prevent denervation changes during direct stimulation (Lømo and Rosenthal, 1972). This paradox was resolved when spontaneous activity in individual mammalian muscle fibers was monitored over periods of a day or more. Although the gross appearance of a denervated muscle suggests continual muscle fiber activity at high rates, *individual* fibers were found to be contracting in a cyclical fashion, with a period of about 24 hours (Purves and Sakmann, 1974). Evidently, spontaneous activity in a muscle fiber gradually inhibits itself so that activity ceases altogether in about 24 hours. The fiber then remains silent for an average of about 48 hours, during which time the inhibition of activity dissipates; the cycle is then repeated. Because a 24-hour period of activity at fibrillatory rates causes only a minor decrease in the ACh sensitivity of denervated fibers, fibrillation does not prevent the development of supersensitivity.

A number of experiments have confirmed Lømo and Rosenthal's initial observation that muscle paralysis induces denervation changes and that direct stimulation of muscle prevents them. Particularly important among these experiments was the demonstration by D. Berg and Z. W. Hall (1975) that chronic *postsynaptic* blockade of nerve-induced activity (produced by curare treatment over several days) also causes denervation changes. This result helped rule out the possibility that action potentials in nerve terminals are required for trophic factor release, a possibility that would have made the effects of activity subsidiary to the trophic hypothesis. Finally, a number of experiments were done to test the effect of activity or its absence on other aspects of the denervation response, such as atrophy, the electrical properties of muscle membrane, and sensitivity to tetrodotoxin (Lømo and Westgaard, 1975, 1976). The upshot of these studies was that most, if not all, denervation effects can be explained by the level of muscle activity.

The belated recognition that muscle activity exerts a major influence on muscle fiber properties stimulated many people to reevaluate the results that had earlier been taken to support the trophic factor hypothesis. A number of studies soon showed that degenerating nerves can

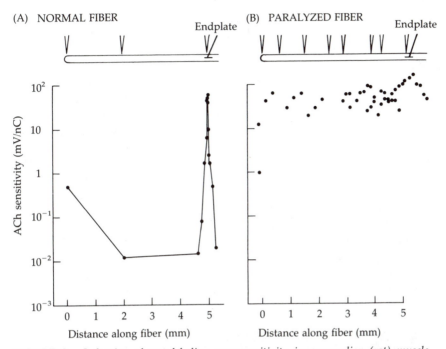

FIGURE 3. *Induction of acetylcholine supersensitivity in mammalian (rat) muscle fibers by chronic application of local anesthetic to the innervating nerve. (A) Typical pattern of acetylcholine sensitivity in a normal soleus fiber measured by the response to local application of acetylcholine at different points along the fiber surface (top). Sensitivity is measured as the depolarization (mV) recorded with an intracellular micropipette per unit charge (nC) delivered through an iontophoretic pipette containing acetylcholine. In normal muscle fibers, significant ACh sensitivity is limited to the endplate region (and, to a lesser degree, the myotendinous junction). In these diagrams only half the fiber length has been examined (the endplate is approximately in the middle of the fiber). Each filled circle represents up to 10 measurements. (B) In contrast, muscle fibers that had been paralyzed for 1 week by application of an anesthetic cuff on the motor nerve showed uniformly high sensitivity along their entire length. (After Lømo and Rosenthal, 1972.)*

induce many of the changes that occur in denervated muscle fibers. For example, muscle membrane becomes supersensitive to ACh simply in the presence of a degenerating nerve (Jones and Vrbová, 1974; Brown et al., 1978; Cangiano and Lutzemberger, 1977, 1980; see also Lømo, 1976). Indeed, this and other denervation changes can even be induced by nonbiological stimuli such as a thread placed on the muscle fiber surface (Jones and Vrbová, 1974). These results suggested that some earlier experiments might be explained by a local effect of degenerating axon terminals on the muscle fiber membrane. If this were so, nerve degeneration could explain the local supersensitivity after the partial denervation of frog sartorius fibers and the slower onset of denervation effects with longer nerve stumps (see earlier).

To summarize the present status of the neurotrophic factor/activity controversy, there is unequivocal evidence that muscle activity is capable of regulating virtually all the muscle properties that change after denervation. Experiments that were initially taken to support the idea of a trophic factor can, at least in some instances, be explained as effects of degenerating nerve products (or in some other way not requiring postulation of a trophic factor). On the other hand, one should not dismiss the idea that neurotrophic agents are involved in the regulation of muscle fiber properties. The fact that degenerating nerves can induce denervation changes shows that these effects can also be regulated by chemical signals. Moreover, there is considerable evidence that factors normally released from developing nerves elicit some of the postsynaptic responses essential for the formation of the neuromuscular junction (Chapter 9). As for denervation changes in adult animals, however, it is fair to say that the onus of establishing that influences other than activity modulate muscle properties has fallen on the proponents of the trophic factor hypothesis.

This largely historical account of the trophic factor/activity controversy in muscle highlights two general points. First, it introduces the

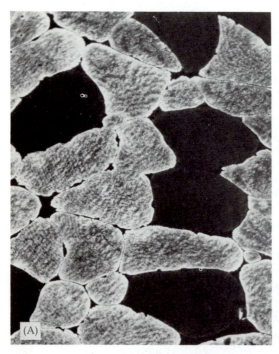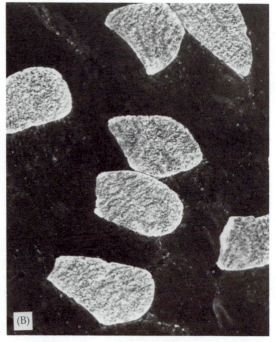

FIGURE 4. *Muscle fiber types in avian muscles. These two panels show adjacent cross sections of a chicken pectoralis muscle. (A) This section has been stained with an antibody to myosin from fast-twitch fibers; black areas indicate fibers that do not stain. (B) Most of the muscle fibers that did not stain in A are stained with an antibody to myosin from slow fibers.* *The majority of the unreactive muscle fibers in A are presumably of the slow variety, whereas the reactive fibers represent fast-twitch fibers. Such staining patterns provide striking evidence of the heterogeneous fiber-type composition of many muscles. (From Gauthier et al., 1982.)*

quite plausible idea that chemical signals operate in the anterograde direction to control postsynaptic cell properties. Second, it indicates that presynaptic influences thought to be chemically mediated must always be carefully distinguished from effects due to electrical activity.

Muscle fiber properties that depend upon motor neuron type

Some muscle fiber properties also depend on the *type* of nerve cell that provides the innervation. Vertebrate muscle fibers are generally categorized according to their contractile, histochemical, antigenic, and metabolic qualities (Figure 4). These detailed fiber type designations can be confusing because there are many fiber types classified in different ways; in consequence, the nomenclature of fibers is somewhat baroque. During the first several months of postnatal life, mammalian muscle fibers gradually differentiate into two broad categories, fast-twitch and slow-twitch (Denny-Brown, 1929; Buller et al., 1960a; Yellin, 1967a,b; Jolesz and Sréter, 1981). Subsequent denervation or paralysis transforms muscle fibers into a type intermediate between fast and slow (Romanul and Hogan, 1965; Hogan et al., 1965; Drachman and Romanul, 1970). A. J. Buller, J. C. Eccles, and their collaborators first showed that when mammalian slow-twitch and fast-twitch muscles are cross-reinnervated, the muscle fiber properties are altered (Figure 5); conversely, reinnervation by the native nerve causes a reappearance of the original muscle fiber properties (Buller et al., 1960b; Close, 1965; Romanul and van der

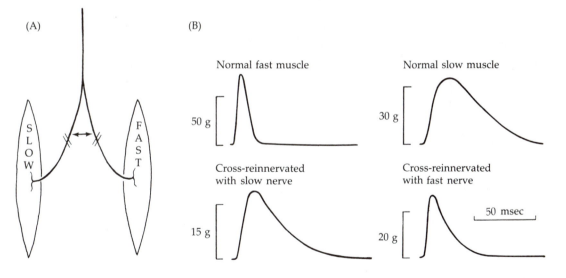

FIGURE 5. *Change in the contractile properties of muscle fibers induced by reinnervation with nerves of another class. (A) In a typical cross-reinnervation experiment, the nerves to two different muscles are transposed; in this case the nerve to the slow-twitch soleus muscle in a rat has been made to innervate the fast-twitch extensor digitorum longus muscle, and vice versa. (B) The contractile responses observed several months later indicate that crossed innervation tends to increase the speed of contraction of the slow muscle and to slow the contraction of the fast muscle. (After Close, 1965.)*

Meulen, 1967; Yellin, 1967b; Karpati and Engel, 1967; Close, 1969). These experiments show that fast-twitch muscles are slowed when reinnervated by the motor neurons that normally innervate slow-twitch muscles, and vice versa. Biochemical measurements confirm that these effects on contraction are expressed in the composition of muscle fiber proteins (Guth and Watson, 1967; McPherson and Tokunaga, 1967; Close, 1972; Pette et al., 1976; Jolesz and Sréter, 1981).

Quite naturally, the question arises of whether these cross-reinnervation effects are due to a chemical (trophic) influence of nerve on muscle or to different patterns of nerve-induced activity. Although this issue is not completely settled, chronic stimulation experiments show that many of the effects of cross-reinnervation are the result of the patterns of activity generated by different types of motor neurons (Figure 6) (Salmons and Vrbová, 1969; Lømo et al., 1974; Pette et al., 1976; Salmons and Sréter, 1976; Buller and Pope, 1977; Lømo et al., 1980; Govind and Kent, 1982). On the other hand, it should also be borne in mind that muscle fiber types can differentiate in the absence of nerves (Butler et al., 1982).

All told, these experiments on cross-reinnervation add considerable strength to the view that neural activity provides a crucial influence on

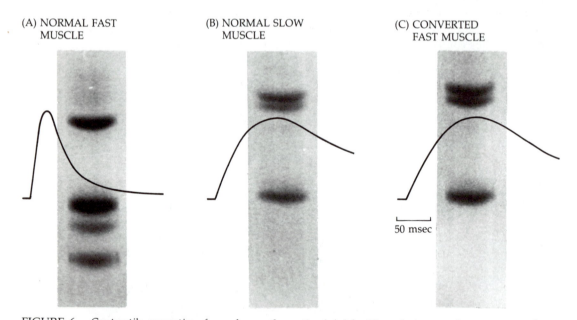

(A) NORMAL FAST MUSCLE

(B) NORMAL SLOW MUSCLE

(C) CONVERTED FAST MUSCLE

50 msec

FIGURE 6.   Contractile properties of muscles can be changed by patterns of electrical stimulation through implanted electrodes. (A) Contractile response of normal rabbit fast muscle (extensor digitorum longus; cf. Figure 5). The SDS-polyacrylamide gel electrophoretogram of the myosins from such a muscle is shown in the background. (B) Contractile response and myosin distribution of a normal slow muscle (soleus). (C) Contractile response and myosin distribution of a fast muscle (EDL) stimulated for 20 weeks in a continuous pattern chosen to mimic the pattern of slow motor neuron discharge. The contractile response of the fast muscle is slowed; in accord with this, the electrophoretic pattern of myosin light chains is shifted toward the pattern seen in normal slow muscles (cf. B and C). This suggests that the effects of cross-reinnervation (Figure 5) are largely a result of altered activity patterns (After Salmons and Sréter, 1976.)

postsynaptic muscle fiber properties. Equally important, they show that the properties of target cells depend not just on the presence or absence of innervation, but on the kind of innervation received.

Effects of neurons on muscle survival during limb regeneration

In addition to modulation of postsynaptic properties, innervation can in some instances determine the survival of muscle, or indeed of an entire structure such as the limb! These latter effects are difficult to explain simply on the basis of target cell activity.

In amphibian or chick embryos, limbs without nerves can be created by preventing axon ingrowth (Hamburger, 1939). In these circumstances, limb morphogenesis is generally normal, although the muscles become atrophic and the number of fibers in each muscle is reduced (Harris, 1981; Butler et al., 1982). An even more profound effect is observed if nerves are prevented from entering the stump of an amputated limb in some urodeles and lizards (Schotté and Butler, 1941; Needham, 1952; Singer, 1952, 1974). Following limb amputation in an animal like the newt, the wound becomes covered within a few days by a specialized epidermis. A terminal bud, called the blastema, appears at the healed surface within 2 weeks and eventually gives rise to all of the normal limb tissues. Over a period of a month or more, joints and digits can be recognized, and eventually the animal regenerates a reasonably well formed limb (Figure 7). T. J. Todd recognized in 1823 that in some amphibian species the ingrowth of nerves is essential to successful regeneration of the limbs (see also Schotté and Butler, 1941; Piatt, 1942). "If the division of the nerve be made after the healing of the stump," Todd summarized for the salamander, "reproduction [regeneration] is either retarded or entirely prevented. And if the nerve be divided after reproduction has commenced, or considerably advanced, the new growth either remains stationary or it wastes, becomes shrivelled and shapeless, or entirely disappears. This derangement cannot, in my opinion, be fairly attributed to the vascular derangement induced in the limb by the wound of the division, but must arise from something peculiar in the influence of the nerve" (Todd, 1823, p. 91). In other amphibians such as frogs, which do not normally regenerate an amputated limb, regeneration can be induced by implantation of extra nerves (Singer, 1954). The importance of nerves for successful limb regeneration is also apparent in the regrowth of lizard tails (Hughes and New, 1959). This is of some interest because lizards develop within an amnion and are therefore phylogenetically closer to mammals than are amphibians.

M. Singer carried out a number of studies in the 1940s and 1950s to explore the quality of nerve essential for successful limb regeneration (Singer, 1952, 1965, 1978). He found that the neural effect on regenerating limbs does not depend on the type of nerve fibers present: either sensory or motor fibers can support regeneration. Nor does limb regeneration depend specifically on limb nerves, because rerouting other

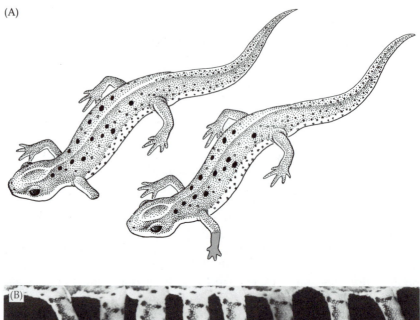

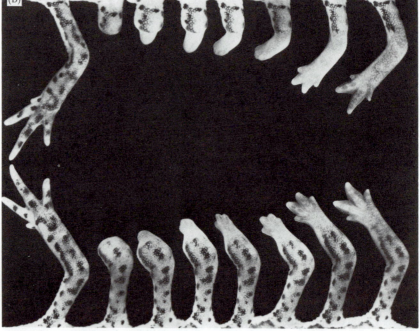

FIGURE 7.   *Regeneration of an amputated forelimb in an adult vertebrate. (A) Some species of lower vertebrates, such as the newt, have the ability to regenerate a complete limb following amputation. (B) Stages of limb regeneration after proximal (above) and distal (below) limb amputation. By about 10 days after amputation, the wound is covered by epidermis. Within a few additional days an apical blastema forms, and within a few weeks rudimentary digits are apparent. The entire regenerative process takes about 8 weeks. The success of this feat depends on the presence of innervation. (A after Singer, 1973; B from Goss, 1969.)*

nerves into the regenerating stump also sustains regrowth (Singer, 1952). Rather, the influence of nerve appears to be quantitative: success evidently depends on a "threshold" number of axons present in the regenerating stump. Singer also attempted to define the biochemical basis of this neural influence in salamander limbs (Singer, 1978). Although he found that a variety of metabolic phenonomena are influenced by the presence of nerve, which, if any, of these effects are specifically important in limb regeneration (or limb stump regression after nerve section) is unclear.

More recent studies have demonstrated a neural influence on the mitotic index of blastemal cells (Tassava and McCullough, 1978). The observation that some neural tissues produce factors that stimulate glial mitogenesis (Brockes et al., 1980; Salzer and Bunge, 1980; Salzer et al., 1980a,b; Lemke and Brockes, 1984) may provide a clue to this puzzle, but no clear understanding has yet emerged (see also Chapter 6).

LONG-TERM EFFECTS OF NEURONS ON SENSORY RECEPTORS

In addition to effects on muscle, nerves also maintain the properties (and integrity) of many sensory structures. Perhaps the best-studied example of a trophic effect of innervation on sense organs is the dependence of taste buds on the nerve fibers that normally contact them (Guth, 1971; Werner, 1974). In mammals, the taste buds are located in papillae on the tongue, soft palate, and epiglottis (Figure 8). Each of

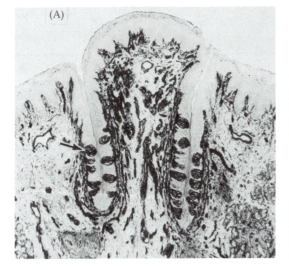 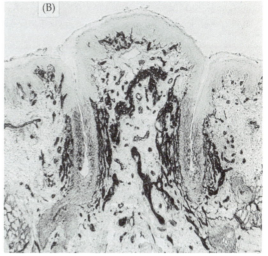

FIGURE 8. *Dependence of taste buds upon innervation. (A) Photomicrograph of a normal vallate papilla from the tongue of an adult rat. The taste buds (arrow) are in the epithelium of the "trench" walls. The section has been treated with an ATPase stain to make the taste buds stand out. (B) A similar photomicrograph 14 days after bilateral transection of the glossopharyngeal nerves. The taste buds have disappeared completely. ×72. (From Zalewski, 1969b.)*

Effects of Innervation on the Morphology of Crustacean Claws

In addition to the trophic effects of nerves on the survival and differentiation of various classes of target cells, more complex effects on morphogenesis have been described in crustaceans (Mellon, 1981). Anyone who has eaten a lobster will have noticed that one claw (the crusher) is larger and stronger than the other (the cutter). This lateral asymmetry is common in crustaceans and reflects the quite different uses of the two claws in feeding and sexual display.

F. Lang, C. K. Govind, and their collaborators (Lang et al., 1978) found that in the lobster each of the two claws has an equal chance of becoming a crusher or a cutter. Up to a certain point in development, removal of one claw induces the other to become the larger crusher claw. However, lobsters raised in tanks without objects to manipulate usually failed to develop a crusher claw (Lang et al., 1978). This finding suggests that use is involved in this asymmetry, as indeed E. B. Wilson had suggested many

(A)

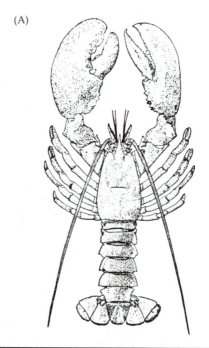

these organs consists of a number of specialized epithelial cells; the apices of the specialized cells bear chemoreceptors and their basal ends are synaptically linked to nerve fibers. Taste buds also contain taste cell precursors (and supporting cells of unknown function). As is true of some other sensory structures in epithelia, there is a continual turnover of the taste cells, which have an average life of about 10 days (Walker, 1960; Beidler, 1963; Beidler and Smallman, 1965). As the taste cells mature, they tend to move from the edge of the bud to its center (May, 1925; Robbins, 1967; Beidler and Smallman, 1965; Farbman, 1971).

The taste buds of mammals (and some other vertebrates) degenerate within a few days of cutting their innervation (Von Vintschgau, 1880; Olmsted, 1920a,b; May, 1925; Torrey, 1934; Guth, 1957, 1971; Zalewski, 1974, 1981) and do not reappear until the sensory axons regenerate (Olmsted, 1920a; Zalewski, 1969a,b, 1972). As after motor nerve section, the latent period before the onset of degenerative changes depends on the length of the distal stump (Parker, 1932; see also Torrey, 1934). In this case, nerve-dependent regeneration is specific in that only certain

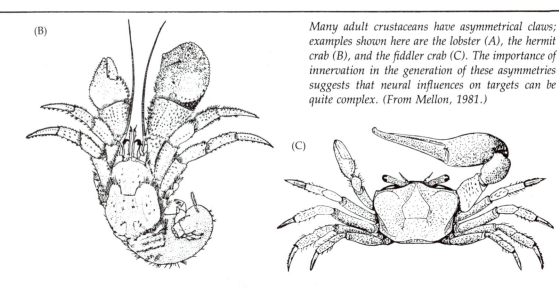

(B)

Many adult crustaceans have asymmetrical claws; examples shown here are the lobster (A), the hermit crab (B), and the fiddler crab (C). The importance of innervation in the generation of these asymmetries suggests that neural influences on targets can be quite complex. (From Mellon, 1981.)

(C)

decades earlier based on the observation that nerve section prevented claw transformation in the snapping shrimp (Wilson, 1903). In confirmation of this view, D. Mellon and P. J. Stephens (1978) found that simply cutting the nerve to the snapper claw of a shrimp (equivalent to the lobster's crusher claw) induced the remaining pincer claw to become a snapper.

These results are, of course, consistent with the influence of nerves (and patterns of neural activity) on target cells observed in a variety of neural systems. Especially remarkable in the development of crustaceans, however, is that these neural effects generate gross morphological differences. Thus, anterograde trophic influences may go beyond simple determination of target cell properties to influence more complex aspects of development. Presumably, nerves influence muscles, and muscles influence the exoskeletal elements to which they attach.

sensory nerves are able to induce the formation of new receptors (Guth, 1958; Zalewski, 1969a,b; Oakley, 1974). Thus, the vagus nerve, a foreign nerve that contains gustatory fibers, is able to maintain taste buds; in contrast, the hypoglossal nerve (which is largely motor) is ineffective. Maintenance of taste buds by nerves appears to depend on the integrity of axoplasmic transport (Sloan et al., 1983).

Other examples of the maintenance of sensory organs by nerve fibers are the sensory specializations in the bill of some aquatic birds: the corpuscles of Herbst, Grandry, and Merkel. The Herbst corpuscles— the receptors studied in greatest detail—are laminated structures just below the bill epithelium (Figure 9); the corpuscles respond to vibrations in the water and presumably help ducks and other water fowl find food. When the epidermis of the bill is denervated, these sensory structures degenerate (Saxod and Sengel, 1968; Saxod, 1972, 1978). Nor will Herbst corpuscles develop in the absence of nerves: when embryonic skin from the beak is transplanted to the chorioallantoic membrane, the skin grows quite well, but no corpuscles form (Saxod, 1978). As in the

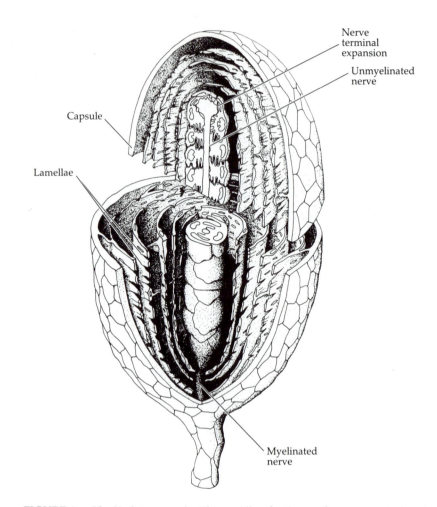

Nerve terminal expansion

Unmyelinated nerve

Capsule

Lamellae

Myelinated nerve

FIGURE 9.   *The Herbst corpuscle. This rapidly adapting mechanoreceptor is found in the epidermis of the bill of many water fowl; the receptor consists of layers of specialized lamellar cells surrounding a nerve terminal that ends in a bulbous expansion. In the absence of the neural component, this elaborate structure is not maintained; nor will it form without innervation. (After Saxod, 1978.)*

case of taste buds, corpuscles can be maintained by other sensory nerves but not by motor or sympathetic axons (Saxod, 1972, 1978). When the skin of the bill is transplanted, the corpuscles develop normally when innervated by a cutaneous limb nerve but are not induced by postganglionic or motor fibers (Dijkstra, 1933; Saxod, 1978).

The same dependence of sensory structures on their innervation occurs in the lateral line organs of some fish (Parker, 1932). These sense organs also respond to vibration in the water and are used in movement detection. When the sensory nerves that supply the lateral line organs are cut, the organs nearest the lesion degenerate first, with more distant receptors degenerating progressively, as if in response to depletion of a neural signal. Like taste buds and corpuscles, when the sensory nerves regenerate, the lateral line organs are reestablished. In other species, however, the dependence of these sensory structures on innervation is more subtle. The lateral line organs of salamanders, for example, are to a degree independent of the innervation they receive, because they reappear in a regenerating salamander tail whether or not innervation is present (Wright, 1947; Speidel, 1947; Jørgensen and Flock, 1976). Only when reinnervation is prevented over a longer time do the sensory organs degenerate (Speidel, 1948).

These and other examples suggest that a dependence of sensory specializations on innervation may be rather general. Because sensory targets are not usually activated by synapses, the influence of nerve cannot be mediated by activity but must be based on a chemical (trophic) signal. An interesting possibility is that some sensory receptors acquire trophic support from their associated axons in the same general way that neurons acquire maintenance factors like NGF from their targets (Chapter 7).

LONG-TERM EFFECTS OF NEURONS ON OTHER NERVE CELLS

Because the examples considered in the preceding sections involve effects of nerves on nonneural targets such as muscle fibers and sensory receptors, it might appear that such trophic phenonoma are limited to highly specialized end organs. In fact, similar maintenance effects are evident when the target cells are other central or peripheral neurons (see also Chapter 6).

Effects of innervation on peripheral nerve cells

The study of trophic effects of neurons on other nerve cells is in many ways a more difficult proposition than assessing neuronal effects on peripheral targets such as muscle fibers. Nonetheless, such experiments were undertaken in the early 1970s by S. W. Kuffler and his collaborators (McMahan and Kuffler, 1971; Harris et al., 1971; Dennis et al., 1971; Kuffler et al., 1971; see Box C). Their approach depended on the advantages provided by Nomarski interference-contrast microscopy and the fact that some autonomic ganglion cells are deployed in thin sheets. The advantage of Nomarski optics—a technique now widely used for a variety of neurobiological studies—is a sharp, high-contrast image of structures not normally visible with ordinary bright-field optics (see Box D). In ganglia in which nerve cells occur singly or in small clusters, detailed observations can thus be made on living neurons.

Using the parasympathetic ganglion in the heart of the frog, U. J. McMahan and Kuffler (1971) found that they could actually see synaptic boutons on the surface of ganglion cell bodies in much the same way that synaptic endings can be identified on muscle fibers (Figure 10). Kuffler and his colleagues found that the sensitivity to acetylcholine is

BOX

C

Stephen William Kuffler (1913–1980)

Stephen Kuffler was born in Tab, Hungary, where he was brought up on a small country estate. He received no formal schooling until he was about 10 years old, when he was sent to a Jesuit boarding school near Vienna. Although steeped in religion, Latin, and Greek for 9 years, he nevertheless entered the medical school in Vienna and graduated in 1937. In 1938, several months after beginning his internship, the Germans invaded Austria. Kuffler emigrated to Australia (via England), where he began working as a pathologist in the Kanamatsu Hospital in Sydney. Through a mutual interest in tennis, he came to know J. C. Eccles, who eventually offered him a position in his neurophysiology laboratory at Sydney Hospital. In Eccles' lab, Kuffler began a series of studies on the muscle endplate, a life-long interest. Kuffler was the first to show (before the advent of intracellular recording) that acetylcholine sensitivity is localized to the endplate region (Kuffler, 1943). This observation then provided the basis for assessing acetylcholine receptor distribution, an approach that has figured heavily in studies of synaptic development (Chapter 9), as well as in the long-term interactions of nerve and muscle discussed in this chapter.

When the war ended in 1945, Kuffler came to the United States where he joined R. Gerard's laboratory at the University of Chicago. Then, in 1947, he moved to the Johns Hopkins Medical School where he spent 12 years in the Wilmer Institute of Ophthalmology. The range of work that he carried out during this time is remarkable, including fundamental studies of muscle spindles and their γ-efferent innervation, studies of sensory transduction in invertebrate stretch receptors, an analysis of fast and slow muscle fibers, and studies on the nature of retinal ganglion cell receptive fields. These latter studies initiated the work pursued by D. H. Hubel and T. N. Wiesel described in Chapters 12 and 14.

In 1959 Kuffler moved to Harvard Medical School where in 1966 he established a department of neurobiology, for many years regarded as the leading department of neuroscience in

FIGURE 10. *Nerve terminals on living neurons can be seen with Nomarski optics. (A,B) Photomicrographs of a living frog cardiac ganglion cell showing the location of three synaptic boutons (arrows). A and B show two different focal planes of the same cell. (C) The cell has been fixed and treated with zinc iodide-osmium; this procedure stains synaptic boutons. Comparison of the images confirms that the structures visualized on the living neuron were actually synapses. (From McMahan and Kuffler, 1971.)*

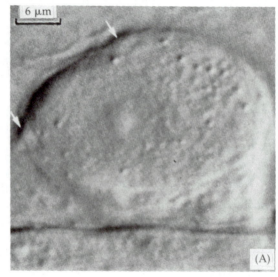

the United States. When he first came to Harvard, Kuffler pursued an earlier observation made with B. Katz concerning the basis of cellular inhibition at the crustacean neuromuscular junction; this work ultimately led to the direct demonstration that γ-aminobutyric acid is an inhibitory neurotransmitter and to important studies on presynaptic inhibition. He also initiated research with D. D. Potter and J. G. Nicholls on the physiology of glial cells in the leech, which led, incidentally, to a concerted effort to understand the central nervous system of this simple invertebrate. Finally, Kuffler continued to unravel the micropharmacology of synapses, including work just before his death on slow synaptic effects mediated by peptides. A detailed summary of Kuffler's scientific contributions can be found in his obituary for the Royal Society (Katz, 1982).

A partial list of Kuffler's protégés includes C. C. Hunt, D. H. Hubel, T. N. Wiesel, D. D. Potter, E. J. Furshpan, E. A. Kravitz, J. G. Nicholls, U. J. McMahan, and L. and Y.-N. Jan. Although the synapse is a theme that runs throughout his work, the hallmark of Kuffler's style was always to explore a new area (usually with a novel preparation), make a critical contribution, and move on to another aspect of the field. The success of his style is perhaps most obvious in the subsequent successes of his collaborators and the high esteem in which they held him (see Benjamin et al., 1983).

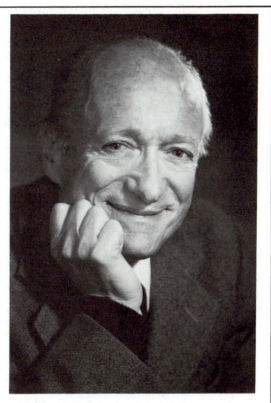

Stephen W. Kuffler. (© Bachrach. Courtesy of The Royal Society.)

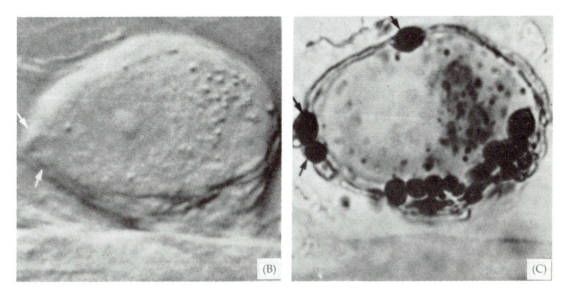

greatest in the vicinity of the synaptic bouton (Figure 11). It is unclear whether a sharp drop-off between junctional and extrajunctional sensitivity exists for synapses on nerve cells. There are as yet no good markers for acetylcholine receptors in autonomic ganglia, and the proximity of terminals on the surface of individual ganglion cells prevents sharp resolution of iontophoretic acetylcholine application. Nevertheless, it is possible to denervate ganglion cells and to ask whether the extrasynaptic membrane shows an appreciable increase in ACh sensitivity in the absence of innervation. Kuffler's group reported that, over a period of a few weeks, the entire surface of denervated autonomic ganglion cells in the frog attains approximately the same level of sen-

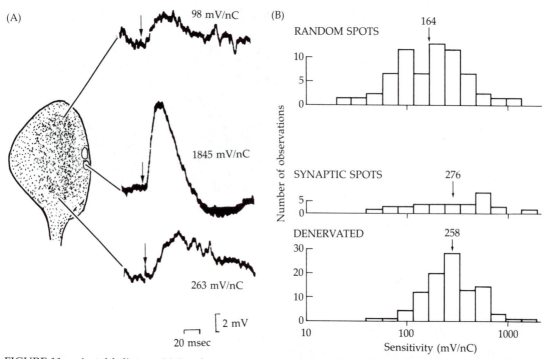

FIGURE 11.   *Acetylcholine sensitivity of synaptic and extrasynaptic regions on the surface of normal frog parasympathetic ganglion cells, and the response to denervation. (A) Using Nomarski optics, two synaptic boutons could be seen along the right-hand margin of this cell (diagram on left; cf. Figure 10). Iontophoretic application of acetylcholine while recording with an intracellular micropipette caused a large depolarization when ACh was applied to the cell surface in the vicinity of the boutons (middle trace on right; sensitivities are measured in millivolts per nanocoulomb, as in Figure 3). Arrows indicate the application of a 1-msec pulse of ACh. Similar iontophoretic application of ACh to extra-* *synaptic regions showed much less sensitivity (upper and lower traces). (B) After denervation, high levels of sensitivity were recorded everywhere on the cell surface. The uppermost histogram shows the sensitivity of randomly tested spots on normal (innervated) cells. The average sensitivity was 164 mV/nC. The middle histogram shows that spots near synaptic boutons are more sensitive on average (276 mV/nC). Two to three weeks after denervation (lower histogram), the average sensitivity of randomly tested spots (258 mV/nC) approaches the average sensitivity of synaptic spots. (After Harris et al., 1971; and Kuffler et al., 1971.)*

Differential Interference Contrast (Nomarski) Microscopy

Among the techniques that have been particularly useful in developmental neurobiology is Nomarski optics. For example, Nomarski microscopy was essential in studies of individual cell lineages in living embryos (Chapter 2), and in the identification of synaptic boutons on living neurons described in the present chapter. Because this method is so widely used, it is useful to outline the principles of differential interference contrast optics (see Allen et al., 1969).

Seeing living cells in any detail with ordinary light microscopy is difficult because cells are transparent (i.e., their constituents lack sufficient contrast). A partial solution to this problem is phase-contrast microscopy, which takes advantage of the fact that the phase of light that passes through a living cell varies because of differences in specimen thickness and refractive index. Because our eyes are insensitive to phase differences, phase-contrast microscopy converts these differences into contrast differences that we can see. Unfortunately, this approach sacrifices resolution, requires very thin specimens, and tends to generate halos around objects. Like phase-contrast, differential interference optics converts phase information into contrast information but utilizes a different strategy that does not sacrifice resolution. A special prism (called a Wollaston prism) splits the incident light beam by a fraction of a micron, an amount just below the resolution of the light microscope. The beams pass through the specimen and are recombined by a second prism. Any phase difference between the two beams causes interference when they recombine. As a result, the intensity of light at each point is proportional to the differences in phase generated by the specimen. The result is an enhancement of the edges of organelles (and other details), where the thick-

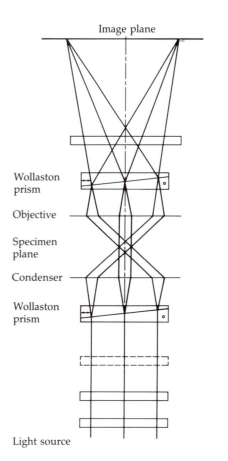

Diagram of the arrangement of the major optical components of a Nomarski microscope.

ness or the refractive index of the specimen changes abruptly. This method yields a remarkably detailed image, which, by virtue of a shadowing effect, also appears to have height and depth. The recent application of Nomarski to video microscopy has added further to its usefulness (Allen et al., 1981).

sitivity as synaptic regions (Kuffler et al., 1971; see also Roper, 1976b, Dennis and Sargent, 1979). Thus, ACh receptors on neurons may be regulated by the innervation they receive in much the same way as receptors on muscle fibers.

Of course, a number of other denervation effects in muscle can be examined in autonomic ganglion cells; some other neuronal properties also change in a manner similar to those of denervated muscle fibers (Purves, 1976). The most instructive of these observations comes from the work of I. B. Black and his collaborators, who examined the influence of innervation on the levels of tyrosine hydroxylase and other enzymes in autonomic ganglia (Black et al., 1972a, 1976; Black and Geen, 1973; Hamill et al., 1977; Black, 1978). Tyrosine hydroxylase is the rate-limiting enzyme in the biosynthetic pathway for norepinephrine in sympathetic ganglion cells. Both in development and in maturity, denervation of ganglion cells causes a marked fall in the level of this enzyme. This sequence of events bears some similarity to atrophic changes in denervated muscle fibers. Black and his collaborators also addressed the question of whether such regulation depends on a neu-

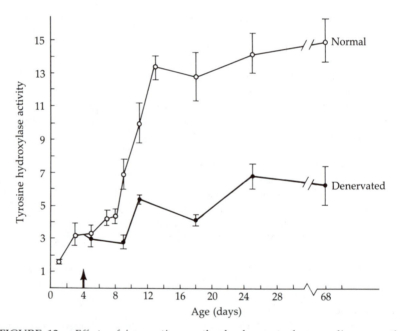

FIGURE 12. *Effects of innervation on the development of mammalian sympathetic ganglion cells. Normally, the level of tyrosine hydroxylase activity in the rat superior cervical ganglion rises progressively during the first month of postnatal life. This enzyme catalyzes an important step in the synthesis of the normal ganglion cell transmitter, norepinephrine. When the superior cervical ganglion is denervated by cutting the cervical sympathetic trunk on the fourth day of life (arrow), the usual rise in enzyme activity is sharply curtailed. This indicates that the development of ganglion cells in this respect depends upon some aspect of preganglionic innervation. Bars indicate the standard error of six determinations. (After Black et al., 1972.)*

rotrophic agent or on activity elicited in ganglion cells by the preganglionic nerves (Black et al., 1972a, 1976). They found about the same fall in tyrosine hydroxylase after spinal cord transection as when the preganglionic nerves were cut (Figure 12). Because the effect persisted when preganglionic projections were present but quiescent after cord transection, the ganglionic enzyme levels are apparently influenced by neural activity. In related experiments, blocking neural activity with drugs also reduced the levels of tyrosine hydroxylase in sympathetic ganglia (Black and Geen, 1973). Thus, neural activity influences the properties of nerve cells as well as those of muscle fibers.

Effects of innervation
on neurons in the central nervous system

Trophic effects between neurons are not limited to the peripheral autonomic system but also occur centrally (Cowan, 1970). Evidence comes from a number of systems including the auditory and vestibular nuclei (Levi-Montalcini, 1949; Powell and Erulkar, 1962), the olfactory system (Matthews and Powell, 1962), the pontine and inferior olivary nuclei (Torvik, 1956), the somatosensory cortex (Woolsey and Van der Loos, 1970; Van der Loos and Woolsey, 1973), and the visual system (Cook et al., 1951; Kelly and Cowan, 1972). In each case, removal of innervation leads to pronounced effects on the target neurons. The most instructive of these systems is the lateral geniculate nucleus in cats and monkeys. Normally, the layers of the lateral geniculate are innervated alternately by inputs from the right and the left eyes. It is thus possible to remove one eye and compare innervated and deprived neurons within the same nucleus. Over a period of a few weeks following eye removal in adult animals, the size of deprived geniculate cells decreases sharply (Figure 13) (Cook et al., 1951; Guillery, 1973b; Kupfer and Palmer, 1964; Hubel et al., 1977). The layers supplied by the intact eye, however, remain normal. Similar atrophic changes in the lateral geniculate are produced simply by sewing the lid of one eye shut (Wiesel and Hubel, 1963a, 1965; Guillery, 1972, 1973a). The layers of the lateral geniculate nucleus deprived of visual stimulation show marked atrophy, even though the geniculate inputs from the covered eye remain intact. When enucleation is carried out in younger animals, not only do the cells shrink, but many of them actually die (Kupfer and Palmer, 1964; see also Torvik, 1956). Thus, innervation influences not only the properties of target cells but also their survival in early life (see also Chapter 6).

Another central system in which long-term anterograde effects have been examined in a developmental context is the neural pathway between sensory hairs (whiskers) on the snouts of rats and mice, and cortical barrels (Figure 14) (Woolsey and Van der Loos, 1970; Van der Loos and Woolsey, 1973; Welker, 1976). Each of these intriguing agglomerations of neurons in the cortex appears to respond to a single whisker, even though three synaptic relays are interposed (Woolsey et

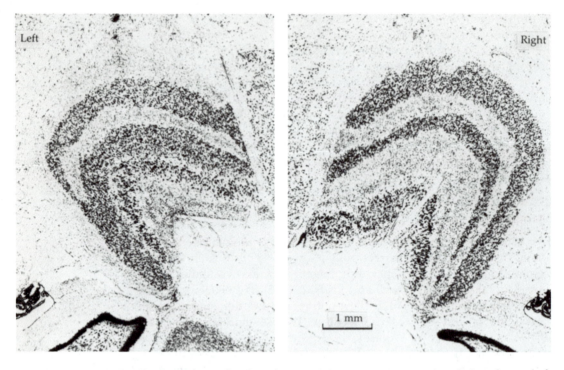

FIGURE 13. *Atrophy of cells in the monkey lateral geniculate nucleus following unilateral eye removal. These photomicrographs show coronal sections through the lateral geniculate bodies of a monkey whose right eye was removed at 2 weeks of age; the sections, which are stained with cresyl violet, were prepared 18½ months later. There is marked atrophy of those layers (pale regions) in each lateral geniculate normally innervated by axons from the missing eye. Axons from the nasal retina of each eye cross at the optic chiasm—therefore, some layers in each lateral geniculate are supplied by the right eye. (From Hubel et al., 1977.)*

al., 1981). The cortical ensembles related to each hair are called barrels because tangential sections through the appropriate region of sensory cortex show a more or less circular arrangement of the sensory neurons serving each whisker. The overall arrangement of barrels in the cortex corresponds to the distribution of whiskers on the snout. When a particular group of hair follicles is injured at birth, the corresponding barrels in the cortex are later missing (Figure 14C) (Van der Loos and Woolsey, 1973; Woolsey et al., 1981; Jeanmonod et al., 1981). Follicle injury at a slightly later stage, however, has little effect (Weller and Johnson, 1975; Woolsey and Wann, 1976). A related observation is that when rodents bear an extra whisker on their snouts there is an extra barrel in the appropriate place in the contralateral somatosensory cortex (Van der Loos and Dörfl, 1978).

The effects of early peripheral ablation in both the visual system and the somatosensory system suggest that central neurons also depend on innervation for normal development. The disappearance of barrels after

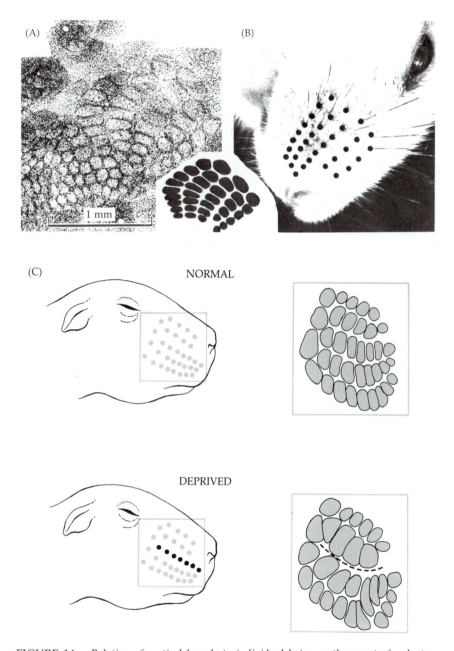

(A)

(B)

1 mm

(C)   NORMAL

DEPRIVED

FIGURE 14.   *Relation of cortical barrels to individual hairs on the snout of rodents.*
(A) Photomicrograph of a Nissl-stained tangential section through the relevant region
of somatosensory cortex. Each barrel is outlined by a ring of darkly staining neurons.
(B) Photograph of the right face of a mouse showing the mystacial vibrissae; the position
of each major hair is indicated by a black dot (axons from the hairs on the right face
project to the left cortex). In normal animals each vibrissa corresponds to an individual
barrel. The inset between A and B shows the overall arrangement of barrels in the cortex.
(C) When a row of hairs is removed in early development, the corresponding barrels are
later missing (dotted line). (A,B from Woolsey, 1978; C after Woolsey et al., 1981.)

whisker removal makes the further point that this influence can be exerted transsynaptically.

CONCLUSIONS

Long-term effects of neurons on the cells they innervate are in many instances as impressive as the retrograde action of target cells on neurons. Innervation is essential in maintaining the properties of muscle fibers, sensory end organs, and targets comprising other nerve cells. Indeed, innervation often determines the very survival of target cells. Thus, the retrograde effects described in Chapter 7 and anterograde influences outlined in this chapter and in Chapter 6 are probably equally important in the formation of neural circuits.

Whereas the mechanism of retrograde effects appears to be a chemical signal provided by trophic agents such as nerve growth factor, the basis of anterograde effects is more complex. In some instances—the innervation of sensory receptors provides an example—the target dependence is presumably based on a chemical signal in much the same style as retrograde trophic effects. On the other hand, many long-term anterograde effects are strongly influenced by neural activity. This influence is particularly clear in muscle where denervation changes can be elicited by paralysis and forestalled or reversed by direct stimulation.

In short, neurons affect the properties of their targets, and targets affect the properties of the nerve cells that innervate them. The agents of these long-term effects are chemical signals and neural activity.

Formation of Synapses

INTRODUCTION

It is probably fair to say that work on synapses dominates present-day neurobiology. The reason for this is the consensus that connections between specific groups of nerve cells are the basis of the immense computational power of nervous systems. By the same token, changes in synapses and synaptic connections are almost certainly the basis for storing information and modulating behavior. In spite of these grand motives for finding out how and why synapses are made between particular cells, most information about the morphology, biochemistry, and physiology of synapse formation comes from work on relatively simple synapses outside the central nervous system, preeminently the vertebrate neuromuscular junction (Figure 1).

Several basic questions about synaptogenesis have been explored in such simple systems: (1) Do specialized regions destined to become postsynaptic sites exist on the surface of target cells before innervation occurs or do nerve endings induce postsynaptic specializations? (2) To what degree do postsynaptic cells induce differentiation of presynaptic elements? (3) How does the structure and function of synapses change as development proceeds? That the answers to these questions have been derived largely from experiments on muscle has both advantages and disadvantages. A disadvantage is that the neuromuscular junction is only a model for central synapses. An important advantage is that the wealth of information about the structure and function of the normal neuromuscular junction allows considerable confidence in the conclusions that have been reached. Although analogous studies in the central nervous system are still at an early stage, there is no compelling reason to imagine that synapse formation in relatively simple circumstances is fundamentally different from synaptogenesis in the brain and spinal cord.

TIME OF SYNAPSE FORMATION

Two generalizations about the timing of synapse formation are probably justified: synaptogenesis begins very early in development, and it continues for a long time.

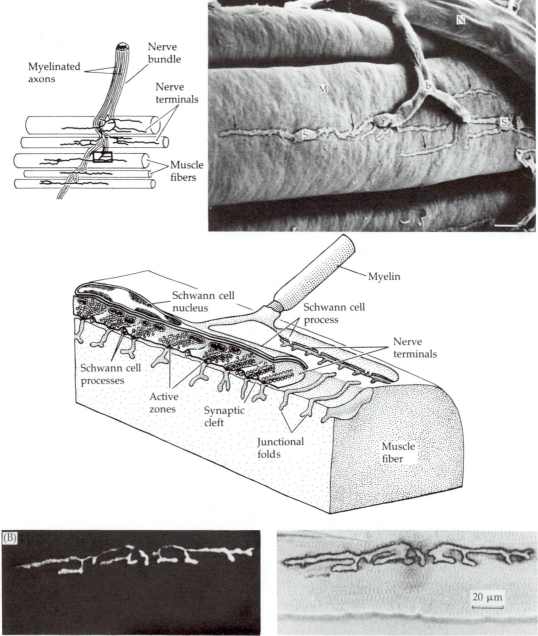

(A) FROG NEUROMUSCULAR JUNCTION

Myelinated axons

Nerve bundle

Nerve terminals

Muscle fibers

Myelin

Schwann cell nucleus

Schwann cell process

Nerve terminals

Schwann cell processes

Active zones

Synaptic cleft

Junctional folds

Muscle fiber

(B)

20 μm

Synapse formation usually starts as soon as axons reach the vicinity of postsynaptic cells. In the developing limb bud of chicks, for example, neural stimulation causes muscle twitching even before the primordial muscle masses have cleaved to form discrete muscles (Landmesser and Morris, 1975). In the frog, axonal processes emerge from the spinal

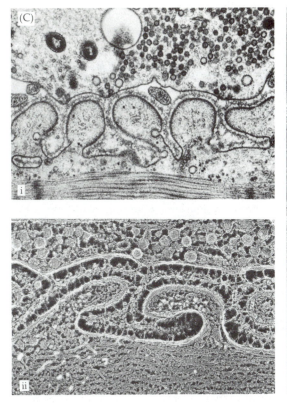

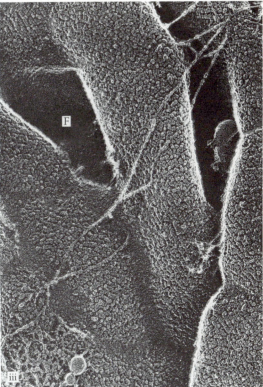

FIGURE 1. *The vertebrate neuromuscular junction. (A) Diagram of a frog neuromuscular junction; the region drawn in detail is shown at the upper left. The accompanying scanning electron micrograph shows the actual appearance of the nerve ending. The cutaway shows that synaptic vesicles are clustered in the nerve terminal opposite postsynaptic folds. These so-called active zones are sites where the contents of vesicles containing acetylcholine are released into the synaptic cleft. (B) Fluorescence staining of acetylcholine receptors with α-bungarotoxin (left), and histochemical cholinesterase staining (right) of the same muscle fiber. The toxin, derived from snake venom, binds specifically and irreversibly to ACh receptors; it is made visible by conjugation with a fluorescent dye. The detailed correspondence of postsynaptic receptors and the distribution of cholinesterase (the enzyme that terminates the action of* acetylcholine on muscle fibers) *indicates the immense precision of the cellular events that underly the formation (and maintenance) of synapses. (C) Ultrastructure of the frog neuromuscular junction. (i) Electron micrograph of the presynaptic terminal (above) and the postsynaptic folds and contractile filaments of the muscle fiber (below). The plane of section is the same as in A. ×29,000. (ii) A quick-frozen, fractured, and deep-etched image of a similar junction showing cytoskeletal elements and synaptic cleft material that is not fully apparent with conventional fixation. ×42,300. (iii) En face view of the postsynaptic membrane (the nerve terminal has been removed). The rosettes are acetylcholine receptors on the apices of the synaptic folds (F). ×80,500. (A after Kuffler and Nicholls, 1976; inset photo from Desaki and Uehara, 1981; B from Anderson and Cohen, 1974; C from Hirokawa and Heuser, 1982.)*

cord, cross the space between the cord and the nearby myotomes (which will form the axial musculature), and immediately begin to establish synaptic contacts with the developing myotubes (Kullberg et al., 1977). Spontaneous miniature endplate potentials can be recorded from individual *Xenopus* muscle fibers at stage 22 (within a day of fertilization

What Is a Synapse?

S. Ramón y Cajal first proposed that cellular contiguity rather than syncytial continuity is the basis of neural function (see Box B). Although Cajal described what he took to be contacts between nerve cells in the cerebellum in 1888, a distinctive terminal apparatus was not observed until 1897. In that year, L. Auerbach and H. Held described so-called end-feet at the tips of axons that contacted cell bodies and dendrites in the mammalian olfactory bulb (see Palay and Chan-Palay, 1975, for a more complete historical account). In spite of these and subsequent descriptions of what are now called synaptic boutons, it was not until the advent of the electron microscope and its application to the nervous system in the mid-1950s that the detailed morphology of synapses was appreciated.

The term *synapse* was coined by C. S. Sherrington in 1897. "So far as our present knowledge goes," Sherrington wrote, "we are led to think that the tip of a twig of the [axonal] arborescence is not continuous with, but merely in contact with the substance of the dendrite or cell body on which it impinges. Such a special connection of one nerve cell with another might be called a synapsis" (Foster and Sherrington, 1897). Years later, J. F. Fulton (1949) remarked that the term *synapse* was actually suggested to Sherrington's collaborator, M. Foster, by a Greek scholar at Cambridge named Verrall. The original *synapsis* (from Greek, meaning "to clasp") was apparently modified to *synapse* quite early (Sherrington used the modern form in his Silliman lectures in 1904).

In spite of the wealth of anatomical information about synapses in various parts of the nervous system, there are a number of persistent problems about the way this word is used.

Because it evolved as a rather general term, *synapse* is still applied in a very broad sense; for example, neurobiologists often speak of *electrical synapses*, even though these intercellular specializations are entirely different from chemical synapses and are in some ways a vindication of the discredited view that cells in the nervous system are continuous with one another. A more subtle problem is the tendency to extrapolate from simple well-studied chemical synapses, such as the neuromuscular junction in vertebrates, to synapses in general. Although many synapses are discrete structures with elaborate and closely aligned presynaptic and postsynaptic specializations (similar to the neuromuscular junction), at other sites in the nervous system the "presynaptic" release of neurotransmitter occurs at a distance from the "postsynaptic" cell, which may in turn show no very obvious specialization in the vicinity of the presynaptic terminals. Examples are the innervation of smooth muscles and glands by the endings of sympathetic or parasympathetic ganglion cells and diffuse projections in the central nervous system (e.g., projections from the locus coeruleus). Should these instances where a nerve terminal affects a target structure at some distance be called synapses? Another point of confusion is that some synapses are reciprocal: both partners have presynaptic and postsynaptic specializations. Finally, in addition to synapses between axon terminals and cell bodies or dendrites, there are numerous examples of dendrodendritic and axoaxonal synapses. Whatever position one takes on the proper nomenclature in these cases, it is clear that some care is required in using the term *synapse*.

and within only a few hours of neural tube closure!); and postsynaptic potentials can be evoked in muscles by nerve stimulation just a few hours later (stage 24) (Blackshaw and Warner, 1976; Kullberg et al., 1977). Similarly, synapses between neurons in the mammalian autonomic nervous system begin to form within hours of axon arrival in the neighborhood of the target cells (Rubin, 1985a,b,c).

In spite of its precociousness, synaptogenesis is surprisingly protracted. In mammalian muscle, this process lasts for many days (Dennis et al., 1981). In rat superior cervical ganglion, the number of synapses gradually increases from about the fourteenth day of gestation (when synapses first appear) well into postnatal life (Figure 2) (Smolen, 1981; Rubin, 1985c). In various parts of the mammalian brain, synaptic numbers also increase gradually over a remarkably long period in early life. In the developing motor cortex (Armstrong-James and Johnson, 1970), somatosensory cortex (Molliver and Van der Loos, 1970), visual cortex (Cragg, 1975; Vrensen et al., 1977; DeGroot and Vrensen, 1978; Blue and Parnavelas, 1983), parietal cortex (Aghajanian and Bloom, 1967; Jones and Cullen, 1979; Jones and Devon, 1980; Adams and Jones, 1982), and cerebellar cortex (Altman, 1972), the numbers of synapses that can be counted in electron microscopical sections increase for weeks to months after birth. Of course, reaching a plateau does not necessarily imply that synapse formation has stopped; synapses might still be turning over at a steady rate (see Chapter 13).

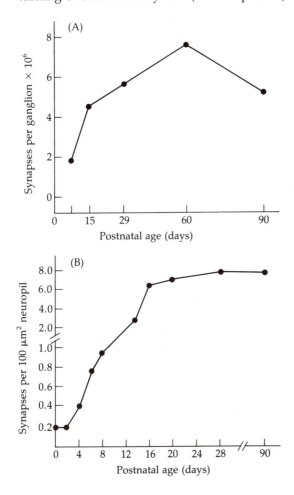

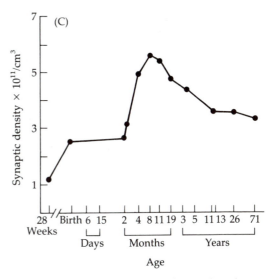

FIGURE 2. *Gradual increase in the number of synapses made between innervating axons and target neurons. Graphs show the postnatal time course of synaptogenesis measured by synapse counts in electron microscopical sections in the rat superior cervical ganglion (A), the rat visual cortex (B), and the human visual cortex (C). A gradual and prolonged elaboration of synapses is typical of many regions of the nervous system that have been examined in this way. Note also that in man, at least, synaptic density eventually begins to fall off significantly. (A after Smolen, 1981; B after Blue and Parnavelas, 1983; C after Huttenlocher et al., 1982.)*

Because of the small number of contacts made and the simple shape of the target cells, most information about the factors that account for the location and spacing of synaptic contacts has come from muscle. In many adult skeletal muscles, synapses are located in a distinct band at about the midpoint of a muscle's length (Figure 3). This characteristic placement of nerve terminals suggests that a specialized region of the postsynaptic cell dictates the initial site of nerve contact. However, M. R. Bennett and A. G. Pettigrew have argued that the adult appearance may be misleading (Bennett and Pettigrew, 1976). The length of developing muscle fibers at the time of innervation is only a few hundred micrometers (Figure 3). Because the growth of muscle fibers probably

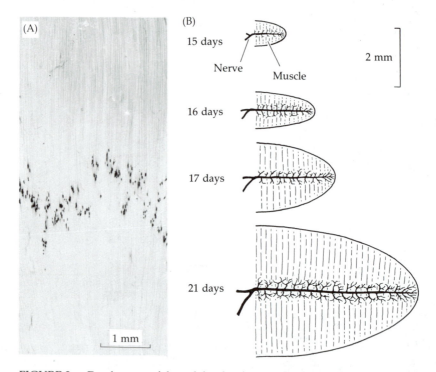

FIGURE 3. *Development of the endplate band in vertebrate muscles. (A) The endplates of many adult muscles are distributed in a discrete band midway along their length. This photomicrograph shows the endplate band in an adult rat muscle; the endplates are stained by cholinesterase histochemistry. (B) These diagrams show the approximate size of a developing rat muscle (the hemidiaphragm) from 15 days gestation until birth. When axons initially grow into the muscle (top), the myotubes that first become innervated are only a few hundred micrometers long. As development proceeds, there is a large increase in the length of muscle fibers, with only a relatively small increase in the width of the zone initially occupied by the nerve endings. This suggests that the characteristic endplate band represents a restriction of synapse formation to the initial length of myotubes. (A from Gordon et al., 1980; B after Bennett and Pettigrew, 1974.)*

occurs by the addition of sarcomeres at the ends of embryonic fibers (Williams and Goldspink, 1971), the band of endplates characteristic of adult skeletal muscles may be the result of more or less random innervation along this initial length, with subsequent fiber growth at the ends (see, however, Harris, 1981).

Most mammalian muscle fibers have a single endplate, which occupies less than 0.1 percent of the fiber surface. Larger muscle fibers may have a second or even a third endplate, but these sites of synaptic contact are usually at some minimum distance from one another (Bennett and Pettigrew, 1975, 1976; Nudell and Grinnell, 1982; see also Chapter 12). Unlike the muscles of mammals, many muscle fibers in birds, reptiles, and amphibians are innervated repeatedly along their length (Zacks, 1974). Here again, however, synapses observe what ap-

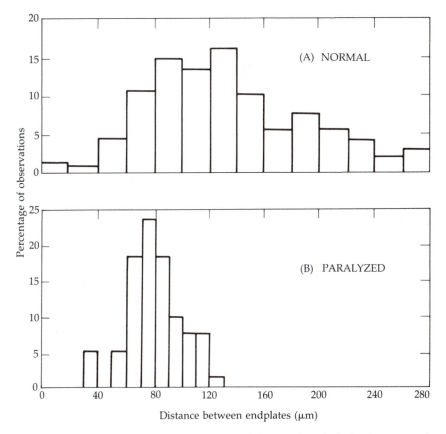

FIGURE 4. *The effect of neural activity on endplate spacing along developing muscle fibers. (A) The distribution of the distances between successive endplates on anterior latissimus dorsi muscle fibers of control 21-day chick embryos. The average endplate separation is about 130 μm. (B) Paralysis for several days reduces the average spacing between endplates to about 80 μm. The embryos were paralyzed by curare injection in ovo from the eleventh to the fourteenth day of incubation. This result suggests that the distribution of innervation is related to electrical activation of the postsynaptic cell. (After Gordon et al., 1974.)*

pears to be a rule of minimum separation (Hess, 1961; Bennett and Pettigrew, 1976).

These observations imply that the single innervation of most mammalian muscle fibers and the minimum separation of synaptic sites along the length of multiply innervated muscle fibers is caused by a region around each contact site that is refractory to additional innervation. The basis of this apparent refractoriness surrounding a point of nerve contact could be a chemical influence derived from the nerve, a change in the composition of the postsynaptic membrane or extracellular matrix, or a local inhibition imparted by the effect of electrical activity. These distinctions have not been resolved. The only evidence in this regard concerns the influence of postsynaptic activity: when developing muscle fibers are paralyzed by curare or some other agent that blocks neuromuscular transmission, the space between endplates is reduced (Figure 4) (Gordon et al., 1974; see also Oppenheim and Chu-Wang, 1983). Whether this is due to a specific effect on spacing is not yet known.

STRUCTURE AND FUNCTION OF NEWLY FORMED SYNAPSES

Once a synapse has formed, the attainment of fully mature characteristics still takes many days or even several weeks (Figures 5 and 6) (Kelly and Zacks, 1969; Rees et al., 1976; Pfenninger and Rees, 1976; Kullberg et al., 1977; Dennis et al., 1981). The first contacts between the presynaptic and postsynaptic elements in skeletal muscle show little evidence of specialization: the growing axon endings have, not surprisingly, the appearance of growth cones (Chapter 4), and the point of initial postsynaptic contact has no obvious distinguishing feature (Kelly and Zacks, 1969; Atsumi, 1971, 1977; Sisto-Daneo and Filogamo, 1974, 1975; Kullberg et al., 1977). Over the next day or so, the glycogen content of the nerve terminals falls and synaptic vesicles begin to appear. The postsynaptic surface becomes perceptibly thickened in the region of contact, and a characteristic basal lamina forms in the synaptic cleft. Gradually the synaptic junction enlarges and becomes more com-

FIGURE 5. *Diagram of the morphological development of synapses. (A) Overall appearance of a developing frog neuromuscular junction as seen by staining both the motor nerves and postsynaptic acetylcholinesterase. (1) The initial nerve contacts are quite small and lack the postsynaptic acetylcholinesterase activity characteristic of the adult junction. As the nerve ending grows, junctional sites become multiply innervated (see Chapter 12), and patchy cholinesterase appears around the perimeter of the junction (2–4). During synaptic growth, sprouts ending in growth cones often extend away from the junctional region, apparently exploring the nearby surface membrane (4,5). As terminal growth proceeds (6,7), multiple innervation is eliminated, the motor axons become ensheathed by myelin, and the presynaptic and postsynaptic constituents of the synapse take on their adult appearances (see Figure 1). (B) Diagram of some of these events at the ultrastructural level. The initial contacts (1–3) are unspecialized and have the fine structure of growth cones. No synaptic vesicles are present, and the characteristic basal lamina between presynaptic and postsynaptic elements is absent. As development proceeds (4–7), vesicles and basal lamina appear, and active zones (see Figure 1) are gradually defined. (A after Letinsky and Morrison-Graham, 1980; B after Kullberg et al., 1977.)*

plex, and active zones appear as vesicles cluster against the presynaptic membrane. A similar sequence of events has been described in the development of synaptic boutons on mammalian neurons (Figure 6).

The best-studied feature of synaptogenesis at the neuromuscular junction is the distribution of acetylcholine (ACh) receptors. Initially, mammalian muscle fibers are sensitive to ACh along their entire length (Figure 7) (Diamond and Miledi, 1962; Bevan and Steinbach, 1977; Den-

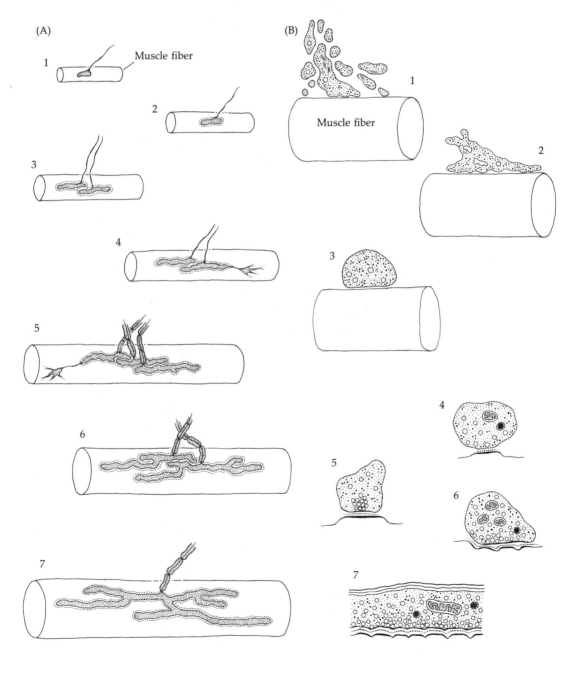

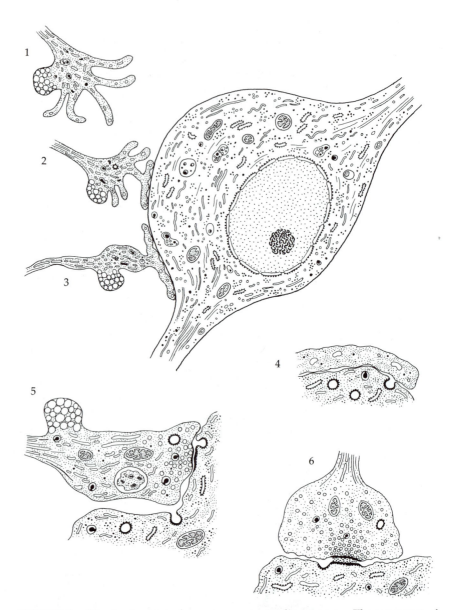

FIGURE 6. *The development of synapses on mammalian neurons. The upper part of the diagram shows an isolated superior cervical ganglion cell after 2 or 3 days in culture; diagrams 1, 2, and 3 show progressive stages of the approach and contact by a presynaptic growth cone arising from a spinal cord explant. As at the neuromuscular junction, vesicles accumulate, synaptic cleft material appears, and the postsynaptic membrane thickens as the growth cone is gradually transformed into a synaptic bouton (4–6). (After Rees et al., 1976.)*

nis et al., 1981; see also Burden, 1977a,b; Weinberg et al., 1981). By about 16 days of gestation in the rat, clusters of ACh receptors at synaptic sites are apparent, even though extrajunctional ACh sensitivity is still high (Bevan and Steinbach, 1977; Steinbach, 1981). These rudimentary postsynaptic specializations gradually enlarge in the succeeding days and weeks: the endplate becomes more elaborate as muscle fibers elongate over the first several months of life (Figure 8) (Gutmann and Hanzliková, 1965; Terävainen, 1968; Nyström, 1968a,b; Steinbach, 1981). The significance of these changes is presumably to allow the efficacy of transmitter release and reception to keep pace with the decreasing input resistance and other changes that accompany the growth of muscle fibers (Kuno et al., 1971; Kelly, 1978). As ACh receptors accumulate at the definitive endplate site, extrajunctional receptors gradually disappear.

The metabolism and function of acetylcholine receptors also change as the endplate forms. Perhaps most important, the rate of turnover of receptors at the endplate decreases. In chick muscle, the half-life of both junctional and extrajunctional receptors 1 week after hatching is about 30 hours; several weeks later, however, the half-life of endplate receptors has increased to 5 days, although the half-life of the dwindling extrajunctional receptors remains about a day (Burden, 1977a,b; see also Brockes and Hall, 1975). A similar stabilization occurs at newly formed synapses in mammalian muscle (Reiness and Weinberg, 1981). The

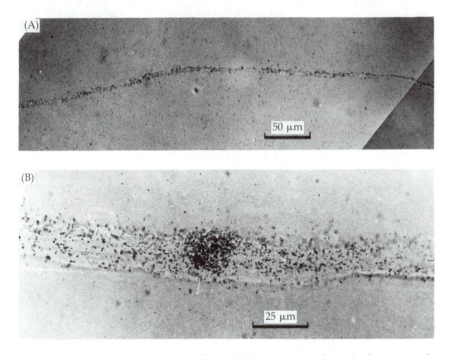

FIGURE 7.   *Changing distribution of acetylcholine receptors along developing muscle fibers. (A) Autoradiograph of a single sternomastoid muscle fiber from a 15-day rat embryo incubated with radiolabeled α-bungarotoxin, a specific ligand for ACh receptors. The silver grains are evenly distributed along the fiber length. (B) Similar autoradiograph of two adjacent fibers from a 16-day embryo; at this stage many fibers show a characteristic accumulation of silver grains in their midregion, presumably at the site of nerve–muscle contact. (From Bevan and Steinbach, 1977.)*

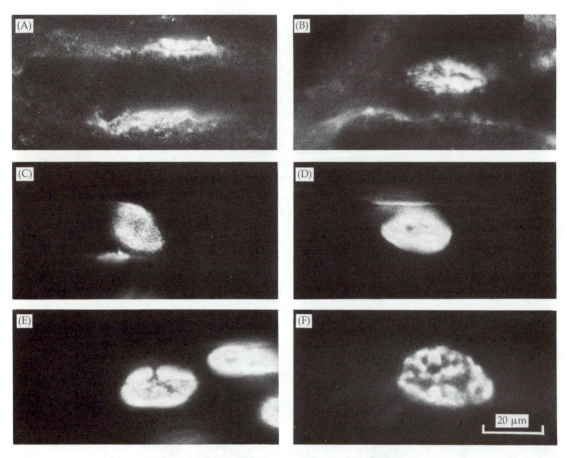

FIGURE 8.   *Progressive changes in the configuration of the endplate at the developing mammalian neuromuscular junction. (A) Poorly defined aggregates of acetylcholine receptors labeled with fluorescent α-bungarotoxin on two muscle fibers from the sternomastoid muscle of a 16-day rat embryo (cf. Figure 7B). (B) A similar but somewhat tighter aggregate from another fiber from a 16-day embryo. (C) By 20 days the receptors have aggregated to form a plaque that has a speckled appearance but shows little structure within the staining pattern. (D–F) Early postnatal fibers show increasing organization of the labeled endplate site, which reaches the fully mature appearance only after several weeks. Note that the configuration of the mammalian endplate is somewhat different from that of the frog (cf. Figure 1). (From Steinbach, 1981.)*

function of receptors in developing muscle also changes during this period. Thus, the average channel open-time of embryonic receptors is curtailed (Sakmann and Brenner, 1978; Fischbach and Schuetze, 1980; Michler and Sakmann, 1980), the response of receptors to curare alters dramatically (Ziskind and Dennis, 1978), and the immunological properties of the receptors change (Hall et al., 1983).

Synaptic function can be recorded in developing target cells before synapses are evident in electron microscopical sections (Dennis et al., 1981; Dennis, 1981; Rubin, 1985c). Not surprisingly, the release of transmitter from these immature terminals is appreciably different from the adult: spontaneous miniature endplate potentials are unusually small

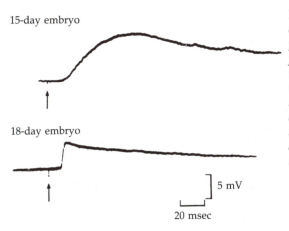

15-day embryo

18-day embryo

5 mV

20 msec

FIGURE 9. *Electrophysiological responses of developing muscle fibers to synaptic activation. Endplate potentials recorded with an intracellular microelectrode from muscle fibers in 15-day (above) and 18-day (below) rat embryos (intercostal muscle). Typically, postsynaptic responses recorded shortly after innervation have slow rise times; the rate of rise gradually increases as development proceeds. Arrows indicate the time of nerve stimulation; the bathing solution contained a small amount of curare to block suprathreshold responses and subsequent contraction. (After Dennis et al., 1981.)*

and infrequent, and evoked release has a lower quantal content and is more apt to fail (Bennett and Pettigrew, 1974, 1975; Letinsky, 1974; Kullberg et al., 1977; Dennis et al., 1981; see also Dennis and Miledi, 1974; Dennis, 1975). Other characteristic features of newly formed synapses are the slow rise-time of the postsynaptic response and its relatively long duration (Figure 9) (Kullberg et al., 1977; Dennis et al., 1981).

The upshot of all this is twofold. First, presynaptic and postsynaptic specializations develop gradually, at least in vertebrates. Second, synapses function long before they have acquired mature structural characteristics.

SOME GENERAL QUESTIONS ABOUT SYNAPSE FORMATION

Are postsynaptic membranes regionally specialized before innervation?

A remarkable aspect of most synapses is that the sites of transmitter release and reception are precisely aligned: the nerve terminal overlies a portion of the postsynaptic membrane that is enriched in receptors and other specializations (Figure 1).

One way that this colocalization might be achieved is by apposition of the nerve to a preexisting specialization on the target cell surface (see also earlier). This possibility has been examined by studying the relation between acetylcholine receptors and sites of nerve contact in cultures of vertebrate skeletal muscle. The initial distribution of ACh receptors on cultured muscle fibers is not entirely uniform: the receptors are often clumped in high-density patches ("hot spots") on the myotubes (Sytkowski et al., 1973; Fischbach and Cohen, 1973; Frank and Fischbach, 1979; Fischbach et al., 1979). Interestingly, acetylcholinesterase, junctional folds, and certain antigens are also localized at these same receptor patches (Moody-Corbett and Cohen, 1981; Sanes et al., 1984). These various observations raise the possibility that receptor clusters (or other localized specializations) induce synapse formation at specific sites along the muscle fiber surface.

M. W. Cohen, M. J. Anderson, and their collaborators (Anderson et

Santiago Ramón y Cajal (1852–1934)

Santiago Ramón y Cajal was born in a village in Navarre, Spain, the eldest son of a farmer who had become a country surgeon rather late in life. The father, clearly an ambitious man, insisted that his son pursue a medical career and made a strenuous effort to educate him. Although Cajal (as he is usually referred to) must have absorbed a great deal of his father's enthusiasm, he was by no means a willing student and was in continual trouble with the monks who sought to instruct him (Ramón y Cajal, 1937). As a teenager, Cajal's ambition was to become an artist, and at this stage in his life he was a thoroughgoing romantic. Nevertheless, he matriculated at the University of Saragossa, and in 1873, at the age of 21, received his licentiate in medicine. Shortly after graduation he was drafted into the army and dispatched to Cuba as a medical officer. This was a disheartening experience that led to a dampening of his romanticism (and to severe malaria). His only positive impression of this period seems to have been the Cuban women of whom he wrote: "When they speak, they sing, and when they look, they caress." Demoralized by his tour of duty, he returned to his studies at the University of Saragossa in the dubious post of "temporary auxilliary professor." This enabled him, however, to get a doctoral degree, which was a prerequisite for the pursuit of academic medicine in Spain.

The next few years were also disappointing ones as he failed in the competition to gain various academic posts that fell vacant. Finally, however, at the age of 32, he was appointed professor of anatomy at the University of Valencia. During this time his own research consisted of relatively pedestrian studies of inflammation and the anatomy of nerve endings in muscle. It was not until 1887, when he was 35 years old, that he embarked upon his life's work. The issue that fired his imagination was whether the nervous system is a syncytium of continuous elements or is made up of billions of separate nerve cells. Cajal settled this controversy over the course of the next few years by using the chrome–silver technique discovered by the Italian neurologist C. Golgi some years earlier. Cajal found that the technique worked especially well in the developing nervous system, and he carried out many of his studies on embryonic material. Cajal described his calling in the following way:

Since the full grown forest turns out to be impenetrable and indefinable, why not revert to the study of the young wood, in the nursery stage, as we might say? Such was the very simple idea which inspired my repeated trials of the silver method upon embryos of birds and mammals. . . . Realizing that I had discovered a rich field, I proceeded to take advantage of it dedicating myself to work, no longer merely with earnestness, but with fury. In proportion as new facts appeared in my preparations, ideas boiled up and jostled each other in my mind. A fever for publication devoured me (Ramón y Cajal, 1937, pp. 324–325).

Indeed, he published 12 papers and monographs in 1889 and a further 16 in 1890, the years that probably represent the apex of his scientific work.

Cajal's contributions to neurology are so numerous and important that they defy easy categorization. At least five avenues of research assured his reputation. First was the work already alluded to, which led to the conclusion that individual cells are the basic units of the nervous system. Although A. Forel and W. His had provided some evidence for this idea, it was Cajal who proved that axons and dendrites are outgrowths of individual cells: with the silver stain he established the critical point that the nervous system operates by contiguity of discrete elements. His second major discovery was the synapse, which he first described in 1888 (see Box A); this, of course, provided a potential mechanism for the interaction of contiguous nerve cells (including, in Cajal's view, long-term trophic interactions). His third major contribution was the assertion that nerve cells are polarized, receiving information on their cell bodies and dendrites, and conducting information to distant locations via axons. Fourth was his discovery and description of the growth cone and its function (see Chapter 4). Finally, and in some ways most important, his detailed description of nerve cell organization in the central and peripheral nervous systems of a host of different animals provided the foundations of modern neuroanatomy. This work is summarized in his two-volume opus, *Histologie du Système Nerveux de l'Homme et des Vertébrés*, written in 1904 (Ramón y Cajal, 1911). Two other important books are *Degeneration and Regeneration of the Nervous System* (1928) and *Studies on Vertebrate Neurogenesis* (1929). Reproductions from these volumes are found in virtually all modern textbooks and in numerous contemporary papers. The continued currency of Cajal's work is almost unique in modern biology—how many other observations of a hundred years ago are still fresh and useful in their original form? Perhaps the reason is that the Golgi technique, which Cajal used so effectively, continues to be used by anatomists in essentially the same manner. The advent of horseradish peroxidase and other modern tracing methods have finally begun to consign Cajal's work to history, but even this will take some time more.

Recognition did not come quickly to Cajal, who initially wrote in Spanish and suffered from residence in a country that at that time was out of the mainstream of European science. What fame he had gained by the time he was 40 was largely a result of the patronage of the anatomist R. A. von Kölliker, professor of anatomy at the University of Würzburg. By the turn of the century, however, Cajal was widely recognized by neurologists and in Spain was already a national figure. In 1905 he won the Helmholtz medal from the Royal Academy of Sciences in Berlin and, in 1906, together with C. Golgi, was awarded the Nobel prize for physiology and medicine. Cajal continued to work productively in his institute in Madrid until his death in 1934.

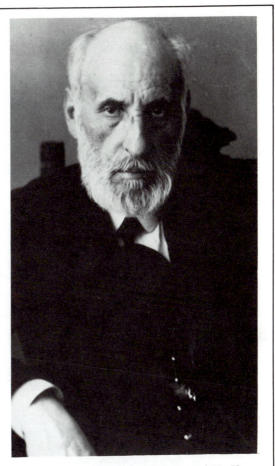

Santiago Ramón y Cajal. (Courtesy of V. Hamburger.)

Although modern students can hardly be expected to wade through his original work, or even his 1904 summary, which, regrettably, has never been translated from the French (this work is now being undertaken), every student of developmental biology should certainly read his marvelous autobiography, which is available in excellent English translation (Ramón y Cajal, 1937). Translations of two other major works are also available (Ramón y Cajal, 1928, 1929). His autobiography not only gives an absorbing account of the major events in his scientific career but also vividly conveys the intensity and brilliance that combined to make him the greatest neurologist of his time.

al., 1977; Anderson and Cohen, 1977; Cohen et al., 1979; Moody-Corbett and Cohen, 1982), and independently E. Frank and G. D. Fischbach (1979), explored this possibility in experiments in which embryonic muscle fibers were cocultured with appropriate neurons. This work showed that nerve terminals do not innervate preexisting hot spots, at

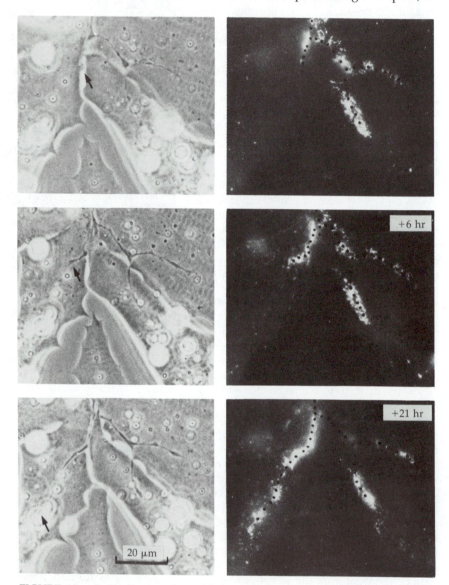

FIGURE 10. *Redistribution of acetylcholine receptors on the surface of cultured frog (Xenopus) myotubes following nerve contact. The left-hand panels show the progress of a neurite over a myotube during a period of about a day (phase-contrast optics). At the beginning of the time in culture, acetylcholine receptors were stained with fluorescent α-bungarotoxin. On the right, the same fields are viewed with fluorescence optics. As the neurite grows, labeled acetylcholine receptors appear along its route (black dots have been added to emphasize the course of the neurite). Arrow indicates the tip of the growing neurite. (From Cohen et al., 1979.)*

least in these circumstances. On the contrary, nerve contact appears to reorganize muscle membrane receptors. Cohen and his collaborators were able to watch this reorganization over a period of 2 or 3 days in cultures of amphibian muscle fibers (Figure 10). Myotube ACh receptors were labeled with fluorescent α-bungarotoxin prior to innervation (see Figures 1 and 8), and the position of receptor patches noted and photographed. When a neurite contacted the fiber, the previously labeled ACh receptors moved in the plane of the membrane to take up positions at the point of contact and along the subsequent route of the neurite across the muscle surface (Figure 10). The same general result was obtained by Frank and Fischbach (1979). Evidently, receptors accumulate at the points of nerve contact and disappear elsewhere. In addition to migration of extant receptors in the plane of the membrane (Anderson and Cohen, 1977), newly formed receptors are probably inserted into these sites preferentially (Frank and Fischbach, 1979). In general, receptor accumulation in culture appears to mimic normal innervation. Although hot spots have not been observed in intact muscle prior to nerve contact, acetylcholine receptors are present before the arrival of nerves and aggregate shortly thereafter (Dennis and Ort, 1977; Chow and Cohen, 1983).

These results imply a neural signal that causes receptor reorganization in muscle. This signal is not related to neural activity because throughout some of these experiments neuromuscular transmission was blocked by an excess of unlabeled bungarotoxin in the medium (Anderson et al., 1977; see also Cohen, 1972). Interestingly, neurites from sympathetic or dorsal root ganglion cells fail to induce receptor aggregates at sites of nerve contact (Cohen et al., 1979). This observation suggests that the neural signal is to some degree specific.

Several groups have joined the search for a neural agent that causes receptor aggregation, and a number of components of neural tissue that can elicit this effect have been partially characterized (Figure 11) (Christian et al., 1978; Podleski et al., 1979; Jessell et al., 1979; Bauer et al., 1981; Salpeter et al., 1982; Buc-Caron et al., 1983; McMahan and Slater, 1984). A problem with this work is that a number of nonbiological stimuli (coated latex beads, for instance) can also cause this effect (Peng and Cheng, 1982). Identification of the physiologically relevant stimulus may therefore be difficult.

In summary, axon terminals, at least in muscle, do not seek out preexisting synaptic sites. Instead, neurons induce acetylcholine receptors to congregate postsynaptically, apparently by means of chemical signals.

Do presynaptic elements induce other postsynaptic specializations?

The fact that nerves cause aggregation of ACh receptors suggests that some postsynaptic aspects of the synapse are induced by signals from the presynaptic cell. Once nerve contact is established, a variety of additional changes occur that also seem to depend on innervation. For

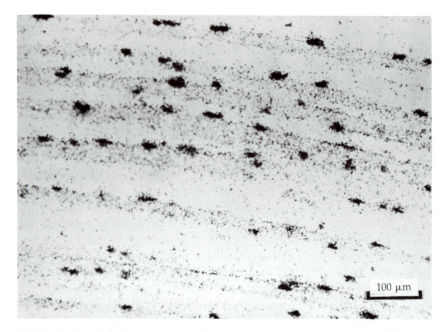

FIGURE 11. *Induction of acetylcholine receptor clustering by treatment with brain extract. Autoradiographs of myotubes grown in culture ordinarily show relatively diffuse labeling with radioactive α-bungarotoxin (see Figure 7A). This autoradiograph shows several chick myotubes after culture for 4 days in the presence of brain extract. Acetylcholine receptors are obviously clustered in patches. (Courtesy of T. Jessell.)*

example, membrane infolding typical of the normal subsynaptic region can be induced at ectopic sites on muscle fibers by implanted nerves (Saito and Zacks, 1969; Korneliussen and Sommerschild, 1976). The accumulation of acetylcholinesterase in the vicinity of the presynaptic terminal is also nerve dependent (Fischbach et al., 1979). Like receptor aggregation, acetylcholinesterase accumulation can be stimulated by nerve extracts (Davey et al., 1979). On the other hand, the aggregation of acetylcholinesterase at endplate sites is also influenced by activity. Whereas the initial aggregation of ACh receptors proceeds in paralyzed muscle fibers, the accumulation of acetylcholinesterase in the vicinity of the endplate in chick fails to occur in the presence of curare (Rubin et al., 1980; see, however, Moody-Corbett et al., 1982; Cohen et al., 1984). In accord with this, direct stimulation of mammalian muscle can induce acetylcholinesterase accumulation at endplate sites (Lømo and Slater, 1980). It seems likely, therefore, that both chemical signals and activity are involved in the initial accumulation of acetylcholinesterase at the neuromuscular junction.

Whether other regions of the nervous system follow the same rules as the innervation of muscle is as yet unclear. In the mouse cerebellum, detailed observations on postsynaptic specializations of Purkinje cells have been made in the presence and absence of their normal innervation

(Hirano and Dembitzer, 1973; Rakic, 1975; Landis and Reese, 1977). This is possible because granule cells (which supply a large portion of the innervation to Purkinje cells) are congenitally absent in some mutants. Normal Purkinje cells, like muscle fibers, show characteristic postsynaptic thickenings at points of synaptic contact in maturity. In mutants lacking granule cell innervation, one can ask whether the postsynaptic thickenings depend on the presence of nerve terminals. Surprisingly, postsynaptic thickenings unapposed by any presynaptic element were often found. Although other explanations are possible in a system as complex as the cerebellum, these observations argue for some caution in extrapolating from observations in muscle to all other types of synapses.

Do postsynaptic cells induce changes in presynaptic neurons?

Because retrograde trophic factors like NGF have important effects on axon terminals (Chapter 7), one might expect postsynaptic cells to influence presynaptic specializations. In fact, a good deal of evidence suggests this sort of interaction.

The most informative work on this issue concerns the ability of motor axons to recognize their former sites of termination on vertebrate skeletal muscle fibers during reinnervation. Although embryonic axons probably form synapses more or less randomly along myotubes, regenerating axons find old endplate sites with uncanny accuracy: reinnervation of former endplates occurs with a precision of greater than 95 percent (Figure 12) (Gutmann and Young, 1944; Saito and Zachs, 1969; Bennett et al., 1973a; Bennett and Pettigrew, 1976; Letinsky et al., 1976). This result is all the more remarkable because denervated muscle is fully capable of receiving additional synapses outside of its original endplate zone. Thus, even though regenerating axons are unable to locate the muscle they originally innervated (Chapter 10), they seem to have a keen sense of the endplate site along the length of each fiber; this ability to sniff out the endplate persists for many weeks, even when the regenerating nerve is delayed by repeated nerve section (Letinsky et al., 1976).

To find out why old endplate sites are so attractive, U. J. McMahan, J. R. Sanes, and L. M. Marshall created segments of muscle lacking myofibers (Marshall et al., 1977; Sanes et al., 1978). When muscle segments are isolated by transection, the fibers degenerate, but the basal lamina—an extracellular coat of collagen and other materials that normally surrounds muscle fibers—remains intact (Figure 13). Because the enzyme acetylcholinesterase is located largely in the basal lamina, the original endplate site can still be iden*ified under these conditions. By crushing the motor nerve at the same time that muscle fibers were caused to degenerate, these workers could ask whether regenerating axons still preferred the original synaptic sites in the absence of the postsynaptic muscle cell. The regenerating axons did, in fact, contact the old sites on the basal lamina "ghosts" and began to elaborate some

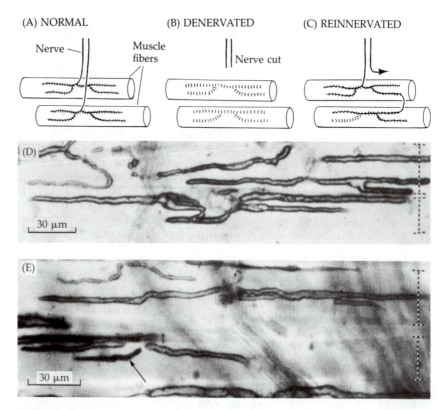

(A) NORMAL   (B) DENERVATED   (C) REINNERVATED

Nerve — | Muscle fibers

Nerve cut

Muscle fibers

(D)

30 μm

(E)

30 μm

FIGURE 12. *Accurate reinnervation of denervated endplates in frog muscle. Diagrams show normal (A), denervated (B), and reinnervated (C) muscle fibers, indicating that the vacated endplate sites are for the most part reoccupied by regenerating axons. Photomicrographs below compare several cutaneous pectoris fibers in a normal muscle (D) and a reinnervated muscle 90 days after nerve crush (E). Nerve terminals are outlined by cholinesterase histochemistry. The railroad track appearance occurs because nerve occupancy of the postsynaptic site excludes the histochemical reagents from the subsynaptic cholinesterase. After reinnervation (E), all but one of the original synaptic gutters of this endplate have been reoccupied by regenerating axons. The evidence for the absence of a nerve terminal at this portion of the endplate (arrow) is the diffuse distribution of the reaction product; this pattern indicates that the cholinesterase is accessible to the reagents. Dotted lines and brackets indicate the width of the two fibers shown in each photo. (A–C after Sanes et al., 1980; D,E from Letinsky et al., 1976.)*

of the specializations characteristic of motor nerve terminals (synaptic vesicles and active zones) (Sanes et al., 1978; Glicksman and Sanes, 1983). Thus, subsynaptic basal lamina appears to contain molecules that induce axon terminals to form synaptic endings (see also Burden et al., 1979). It is already clear that several antibodies made against muscle bind specifically to antigens in synaptic basal lamina (Sanes and Hall, 1979). Although some of these antigens are expected (acetylcholinesterase, for example), other synapse-specific antigens may reflect molecules important in stimulating synapse formation (Sanes and Hall, 1979; Bayne et al., 1981; Chiu and Sanes, 1984).

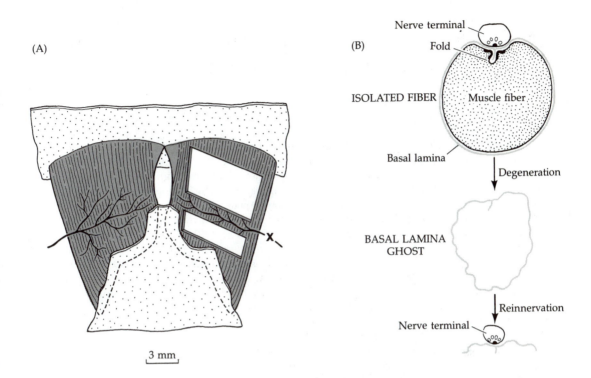

(A)

3 mm

(B)

Nerve terminal

Fold

ISOLATED FIBER — Muscle fiber

Basal lamina

Degeneration

BASAL LAMINA
GHOST

Reinnervation

Nerve terminal

FIGURE 13. *Evidence that the basal lamina surrounding muscle fibers participates in the establishment of synaptic contacts. (A) Diagram of a normal frog cutaneous pectoris muscle (left) and the contralateral muscle in which a central bridge has been surgically isolated. (B) Individual myofibers in such isolated bridges degenerate, leaving a basal lamina "ghost." If the nerve is cut at the same time (at the X in diagram A), then regenerating axons will grow out to the basal lamina ghost. Because the old endplate site can still be identified by the presence of cholinesterase and the infolding of the basal lamina, it is possible to ask whether regenerating axons "reinnervate" original synaptic sites. The evidence is that they do: even though muscle cells are no longer present in the bridge, the outgrowing nerve terminals reoccupy former endplate sites with remarkable accuracy. This implies the presence in synaptic basal lamina of molecules that are recognized by regen-*

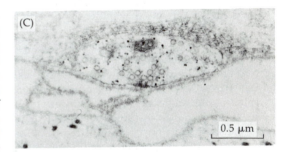

(C)

0.5 μm

erating axons. (C) Electron micrograph of a nerve terminal reoccupying an original synaptic site on a basal lamina ghost. Note that the presynaptic specialization (vesicles and an active zone) overlies a postsynaptic fold. (A after Sanes et al., 1978; B after Sanes, 1983; C from Glicksman and Sanes, 1983.)

When the persistence of nerve endings on basal lamina ghosts was examined after the muscle fibers were prevented from regenerating by X irradiation (Sanes et al., 1978), the number of profiles maintained at the old sites gradually diminished over a period of several weeks (Figure 14). Whether the endings would have disappeared altogether had such

BOX
C

Synapse Formation between Mismatched Presynaptic and Postsynaptic Elements

Another class of experiments that sheds some light on the rules that govern the formation of synapses uses deliberate mismatching. Is virtually any pair of presynaptic and postsynaptic elements competent to make synapses, or is there a limit to the disparity that can be tolerated? This question is also relevant to the specificity of neural connections (taken up in the following chapter).

Foreign axons can readily innervate muscle fibers and form functional synaptic contacts with them (Langley and Anderson, 1904; Guth and Frank, 1959; Landmesser, 1971, 1972; Ramirez and Luco, 1973; Bennett et al., 1973b; Grinnell and Rheuben, 1979; Gordon et al., 1980). Similarly, axons can innervate inappropriate neuronal targets (Langley and Anderson, 1904; McLachlan, 1974; Östberg et al., 1976; Purves, 1976; Proctor et al., 1982). In these circumstances, one can ask whether the synapses are normal and, if not, whether the contacts reflect a dominant influence of the target cell on nerve, a dominance of nerve over the target cell, or a compromise in synaptic properties. When frog skeletal muscle fibers are reinnervated by the vagus nerve (Landmesser, 1971, 1972), the synapses that form have many qualities that are quite normal. Endplate responses can be evoked in the muscle cell, innervation appears to have occurred at the old endplate site, and many physiological properties are more or less appropriate. Other aspects, however, are abnormal. For instance, the vagus nerve is incapable of inducing much cholinesterase at sites of nerve–muscle contact (Landmesser, 1972; Grinnell and Rheuben, 1979; see however, Gordon et al., 1980). A further difference is the increased sensitivity of postsynaptic receptors to the blocking agent hexamethonium (which normally blocks ganglionic, but not neuromuscular, transmission) (Land-messer, 1972; Breitschmid and Brenner, 1981; see, however, Grinnell and Rheuben, 1979). On the other hand, the highly specific ligand α-bungarotoxin (which is ineffective at many ganglionic synapses) blocks neuromuscular transmission mediated by vagal axons (Breitschmid and Brenner, 1981). The presynaptic release properties retain the characteristics of autonomic axons (Grinnell and Rheuben, 1979). In general, then, these hybrid synapses have qualities that reflect both component parts—in this sense, they are a compromise.

Even more bizarre are mismatched synapses that can be induced in tissue culture. Sensory neurons do not normally form synapses with each other. However, when rat nodose ganglion cells are cultured in the absence of satellite cells, they readily make cholinergic contacts with nearby neighbors (Cooper, 1984). Dissociated sympathetic ganglion cells also form synapses with one other (O'Lague et al., 1974). Many of these synapses are cholinergic and are therefore functional because ganglion cells normally receive cholinergic innervation. However, adrenergic synapses are also established between these dissociated neurons (Landis, 1980). Because the postsynaptic neurons are not equipped to respond to adrenergic signals, these synapses presumably do not work. Stranger still, some of these cells actually form nonfunctional adrenergic endings on themselves (called "autapses") (Landis, 1976; Furshpan et al., 1976).

The upshot of these various observations is that a wide disparity of individual elements can be tolerated in the formation of a synapse. Although these connections may not work normally (and, in some situations, may not work at all), the implication of these results is that the signals for synapse formation per se must be fairly general.

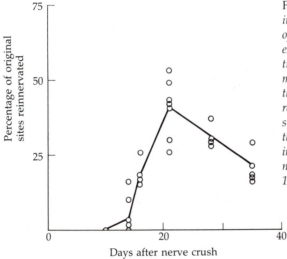

FIGURE 14. *Eventual loss of terminals on basal lamina ghosts in the absence of muscle fibers. The percentage of original sites occupied by regenerated axons in the experiments diagramed in Figure 13 is shown as a function of time after nerve crush. The regeneration of myofibers has been prevented by local irradiation. Although about half of the original sites are reoccupied by regenerating axons within 20 days, this number falls significantly thereafter. This finding suggests that although the original endplate region along the basal lamina ghosts provides some attraction to exploring terminals, it fails to maintain them. (After Sanes et al., 1978.)*

experiments been carried on for longer periods has not yet been studied. Nonetheless, this result suggests that the cues present in basal lamina are gradually used up or otherwise neutralized so that nerve terminals no longer sense the signal they require in order to be maintained.

Even though synapses between neurons lack an obvious basal lamina, it seems likely that these inductive events at the neuromuscular junction have a counterpart in the nervous system generally. For example, preganglionic axons probably reoccupy former synaptic sites during the reinnervation of mammalian sympathetic ganglia (Raisman et al., 1974). Moreover, terminals of preganglionic axons fail to develop significant levels of the enzyme choline acetyltransferase when sympathetic ganglion cells are caused to degenerate by pharmacological or immunological means (Black et al., 1972). Because this enzyme is characteristic of presynaptic (cholinergic) terminals, these results imply that preganglionic terminals do not differentiate normally in the absence of a target-derived signal (see Chapter 7).

CONCLUSIONS

A description of the normal sequence of events during synaptogenesis, of the regulation of postsynaptic receptors by innervation, and of the apparent instructions provided to axons by the postsynaptic cell hardly begins to answer the question of how synapses form. Nonetheless, these experiments lead to some important generalizations. Based on evidence derived largely from cultured muscle and nerve, it seems unlikely that there are specialized postsynaptic sites that attract innervation *before* nerve contact. Once formed, however, the postsynaptic specialization persists and provides a compelling attraction to regenerating axons. A variety of postsynaptic changes that occur during synapse formation indicate that presynaptic axons have a strong influence on the differentiation of postsynaptic specializations. The postsynaptic cell has a similar influence on the presynaptic cell.

In addition to chemical signals acting in both the anterograde and retrograde direction, synapse formation is evidently influenced by electrical activity; the localization of acetylcholinesterase at synaptic sites, for example, is activity dependent. Although the initial accumulation of ACh receptors at the neuromuscular junction occurs independently of nerve activity, the extrajunctional distribution of receptors is also activity-dependent (see Chapter 8). Finally, a variety of mismatched synaptic elements are able to achieve a greater or lesser degree of synaptic differentiation, thereby indicating that synaptogenic signals are rather general.

All told, the formation of synapses appears to be the result of a prolonged two-way conversation between presynaptic and postsynaptic elements during development. In this sense synaptogenesis is a particular manifestation of the trophic interactions described in Chapters 7 and 8.

chapter 10

Selective Synaptic Connections

INTRODUCTION

An abiding concern in neurobiology is the basis of the highly stereo-typed patterns of connections that characterize the mature nervous system, an issue loosely referred to as the problem of "neural specificity." One difficulty in understanding the genesis of neural specificity is that many developmental phenomena—neuronal migration, death, differentiation, and axon outgrowth—make important contributions to the final pattern of nerve cell connections. Thus, the assumption that understanding specificity is equivalent to understanding how neurons choose appropriate synaptic partners from among a variety of target cells is misleading. Nevertheless, selective synapse formation is certainly an important aspect of patterned connections in many parts of the nervous system.

Selective synapse formation has, for a variety of reasons, been difficult to demonstrate directly. The purpose of this chapter is to consider evidence for this phenomenon in some relatively simple systems in which connections between individual cells can be studied. In the following chapter we consider neural specificity and its molecular basis in more complex systems.

SELECTIVE SYNAPTIC CONNECTIONS IN SKELETAL MUSCLE

The innervation of muscles by motor neurons in vertebrates (and invertebrates) is highly patterned: well-defined groups of motor neurons innervate particular muscles. Much of this specificity can probably be accounted for in terms of axon outgrowth (Chapter 5). However, axons that have reached the periphery also have some ability to select between different classes of muscle cells and even different muscles.

Selective innervation of nonmammalian muscles

Most work in muscle has focused on the question of whether individual muscles are identified as such by the nerves that innervate them. In some lower vertebrates and in invertebrates, motor nerves show a preference for their original target muscles during reinnervation (Sperry and Arora, 1965; Mark, 1965; Pearson and Bradley, 1972; Cass and Mark, 1975; Van Essen and Jansen, 1977; Stephenson, 1979). The motor (but not sensory) axons in transected nerves in the salamander, for instance, recapture their original muscles with some precision (Figure 1) (Cass et al., 1973; Cass and Mark, 1975; Johnston et al., 1975). Furthermore, when particular motor axons branch to innervate both a normal and a

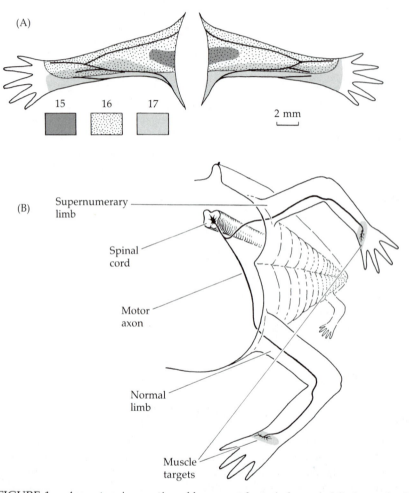

FIGURE 1. *Accurate reinnervation of lower vertebrate (salamander) limb muscles by motor nerves. (A) Segmental innervation of a normal (right) and reinnervated (left) salamander limb. The left motor nerves were cut and intentionally disrupted; 9 months later, however, the segmental pattern of innervation determined by intracellular recording was similar to the unoperated control side. Different patterns of shading correspond to innervation by segments 15–17, as indicated; the flexor surface of the limb is shown. (B) Diagram of motor axon branching to innervate both a normal (below) and a supernumerary limb. Electrophysiological tests showed that single motor axons that innervated musculature in both limbs usually contacted either identical or synergistic muscles in the two extremities (20 out of 26 cases). (A after Cass et al., 1973; B after Stephenson, 1979.)*

supernumerary limb in the salamander, they show a strong tendency to innervate the same muscle in both limbs (Stephenson, 1979).

Although these experiments could be explained by axon guidance, the appropriate reinnervation of muscles by motor neurons in some vertebrates is due at least in part to events at the level of synapse formation. This fact has been demonstrated in the salamander by experiments that have examined competition between native and foreign terminals during muscle reinnervation (Dennis and Yip, 1978; see also Genat and Mark, 1977; Bennett and Raftos, 1977; Bennett et al., 1979). In this work, a particular limb muscle was deprived of its normal innervation and a foreign motor nerve implanted. When the native nerve was prevented from promptly reinnervating the target, the foreign nerve established functional synapses with virtually all of the muscle fibers. However, when the native nerve was subsequently allowed to reach the muscle, the balance of innervation changed over a period of weeks (Figure 2). The amount of transmitter released by the foreign nerve terminals gradually decreased, whereas the quantal content of the native nerve synapses gradually increased. In the end, the foreign axons were, for the most part, unable to activate the muscle fibers. Moreover, all of the nerve terminals on the muscle could be labeled by uptake of the marker horseradish peroxidase when the native nerve was stimulated. This outcome indicates that the remaining terminals were all derived from the native nerve and that the foreign terminals had withdrawn (Dennis and Yip, 1978; see, however, Mark, 1974).

These experiments imply selective synaptogenesis (i.e., motor axons seem to recognize different muscles as such); other explanations, how-

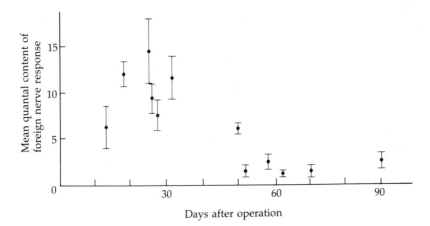

FIGURE 2. *Native nerves can displace foreign neuromuscular synapses in some lower vertebrates. This graph shows the mean quantal content of the response elicited by stimulation of a foreign nerve that had been implanted into a forelimb muscle of an adult salamander (each point represents measurements in 6–10 fibers; vertical bars show standard error). During the period shown, the cut native nerve regenerated and reached the foreign-innervated muscle fibers. The quantal content of the responses elicited by the foreign nerve fell progressively as native nerve synapses became reestablished. (After Dennis and Yip, 1978.)*

ever, are not entirely ruled out. Motor axons that have been induced to make more than their normal complement of synaptic connections give way to regenerating axons during reinnervation (Brown and Ironton, 1978; Wigston, 1980). Similarly, when two foreign nerves are made to innervate the same muscle, each nerve is capable of competition on an apparently equal footing: the foreign nerve that arrives first gives up some of its innervation to a second foreign nerve that arrives later (Grinnell et al., 1979; Wigston, 1980). Indeed, even when a foreign nerve is implanted at the endplate region of an innervated muscle, some foreign synapses manage to establish themselves by successfully competing with native axons for occupied endplate sites (Bixby and Van Essen, 1979). All this suggests that the impetus to make synapses is in part related to the *number* of contacts already established. Therefore, displacement of one set of nerve terminals by another may represent competition on a quantitative rather than a qualitative basis.

Another complication is that motor nerves in some lower vertebrates do *not* show an obvious preference for their original muscles during reinnervation. In the perch, for example, experiments similar to those in salamanders indicate that the muscle fibers remain innervated by both native and foreign axons indefinitely (Frank and Jansen, 1976; see also Sayers and Tonge, 1982). The situation in insects is also confusing. Evidence for selective reinnervation of limb muscles has been found by some workers (Denburg et al., 1977) but not by others (Whitington, 1979; Donaldson and Josephson, 1981).

Selective innervation of mammalian muscles

Whether each muscle as a whole has some special affinity for its native innervation has been tested in mammals by cutting a nerve carrying innervation to two or more different muscles and allowing it to regenerate (Bernstein and Guth, 1961; Brushart and Mesulam, 1980; Brushart et al., 1981; see also Devor and Wall, 1978); a variant of this approach involves surgically rerouting a foreign nerve so that it competes with the native nerve during reinnervation (Figure 3) (Weiss and Hoag, 1946; Gerding et al., 1977). Both of these sorts of experiments have, for mammalian muscles, given the same result: different muscles of similar fiber composition show little or no tendency to become reinnervated by their original motor axons (Figure 4). Thus, by these rather gross tests, reinnervation of mammalian muscle is quite indiscriminate: inappropriate and appropriate axons show an approximately equal ability to make synapses with the target muscle fibers.

More subtle tests, however, show that mammalian motor axons can make a weak discrimination between muscles during synapse formation. D. J. Wigston and J. R. Sanes transplanted rat intercostal muscles from two different segmental levels to the position of the superior cervical ganglion in a host animal in which the ganglion had been extirpated (Wigston and Sanes, 1982, 1985). By this procedure the two muscles were each exposed to cholinergic axons (the preganglionic axons in the cervical sympathetic trunk) that originate from the first six

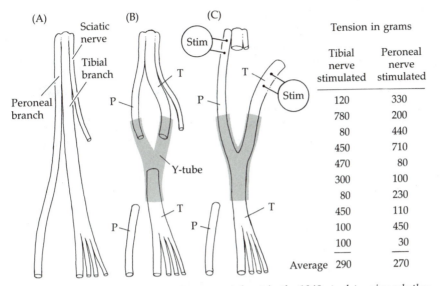

Tension in grams

	Tibial nerve stimulated	Peroneal nerve stimulated
	120	330
	780	200
	80	440
	450	710
	470	80
	300	100
	80	230
	450	110
	100	450
	100	30
Average	290	270

FIGURE 3. *Diagram of an experiment carried out in the 1940s to determine whether motor nerves to different muscles show any preference for their original target. (A) The normal arrangement of the peroneal (P) and tibial (T) branches of the sciatic nerve in the leg of the rat. (B) The motor nerves were cut and placed into the limbs of a Y-tube so that the two proximal nerves grew together into the distal nerve stump to the tibial muscles. The Y-tube is the aortic bifurcation from another animal. (C) To test the result, investigators stimulated the two different motor nerves after regeneration and measured the tension in the tibial muscle. The table shows that no consistent difference was found between the tensions produced by the native and the foreign nerves. (After Weiss and Hoag, 1946.)*

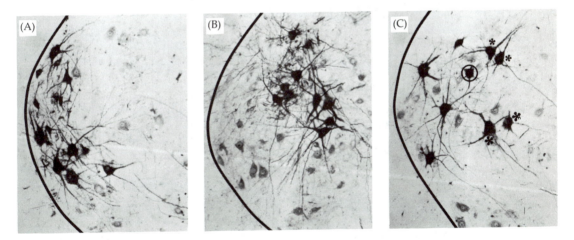

FIGURE 4. *Failure of motor axons to return to their original target muscles during regeneration in higher vertebrates. Representative spinal cord sections from a rat showing the location of the normal peroneal (A) and tibial (B) motor neuron pools. After sciatic nerve section and regeneration (C), the neurons retrogradely labeled by HRP injection into the peroneal muscles are distrib-uted in both pools. Asterisks denote labeled neurons in the position of the tibial pool; the other neurons occupy the region of the peroneal pool. The circled neuron is at the border of the two pools and was not scored in the original experiment. These results show that motor ax-ons in mammals have little or no ability to get back to their original muscles. (From Brushart et al., 1983.)*

thoracic spinal cord segments (Figure 5). By stimulating each of the thoracic ventral roots, they could test whether axons showed a preference for muscles derived from different segmental levels. Although the effect was small, the more rostrally derived segmental muscles were more frequently innervated by axons arising from more rostral levels of the cord; conversely, the caudally derived intercostal muscles showed a slight preference for innervation arising from more caudal segments. It seems unlikely that this effect could, in the course of development, account for the segmental innervation of intercostal or other muscles.

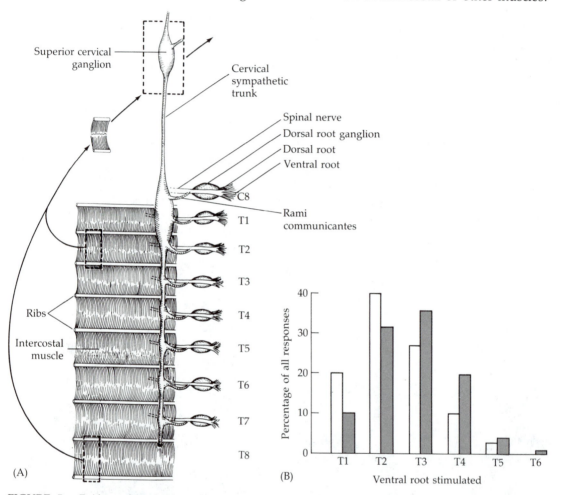

FIGURE 5. *Evidence for selective reinnervation of mammalian intercostal muscles derived from different segments. (A) Small pieces of rat intercostal muscle from two different interspaces (T2 and T8) were taken from a donor animal and implanted in the position of an excised superior cervical ganglion in a host rat. This procedure exposes the transplanted muscles to the pre-ganglionic axons carried in the cervical sympathetic trunk which arise from a number of different spinal segments (T1–T6). (B) When these muscles were tested 2 to 4 weeks later, the more rostrally derived muscle transplants (open bars) responded more often to stimulation of relatively rostral ventral roots than the caudally derived transplants (dark bars). This result implies that axons discriminate weakly between transplants from the two different levels. (After Wigston and Sanes, 1982.)*

Nevertheless, the operation of such weak signals might abet other mechanisms to produce appropriate muscle innervation.

Selective innervation of muscle fiber types

Another class of experiments carried out in muscle has been done to determine whether functionally different fiber types within a particular muscle are selectively innervated. Many nonmammalian vertebrate muscles are composed of both tonic and twitch fibers (Kuffler and Vaughan-Williams, 1953a,b; see also Chapter 8). These fiber types are very different not only in their contraction times but also in the pattern of innervation they receive: twitch fibers have solitary endplates, whereas tonic fibers have smaller, distributed endplates (Cole, 1955; Zacks, 1974; Hoyle, 1983). What makes this pattern interesting from the viewpoint of selective synaptogenesis is that individual motor axons innervate only one type of fiber.

The pyriformis of the frog is an example of a muscle that contains both slow and fast fibers. During reinnervation both classes of fibers are initially contacted by the twitch motor axons (Schmidt and Stefani, 1976). However, when the tonic motor axons (which take longer to regenerate) eventually reach the muscle, they apparently displace the synapses formed by the fast axons on the tonic fibers (Elul et al., 1970; Schmidt and Stefani, 1976, 1977). These experiments depend on the fact that the axons that innervate twitch fibers in the frog normally have greater conduction velocities than axons that innervate the tonic muscle fibers; because the velocities of these two sets of axons remain distinct after nerve section and during regeneration, it is possible to assess the matching of appropriate elements. On the other hand, similar experiments in mammalian muscle show little or no selective reinnervation of slow-twitch and fast-twitch muscle fiber populations (Miledi and Stefani, 1969). Indeed, rather than being selectively reinnervated, mammalian muscle fibers are evidently converted to a different type by the axons that happen to contact them (Kugelberg et al., 1970; see also Figure 5 in Chapter 8).

In summary, observations in invertebrates, lower vertebrates, and mammals all indicate that synapse formation in muscle is not strongly selective, a conclusion in accord with the results of the mismatching experiments described in Chapter 9. Nonetheless, there is apparently some degree of qualitative recognition during the formation of neuromuscular junctions.

SELECTIVE SYNAPTIC CONNECTIONS IN AUTONOMIC GANGLIA

Another relatively simple peripheral system in which selective innervation has been studied is autonomic ganglia. These collections of neurons are found in all vertebrates and, like muscle, have the advantage of being both accessible and anatomically straightforward.

Innervation of superior cervical ganglion cells

An accurate description of the innervation of autonomic ganglia was first provided by the English physiologist J. N. Langley in the 1890s (see Box A). Although Langley had at his disposal only the techniques of surgery and primitive electrophysiological stimulation, he made a series of observations that correctly defined the arrangement of peripheral autonomic innervation and established the basis for a great many subsequent studies in this system.

The ganglion investigated in most detail by Langley was the superior cervical. Some neurons in this most rostral of the chain of segmental sympathetic ganglia innervate sympathetic organs such as the dilator muscle of the iris; others innervate blood vessels; and still others innervate piloerector muscles or salivary glands. This partial list of targets of the superior cervical ganglion in the head and neck makes the point that a variety of functionally and spatially distinct organs are innervated by the relatively small number of cells (a few tens of thousands) that make up the ganglion. Langley found that axons arising from different spinal cord segments in mammals innervate superior cervical ganglion cells in a highly stereotyped way. To summarize Langley's extensive observations, when he stimulated the first thoracic ventral root (T1) (thus stimulating all the preganglionic axons emerging from the segment; Rubin and Purves, 1980), he observed a particular constellation of end organ effects: the pupil dilated strongly, but other sympathetic responses, such as constriction of the blood vessels in the ear or piloerection, were weak or absent (Langley, 1892, 1895, 1897). Conversely, when he stimulated a somewhat lower thoracic segment such as T4, he observed a different set of end organ effects: the blood vessels of the ear constricted strongly, the hair in part of the territory of the superior cervical ganglion stood on end, but pupillary dilation was weak or absent. Langley concluded that there must be a special relationship between preganglionic axons arising from different thoracic segments and different subsets or classes of superior cervical ganglion cells (Figure 6) (Langley, 1895, 1897).

More recent experiments have examined the cellular basis of the specific innervation of mammalian ganglion cells. Intracellular recording from individual ganglion cells while stimulating ventral roots (Figure 7) shows that each neuron in the guinea pig superior cervical ganglion is innervated by a number of different axons (about 12) from several different spinal cord segments (about 4). (Other mammals and birds show a similar arrangement.) The set of spinal cord segments supplying innervation to particular ganglion cells is nearly always contiguous (Figure 8). Moreover, each ganglion cell tends to be innervated most strongly by axons arising from a particular spinal cord segment, with the strength of innervation from other segments falling off as a function of distance from the dominant segment (Njå and Purves, 1977a). Evidently, the criteria for matching presynaptic and postsynaptic elements

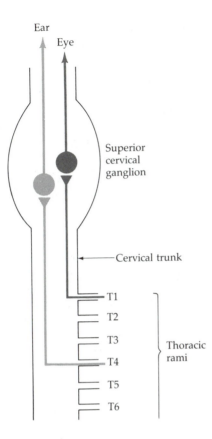

Ear

Eye

Superior
cervical
ganglion

Cervical trunk

T1

T2

T3

Thoracic
rami

T4

T5

T6

FIGURE 6. *Diagram summarizing J. N. Langley's observations on the innervation of the mammalian superior cervical ganglion. Stimulation of the outflow of different spinal segments supplying the ganglion activates different peripheral end organs in the head and neck; in this illustration, T1 stimulation affects the eye, and T4 the ear. This pattern implies a special relationship between classes of ganglion cells and preganglionic axons arising from different levels of the spinal cord.*

are continuously graded. These rules of contiguity and segmental dominance apply equally to other ganglia in the sympathetic chain (Lichtman et al., 1980). Thus, the basis of Langley's observation that the stimulation of a particular preganglionic segment elicits particular postganglionic effects is the preferential innervation of different classes of ganglion cells by a contiguous subset of the segments that supply innervation to the ganglion as a whole.

Because sympathetic end organs like hairs or blood vessels are distributed throughout the entire territory supplied by the superior cervical ganglion, it is possible to ask whether activation of a given target modality (e.g., hairs) varies according to the spinal level stimulated (Lichtman et al., 1979). In fact, progressively more caudal patches of hairs are activated by stimulating progressively more caudal spinal segments (Figure 9). In contrast, stimulation of a given segment stimulates all the end organ types within a given region of the postganglionic territory. These observations show that targets in different parts of the superior cervical territory are innervated by ganglion cells synaptically driven by different spinal cord segments. Evidently the matching of ganglion cells and preganglionic axons obeys a positional criterion:

neurons that send their axons to different locations in the postganglionic territory are, in turn, innervated by preganglionic axons that reside at different rostrocaudal levels of the spinal cord.

An additional criterion for matching presynaptic and postsynaptic elements in this system is functional modality. In the 1930s, P. Heinbecker, G. H. Bishop, and J. C. Eccles found that axons mediating different sympathetic modalities (e.g., pupillary dilation and vasoconstriction) have different conduction velocities (Bishop and Heinbecker, 1932; Eccles, 1935). The conduction velocities of axons innervating a given ganglion cell tend to fall within a particular range of the velocities evident in all the preganglionic fibers (Wigston, 1983). This fact is in accord with findings in nonmammalian vertebrates in which ganglion

FIGURE 7. *Selective innervation of autonomic ganglion cells. (A) In these studies the superior cervical ganglion was dissected together with the sympathetic chain, communicating rami, and ventral roots. The innervation of individual neurons was assessed by impaling superior cervical ganglion cells in vitro while stimulating each of the thoracic ventral roots in turn. (B–D) These oscillographs show three examples of superior cervical ganglion cell responses to stimulation of the various ventral roots. Each cell receives dominant innervation from one or two segments and weaker innervation from several adjacent segments. (From Njå and Purves, 1977a.)*

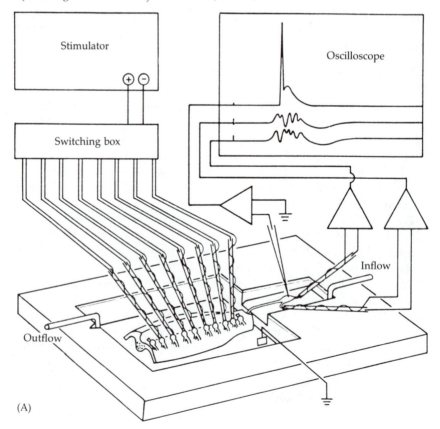

(A)

cells also appear to be specifically innervated according to modality (Nishi et al., 1965; Marwitt et al., 1971; Dodd and Horn, 1983). Taken together, these studies indicate that at least two different criteria—function and position—are relevant during synapse formation.

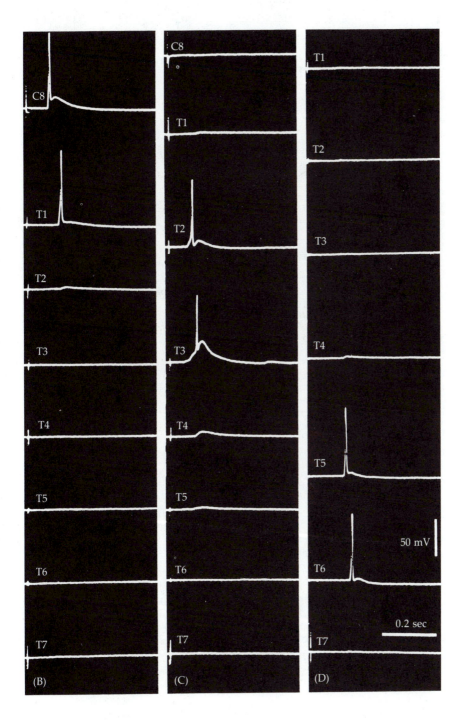

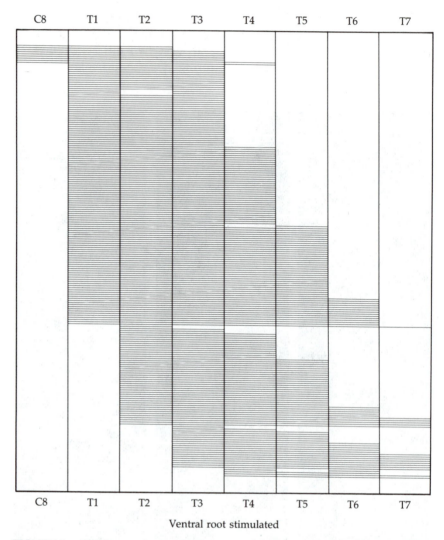

Ventral root stimulated

FIGURE 8. *Contiguous pattern of innervation of superior cervical ganglion cells. Each horizontal line represents the innervation of a different guinea pig superior cervical ganglion cell studied in the manner shown in Figure 7. The integrity of the vast majority of the horizontal lines shows that each neuron is innervated by a contiguous subset of the segments that supply the ganglion as a whole. This pattern implies that individual target cells and axons are preferentially matched during synapse formation (see also Figure 7B-D). (After Njå and Purves, 1977a.)*

Reinnervation of autonomic ganglion cells

There are a number of ways in which matching between ganglion cells and their preganglionic innervation could arise, not all of them involving selective synapse formation. It might be, for example, that different classes of presynaptic and postsynaptic cells were the only ones available at a particular point in development and that connections between

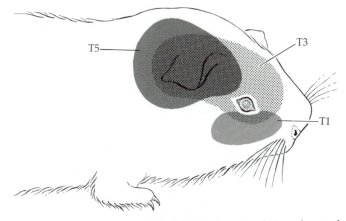

FIGURE 9. *The areas of piloerection elicited by in vivo stimulation of ventral roots T1, T3, and T5 are shown in the guinea pig. As successively more caudal ventral roots are stimulated, the patches of hair that respond occupy progressively more caudal positions in the territory supplied by the superior cervical ganglion. (After Lichtman et al., 1979.)*

partners formed simply as a consequence of availability. Studies of reinnervation argue against this possibility (see Rubin, 1985b,c).

Preganglionic sympathetic fibers, like other peripheral axons, readily regenerate when they are severed. Langley (1895, 1987) found that recovery of end organ responses occurred a few weeks after cutting the preganglionic nerve to the superior cervical ganglion (the cervical trunk; see Figure 6). In general, the end organ responses after reinnervation were organized as before: stimulation of T1 still elicited its particular constellation of largely nonoverlapping end organ effects compared to stimulation of T4. Modern experiments have confirmed Langley's findings and have shown that the normal pattern of innervation observed with intracellular recording (see Figures 7 and 8) is reestablished following regeneration of the preganglionic nerve (Njå and Purves, 1977b; see also Guth and Bernstein, 1961; Purves and Thompson, 1979). Moreover, reinnervation appears to be accurate from the very first contacts that are made by the regenerating axons (Njå and Purves, 1978). Selective reinnervation also occurs in parasympathetic ganglia. In the chick ciliary ganglion, there are two functionally and anatomically distinct populations of ganglion cells, the ciliary cells and the choroidal cells (Marwitt et al., 1971). Because these ganglion cells can be separately identified and are in turn innervated by preganglionic axons with different conduction velocities, one can ask whether these two populations are reinnervated by the same classes of axons that contacted them in the first place. As in the mammalian sympathetic system, appropriate contacts are reestablished during reinnervation (Landmesser and Pilar, 1970).

The accurate reinnervation of different classes of sympathetic neurons is especially remarkable because the ganglion cells innervated by a particular segment (or innervating a particular target) are distributed

John Newport Langley (1852–1925)

John Langley, the second son of a school master, was born in Newbury, England. After an early education at home, he attended Exeter Grammar School, where his uncle was headmaster. In 1871 he matriculated at St. Johns College, Cambridge, intent upon entering the civil service. However, one of his teachers, Michael Foster (an eminent physiologist in his own right and the founder of the *Journal of Physiology*), convinced him to take an interest in the natural sciences. In 1875 Foster made Langley his demonstrator, and for the next 9 years Langley was in charge of most of the course and laboratory work in the college. Langley never left Cambridge, rising from staff lecturer to university lecturer, deputy professor, and finally, upon Foster's retirement, professor of physiology and department chairman in 1903. Aside from occasional jaunts to Paris, Langley's life was quiet and conventional; family, tulips, and roses were evidently his major preoccupations. As W. M. Fletcher remarked in the Royal Society's *Notices of Fellows Deceased,*

"The story of his life is the story of his researches" (Fletcher, 1925).

Langley's early investigations, from about 1875 until 1890, involved primarily work on the mechanism of secretion; a particular interest was the effect of the newly introduced drug pilocarpine (Fletcher, 1926). Although this work was certainly not his major contribution, it was nonetheless substantial. Among other things he showed that cellular granules were stored up at rest and expelled during secretion. These studies led naturally to his interest in the nervous control of visceral functions, which W. H. Gaskell had recently suggested was mediated by a separate subdivision of the nervous system. Using another newly discovered drug—nicotine—Langley began in the late 1880s to define the autonomic nervous system, both anatomically and physiologically (see Langley, 1921). This work established the modern view of the autonomic nervous system as consisting of sympathetic, parasympathetic, and enteric divisions. In the 1890s Langley un-

more or less randomly throughout the ganglion (Lichtman et al., 1980; Purves and Wigston, 1983). This arrangement implies recognition at the level of the target cells. In accord with this view, when preganglionic axons sprout after partial denervation, they also innervate the correct class of ganglion cells (Maehlen and Njå, 1981).

A more direct way to explore the implication that ganglion cells bear some more or less permanent identity is to transplant different sympathetic chain ganglia from a donor animal to a host where the ganglia can be exposed to the *same* segmental set of preganglionic axons during reinnervation (Figure 10) (Purves et al., 1981; see also Figure 5). In this circumstance, one can ask whether two different ganglia (which are ordinarily innervated by different sets of axons) are selectively reinnervated by axons arising from different segments. Different sympathetic chain ganglia (in this case, the superior cervical ganglion and the fifth thoracic ganglion) are indeed distinguished by the preganglionic axons

dertook a further series of studies in the autonomic system in which he investigated ganglionic organization from the point of view of
specificity (see text). The significance of this
work was not appreciated during his lifetime:
his demonstration of selectivity in the autonomic nervous system, his initial statement of
what was later called the chemoaffinity hypothesis (Chapter 11), and his important experiments with H. K. Anderson on mismatching nerves and their targets (Chapter 9) are
hardly mentioned in the tributes at the time of
his death. During the latter part of his career
Langley turned increasingly to the interaction
of nerves and muscle. He showed that nerves
have a local effect on muscle and that they
impinge upon a specifically excitable region of
the postsynaptic membrane (the endplate)
(Langley, 1907; 1908a,b). This set the stage for
later studies of chemical synaptic transmission
and the control of muscle properties by nerves
(Chapter 8).

In addition to these major contributions,
Langley trained A. V. Hill, J. Barcroft, H. H.
Dale, K. Lucas, E. D. Adrian, and T. R. Elliot.
Finally, Langley was for 30 years the senior
editor of the *Journal of Physiology*. Indeed, he
was not only editor, but owner; he purchased
the *Journal* in 1894 when it fell upon hard times.
In spite of these many successes, much of his
work became appreciated only retrospectively

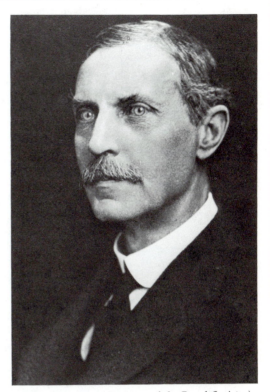

John N. Langley. (Courtesy of the Royal Society.)

when others took up the research that he
initiated.

in the host cervical sympathetic trunk. The superior cervical ganglion
is reinnervated in a manner that approximates its original segmental
innervation; the fifth thoracic ganglion, on the other hand, is reinnervated by an overlapping but caudally shifted subset of the thoracic
spinal cord segments that normally contribute to the cervical sympathetic trunk. This more caudal innervation approximates the original
segmental innervation of the fifth thoracic ganglion. These results indicate that ganglion cells carry with them a property that biases the
innervation they receive.

SELECTIVE SYNAPTIC CONNECTIONS IN THE SPINAL CORD

The innervation of spinal motor neurons in vertebrates provides another
relatively simple system in which intracellular recording has been used
to explore selective synapse formation. The pattern of innervation to

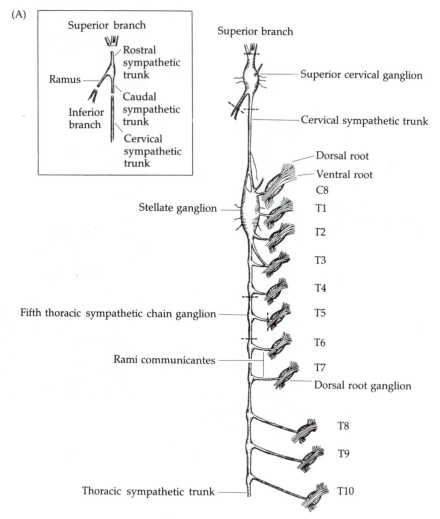

(A)

Superior branch

Rostral sympathetic trunk

Ramus

Inferior branch

Caudal sympathetic trunk

Cervical sympathetic trunk

Superior branch

Superior cervical ganglion

Cervical sympathetic trunk

Dorsal root

Ventral root

C8

Stellate ganglion

T1

T2

T3

T4

Fifth thoracic sympathetic chain ganglion

T5

T6

Rami communicantes

T7

Dorsal root ganglion

T8

T9

Thoracic sympathetic trunk

T10

motor neurons is more difficult to analyze because a variety of axonal classes impinge upon these cells. Moreover, the vast majority of the thousands of synapses on each motor neuron derive from interneurons, a type of cell that is notoriously difficult to study. However, one class of input to motor neurons has proved tractable: the afferent innervation from muscle spindles which forms the central limb of the myotatic or stretch reflex (Liddell and Sherrington, 1924). These sensory–motor synapses are probably more thoroughly understood than any other connections in the vertebrate central nervous system.

In the 1940s and 1950s, D. P. C. Lloyd, J. C. Eccles, and their collaborators showed that the connections between muscle afferents and motor neuron pools are specific in the sense that the afferents from a particular muscle preferentially contact the motor neurons that inner-vate the same muscle (Lloyd, 1943; Eccles et al., 1957). More recently, connections between individual stretch-sensitive afferents and motor neurons have been studied using spike-triggered averaging (Mendell

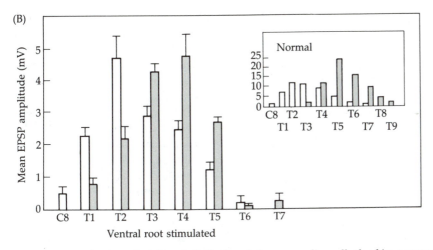

(B)

FIGURE 10. *Evidence for inherent distinctions between ganglion cells that bias synapse formation. (A) Guinea pig ganglia from different segmental levels were exposed to the same segmental set of axons by transplantation to the bed of the excised superior cervical ganglion in a host animal (cf. Figure 5A). An inbred strain was used to minimize rejection; either the superior cervical ganglion (control) or the fifth thoracic (T5) ganglion was implanted. Inset shows details of a T5 implantation. The segmental reinnervation of these two ganglia could be tested several months later in the manner shown in Figure 7. (B) Graph shows the average postsynaptic response of neurons in transplanted cervical (open bars) and T5 (dark bars) ganglia to stimulation of different spinal segments; inset shows the normal distribution of excitatory postsynaptic potential (EPSP) amplitudes. Standard errors are shown. Although there is some overlap both normally and after reinnervation, ganglion cells in transplanted T5 ganglia are reinnervated by a more caudal set of segments than transplanted superior cervical ganglion cells are (cf. Figure 5B) (n ≈ 500). (After Purves et al., 1981.)*

and Henneman, 1971; Scott and Mendell, 1976; Nelson and Mendell, 1978), a technique that allows accurate detection of the very small postsynaptic responses generated by each afferent axon. In accord with earlier results, each sensory axon from a particular muscle in the cat makes stronger synaptic connections with the motor neurons that innervate that muscle (homonymous connections) than with motor neurons that innervate synergist muscles (heteronymous connections; antagonist motor neurons are usually not innervated at all). For example, each of the approximately 60 primary afferent fibers from the medial gastrocnemius elicits a measurable synaptic response in nearly every medial gastrocnemius motor neuron (over 300 cells) (Mendell and Henneman, 1971; Scott and Mendell, 1976). On the other hand, each afferent axon projects to only about 60 percent of the motor neurons in a synergist pool (lateral gastrocnemius). In agreement with this finding, experiments in frogs have shown that the projection frequency and synaptic influence of individual sensory afferents on homonymous motor neurons is greater than on heteronymous motor neurons (Lichtman and Frank, 1984; see also Frank and Westerfield, 1982). This is analogous to selective innervation in the sympathetic system: in both cases preferred innervation is reflected in a greater number of innervating axons and larger synaptic potentials elicited by each axon.

In both the cat and the frog, intracellular staining of individual afferents with horseradish peroxidase consistently shows only a few contacts between homonymous presynaptic and postsynaptic cells (Figure 11) (Iles, 1976; Burke et al., 1979; Redman and Walmsley, 1981; Brown and Fyffe, 1981; Lichtman et al., 1984; Grantyn et al., 1984). The small number of boutons made by each sensory axon on individual motor neurons suggests that correct innervation of the homonymous neurons is achieved in spite of a relatively weak synaptogenic stimulus between the presynaptic and postsynaptic partners. This finding is all the more remarkable as there is no obvious segregation of homonymous, heteronymous, and unrelated motor neuron dendrites within the spinal cord (Figure 12) (Lichtman et al., 1984). As in sympathetic ganglia, appropriate and less appropriate axons and target cells intermingle in the same general region. In both systems, innervating axons evidently recognize different classes of target neurons.

SELECTIVE SYNAPTIC CONNECTIONS IN THE INVERTEBRATE CENTRAL NERVOUS SYSTEM

Studies of reinnervation in the central nervous system of several invertebrate preparations provide additional examples of selective synapse formation in a relatively simple context (Muller, 1979; Anderson et al., 1980). The advantage of invertebrates in this regard is that, in contrast

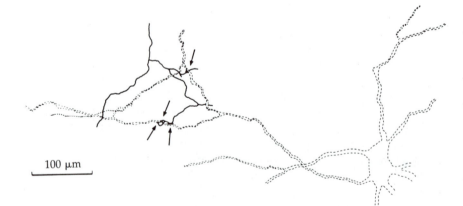

100 μm

FIGURE 11. *Selective innervation of spinal motor neurons by primary sensory terminals ramifying in the spinal cord. Axon of a muscle afferent stained with horseradish peroxidase (solid lines); a motor neuron from the homonymous pool has also been labeled with peroxidase (dotted line). The figure shows a serial reconstruction of the points of contact between the afferent terminals (arrows) and the motor neuron dendrites. Although virtually every motor neuron in the homonymous pool is innervated by each Ia afferent fiber, only a small number of synaptic boutons are established between any one axon and a homonymous motor neuron. (After Redman and Walmsley, 1981.)*

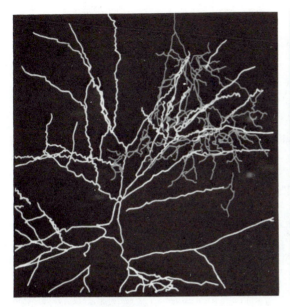 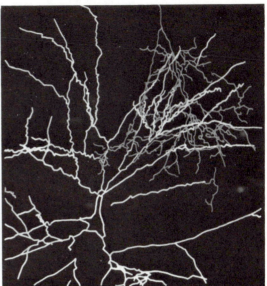

(A) HOMONYMOUS PAIR

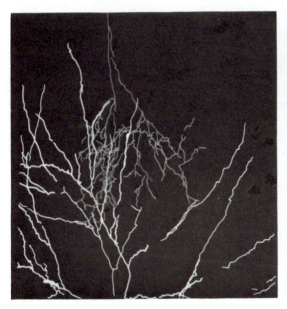

(B) UNRELATED PAIR

FIGURE 12. *Reconstructions of individual sensory axon arbors in relation to homonymous and unrelated motor neurons in the frog spinal cord after peroxidase labeling. (A) Stereo pair of the region of sensory–motor overlap of a triceps sensory axon and a homonymous motor neuron (cf. Figure 11). Because triceps sensory axons ramify in close proximity to the dendrites of both* *homonymous and unrelated neurons, recognition of appropriate target cells is implied. Presynaptic and postsynaptic elements are apposed at several sites. (B) Stereo pair of the region of overlap of a triceps sensory axon and an unrelated motor neuron (subscapularis). No sites of close apposition are seen. (From Lichtman et al., 1984.)*

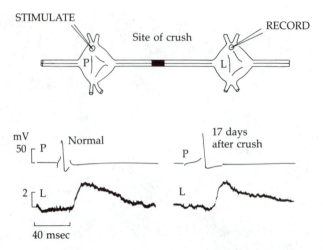

FIGURE 13. *Selective reinnervation of identified neurons in adjacent leech ganglia. Diagram (above) indicates the site of nerve crush in the connective between two segmental ganglia. Seventeen days later, the connection normally seen between an identified neuron pair (a sensory cell called P and a motor neuron called L) is restored. The preparation was maintained in vitro during the period of regeneration. (After Wallace et al., 1977.)*

to vertebrate autonomic ganglia or spinal cord, individual neurons can be reliably identified from animal to animal.

Perhaps the preparation that has been best exploited for studies of selective innervation in invertebrates is the segmental ganglion of the leech (*Hirudo medicinalis*). Each segment in the worm is innervated by a corresponding ganglion comprising several hundred neurons. Much of the normal connectivity between the neurons within each ganglion and between ganglia in adjacent and more distant segments has been established by J. G. Nicholls and his colleagues who have recorded from pairs of identified presynaptic and postsynaptic cells (Muller et al., 1981). When the connections between two adjacent ganglia are

FIGURE 14. *Selective synapse formation between identified leech neurons in vitro.* ▶
(A) Single identified neurons can be dissected by making a slit in the capsule of the ganglion. After an identified cell is teased free, it is lassoed with a loop of hair and placed in culture. The cell has a diameter of about 60 μm. By placing pairs of identified neurons together, the tendency to make selective synaptic connections can be explored in vitro. (B) Intracellular recordings from pairs of cells maintained in vitro show that certain pairs predictably form synaptic linkages, whereas others do not. In this example, a Retzius cell has formed a chemical synapse with a sensory (P) cell after 11 days in culture. Although the synaptic potentials are depolarizing, they are actually inhibitory potentials, the signs of which have been reversed by chloride injection into the postsynaptic cell. (C) Retzius cell has been labeled by horseradish peroxidase injection; after only 3 days in culture, numerous processes cover the P cell, and, as in B, a chemical synaptic connection can be detected electrophysiologically. (A from Fuchs et al., 1981; B after Henderson et al., 1983; C from Fuchs et al., 1982.)

severed by cutting the connective that runs between segments (Figure 13), the cut axons regenerate over a few weeks and reestablish synaptic connections (Baylor and Nicholls, 1971; Jansen and Nicholls, 1972; Wallace et al., 1977; Elliott and Muller, 1983; see also Muller, 1979). By recording intracellularly from one identified cell while stimulating another, Nicholls and co-workers could ask whether original synaptic connections are restored during the process of repair. Although some novel synapses form, the normal pattern of connections between particular neurons in adjacent leech ganglia is generally reestablished (Figure 13).

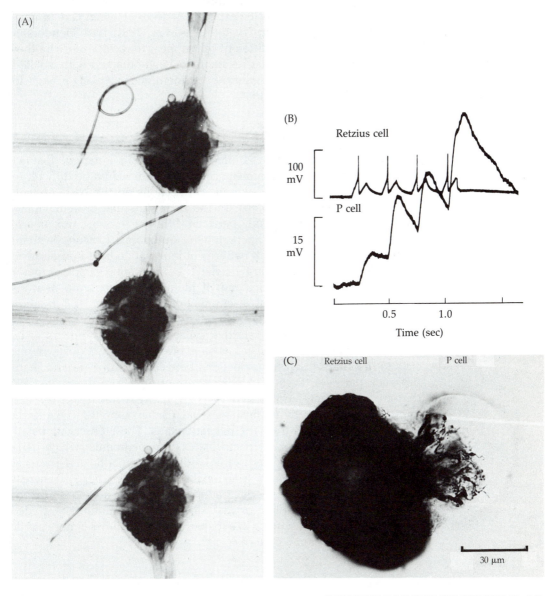

More recently, selective synapse formation between identified leech neurons has been examined among isolated nerve cells in culture (Ready and Nicholls, 1979; Fuchs et al., 1981, 1982; Henderson et al., 1983; see also Kaczmarek et al., 1979; Dagan and Levitan, 1981; Wong et al., 1981; Bodmer et al., 1984). These experiments take advantage of the fact that identified neurons can be dissected from leech ganglia and placed into culture wells in association with another cell of known function (Figure 14). Isolated neuronal pairs survive for some weeks, and the connections that cells make with one another can be studied both electrophysiologically and anatomically. Leech neurons that make electrical junctions with each other in vivo also make such connections in culture (Fuchs et al., 1981; see also Kaczmarek et al., 1979). Chemical synaptic relationships also form predictably between particular neurons, although synapses that might be expected to form between certain neuronal pairs have not been observed (Fuchs et al., 1981, 1982; Henderson et al., 1983). Nonetheless, different cells appear to recognize each other in a selective manner. Similar results have been obtained with isolated neurons from various ganglia of the marine mollusk *Aplysia* (Camardo et al., 1983; Bodmer et al., 1984).

CONCLUSIONS

Selective synapse formation is inferred when axons innervate distinct classes of target cells in circumstances in which it would be difficult to explain the final pattern of synaptic connections on the basis of axon guidance or other mechanisms. In the neuromuscular system, motor axons can discriminate weakly between different muscles and muscle fiber types. Similarly, in the peripheral autonomic nervous system, preganglionic axons establish patterns of innervation based on discrimination at the level of the target cells. The innervation of spinal motor neurons by muscle afferents and of identified invertebrate neurons provide further examples of discrimination during synapse formation in relatively simple systems.

In each of these cases, selective synapse formation appears to be based on relative preferences between presynaptic and postsynaptic cells rather than absolute distinctions between appropriate and inappropriate partners. Particular axons are more likely to innervate cells that are appropriate and to make more synapses with them, but less appropriate cells are by no means excluded; they simply receive fewer (and weaker) contacts from the relevant axons. These observations are in agreement with a variety of mismatching experiments, which demonstrate considerable leeway in the kinds of presynaptic and postsynaptic elements that can form functional synapses (Chapter 9). Whereas axon guidance generates specific patterns on an all-or-none basis (axons either get to the right place or they do not), the continuously graded nature of qualitative accuracy in synapse formation allows a more subtle modulation of synaptic pattern.

The Molecular Basis of Neuronal Recognition

INTRODUCTION

Throughout the course of neuronal differentiation, migration, axon guidance, and selective synaptogenesis, nerve cells respond to environmental cues that have a molecular basis. Most neurobiologists would probably agree that identification of the relevant molecules is an important goal. The part of the nervous system to which most attention has been paid from the point of view of understanding neuronal recognition at the molecular level is the retinotectal system of lower vertebrates. The purpose of this chapter is to review the status of this difficult field.

THE RETINOTECTAL SYSTEM

The aspect of innervation taken to be the hallmark of specificity in the retinotectal system is a topographical map, a feature characteristic of many neural projections. Images of objects on the retina are transferred to the next level in the visual pathway (called the tectum in lower vertebrates) in a highly organized way: the projections of retinal axons to the tectum form a continuous point-to-point map that can be assessed anatomically or, more conventionally, by electrophysiological means (Figure 1). Studies of retinal ganglion cell projections are usually carried out by presenting local images (spots of light) to an anesthetized animal while recording from the exposed tectum with an extracellular microelectrode. In this way, one can determine the region on the retina that activates a particular part of the tectum. These retinotectal maps (Figure 1B) provide the experimental basis for evaluating neural specificity (and by implication, neuronal recognition) in this system.

The investigation of the retinotectal system dates from the 1920s when R. Matthey showed that a newt can see again a few weeks after optic nerve section (Matthey, 1925). This phenomenon is so robust that the same eye can be transplanted repeatedly, with recovery of vision each time (Stone and Farthing, 1942). In the 1940s, L.S. Stone and R.W. Sperry adopted this system for work on neural specificity (Stone and Zaur, 1940; Stone, 1941, 1944; Sperry, 1943a,b, 1944). At that time the prevailing view, championed by P. Weiss (see Box A), was that speci-

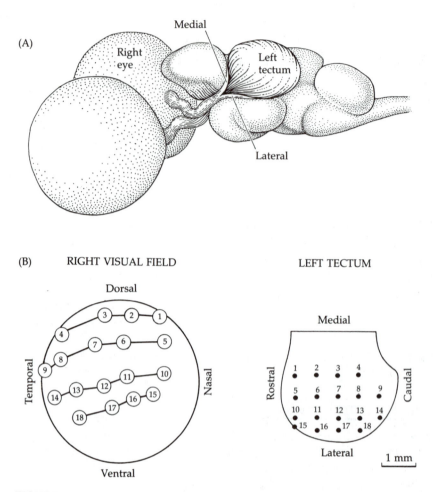

(A)

Medial

Right eye

Left tectum

Lateral

(B)　　RIGHT VISUAL FIELD　　　　　　　LEFT TECTUM

Dorsal

Temporal

Nasal

Ventral

Medial

Rostral

Caudal

Lateral

1 mm

FIGURE 1.　*Topographical projection of retinal axons to the tectum in lower vertebrates. (A) Schematic drawing of the goldfish optic system. The optic nerves cross completely at the optic chiasm and innervate the contralateral tectum. (B) Electrophysiological mapping of the projection of the right eye to the left tectum in a goldfish. Numbered points in the tectum represent electrode positions that were maximally active when a stimulus was presented at the position with the corresponding number in the visual field. An orderly map is apparent. (A after Attardi and Sperry, 1963; B after Schmidt et al., 1978.)*

ficity arose through target responsiveness to only those axons that carried appropriate activity patterns (the resonance hypothesis; see later). "The conclusion was being drawn," Sperry wrote later, "that selective communication in the nervous system must be based not on selectivity among synaptic connections . . . but rather upon some kind of qualitative selectivity among the signals carried by different fiber types . . . the old telephone switchboard analogy was replaced by a radio broadcasting concept of communication" (Sperry, 1965, p. 163). Sperry (see Box B) was unenthusiastic about this explanation because he had found that inappropriate neuromuscular connections failed to induce the sort of compensatory changes that Weiss' ideas predicted; indeed, neural rerouting in mammals appeared to produce permanent defects of motor coordination (Sperry, 1941; see Chapter 10).

To further investigate the merits of the resonance hypothesis, Sperry cut the optic nerve in newts and rotated the eye 180° in an experiment now considered the classic observation in this field (Sperry, 1943a,b; see also Stone, 1944; Stone and Zaur, 1940). After optic nerve regeneration, animals with rotated eyes behaved as if their visual world had been inverted and shifted left for right (Figure 2). This finding suggested that retinal ganglion cells grew back to approximately the same tectal cells they originally contacted, even though these connections were now maladaptive. Furthermore, no amount of practice could reverse the deficit: animals that viewed the world through a rotated eye continued to strike inappropriately at a lure for as long as the experimenter had the patience to continue the "training." Some years later, D. G. Attardi and Sperry (1963) provided additional evidence that axons from particular regions of the retina regenerate preferentially to appropriate regions of the tectum. After removing a large portion of the retina in

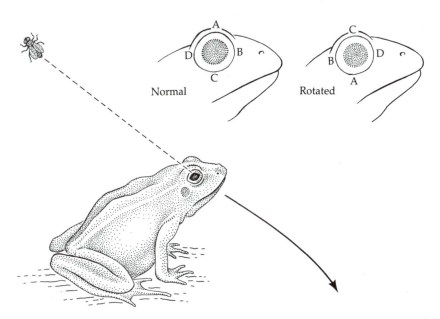

FIGURE 2. *The effects of eye rotation on the visual behavior of a frog following optic nerve regeneration. This picture shows the response of a frog, the right optic nerve of which had been cut some weeks earlier; at the time of surgery the eye was rotated through 180° and sutured in position (inset). Following recovery, the animal was able to see again through the affected eye. However, when a target of interest (a fly) appeared in the visual field, the frog's attack was misdirected by approximately 180° (arrow). This result suggests that retinal axons reinnervate their original target cells in the tectum (or cells near them) and that the central nervous system has little or no ability to compensate for the maladaptive behavior that results. (After Sperry, 1956.)*

Paul Alfred Weiss (b. 1898)

Paul Weiss was born and educated in Vienna, Austria, where he received his doctoral degree in engineering from the University of Vienna in 1922. For the next 8 years he carried out postdoctoral work in several European laboratories under the auspices of the Rockefeller Foundation; in 1930 he accepted R. G. Harrison's invitation to become a Sterling Fellow in the zoology department at Yale University. After several years at Yale he moved to the University of Chicago, where he became professor of zoology, a post he held until 1954. In that year he accepted an appointment at the Rockefeller University, where he remained until his retirement in 1964. In addition to these scientific positions he was dean of the graduate school at the University of Chicago and later at the University of Texas in Houston (1964-1966).

In his early work, for which he is best known by developmental biologists, Weiss showed that "each muscle of an extra limb grafted near a native limb contracted always and without exception exactly together with [its] namesake muscle in the neighboring normal limb, regardless of whether or not the resultant movement of the graft was of any use to the animal" (Weiss, 1968). This so-called homologous response was taken as evidence for Weiss' "resonance principle" (see text).

In the 1930s Weiss became interested in morphogenesis and attacked the problem of how cells take on particular forms. Indeed, it was this interest that brought him to Harrison's laboratory, where he applied the principle of "contact guidance" to nerve fiber outgrowth. These experiments gave rise to the important idea that mechanical forces can determine cell shape and the direction of axon outgrowth (Chapter 5). During the Second World War, Weiss' interest in nerve outgrowth was put to clinical use when he carried out a series of experiments on nerve grafting for the government. In the course of this work he did additional experiments on the selectivity of muscle reinnervation (see Chapter 10) and, by his own account, laid the groundwork for using freeze-dried tissues in clinical medicine (Weiss, 1968).

Shortly after the war, Weiss, together with

goldfish and cutting the optic nerve, regenerating axons from the remaining retinal piece reached the tectum by running in the appropriate division of the optic tract (Figure 3). Moreover, these fractional projections appeared to ignore large areas of the denervated target to contact the part of the tectum in which they originally terminated. Clearly Sperry's experiments argued for some form of recognition between retinal and tectal neurons.

THE CHEMOAFFINITY HYPOTHESIS

Although Ramón y Cajal had emphasized the importance of chemical interactions in forming neural connections (Ramón y Cajal, 1892), the first clear statement of a mechanism that might explain specific reinnervation was made by J. N. Langley in 1895. In his view, axons grew more or less randomly throughout targets, exploring the suitability of

H. B. Hiscoe, made what many consider his major contribution to neurobiology, the discovery of axoplasmic transport (Weiss and Hiscoe, 1948). Even though the idea of materials moving down axons to support distal arborizations had been discussed by Cajal and others, Weiss and Hiscoe's simple experiments in which nerves were mechanically constricted provided the first direct evidence for a transport mechanism. Subsequent studies of axonal transport confirmed the validity of Weiss' interpretation and established transport as a mechanism of tremendous neurobiological importance.

In addition to these major contributions Weiss, who authored some 300 articles and several books, ranged widely into other biological fields, carrying out studies on wound healing, histiotypic cell aggregation, and the nature of collagen.

Many great innovators attract disciples who carry forward their ideas. Other equally effective scientists seem to generate a sense of rebellion in their students and colleagues. Weiss appears to belong in the latter category. In spite of his obvious accomplishments, one senses a lack of enthusiasm for Weiss' work among his contemporaries. Among the reasons were Weiss' high regard for the significance of his own approach, a certain dogmatism about his theories, and the novelty of the work itself.

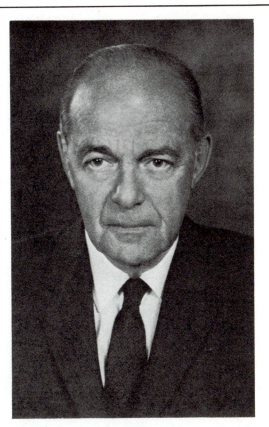

Paul A. Weiss. (Courtesy of the Wakeman Foundation.)

cells that they happened to contact. In reviewing his experiments on ganglion cell reinnervation (see Chapter 10), Langley wrote:

> The only feasible explanation appears to me to be that the [preganglionic] sympathetic fibres grow out along the peripheral piece of nerve—as nerve fibres usually are supposed to grow out—spreading amongst the cells of [the] ganglion, and that there is some special chemical relation between each class of nerve fibre and each class of nerve cell, which induces each fibre to grow towards a cell of its own class and there to form its terminal branches. At bottom then the [phenomenon] would be a chemiotactic one (Langley, 1895, p. 284).

This idea was revived several decades later when Sperry put forward a detailed hypothesis of neural specificity based on apparent recognition in the retinotectal system. Sperry's conception of chemoaffinity underwent some evolution during the 25 years or so that he was concerned

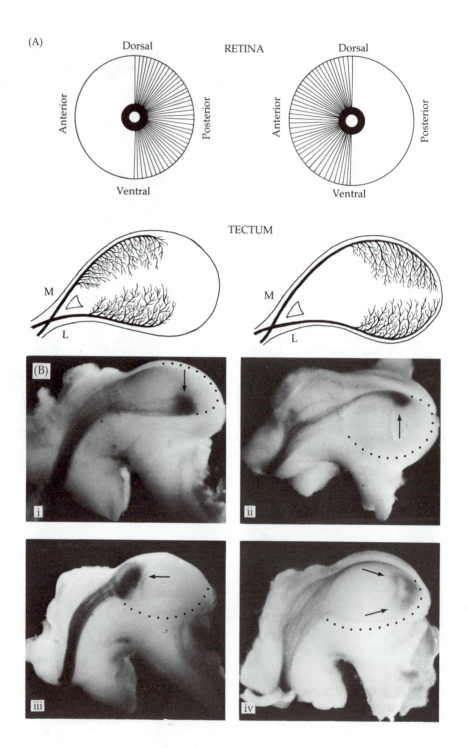

with this issue; his definitive view appears in a brief review in 1963 (Sperry, 1963; see also Meyer and Sperry, 1976). Sperry's notion of chemoaffinity has several elements: (1) neurons are intrinsically different from one another, (2) these differences are position dependent; (3)

FIGURE 3. *Anatomical evidence for retinal axon regeneration to original sites of termination in the optic tectum. (A) Pattern of regenerated fibers in the goldfish optic tract and tectum after removal of the anterior (left) or posterior (right) half-retina; the optic nerve was cut at the time of retinal extirpation. The course and termination of the residual regenerated axons was observed a number of weeks later with silver staining (Bodian protargol). The regenerating axons terminate in appropriate regions. M and L indicate medial and lateral optic tract bundles. (B) A modern demonstration of the preservation of the retinotectal map using horseradish peroxidase (HRP) transport in the adult newt. Each of these photographs (i–iv) shows the trajectory of labeled axons after HRP injection into a different retinal quadrant. In newt, as in goldfish and frog, regenerating axons terminate (arrows) in the same general region of the tectum as their original projections. i, Dorsal quadrant of retina injected; ii, ventral; iii, temporal; iv, nasal; dots outline the tectum. The optic nerve was cut 10 weeks earlier. (A after Attardi and Sperry, 1963; B from Fujisawa, 1981b.)*

the differences are acquired very early in the course of development; (4) the differences are biochemical in nature; and (5) presynaptic and postsynaptic cells with matching biochemical labels connect with one another in a selective and exclusive manner. With regard to this last point, Sperry summarized his work on the retinotectal system as follows:

> It seemed a necessary conclusion from these results that the cells and fibers of the brain . . . must carry some kind of individual identification tags, presumably cytochemical in nature, by which they are distinguished one from another almost, in many regions, to the level of the single neuron; and further, that the growing fibers are extremely particular when it comes to establishing synaptic connections, each axon linking only with certain neurons to which it becomes selectively attached by specific chemical affinities. (Sperry, 1963, pp. 703–704).

TESTS OF SPERRY'S HYPOTHESIS

Subsequent work on the retinotectal system in the 1960s and 1970s was largely aimed at testing the narrowest interpretation of Sperry's idea, namely, that connections are established according to cytochemical labels that provide a rigid, inflexible wiring diagram. Not surprisingly, this interpretation proved false.

One class of tests that was brought to bear involved an extension of the size-disparity experiments first undertaken by Attardi and Sperry (1963). When the entire retinal projection was allowed to regenerate to a tectum half of which had been surgically removed, the retinotectal map was compressed (Figure 4). Although the regenerating axons at first showed some tendency to project appropriately, the half-tectum ultimately accommodated fibers from the entire retina (Gaze and Sharma, 1970; Yoon, 1971, 1976; Schmidt et al., 1978). Conversely, when half the retina was extirpated, the residual retinal axons mapped across the entire tectum (Horder, 1971; Yoon, 1972; Schmidt et al., 1978). Again, the initial projections tended to be appropriate (Schmidt et al.,

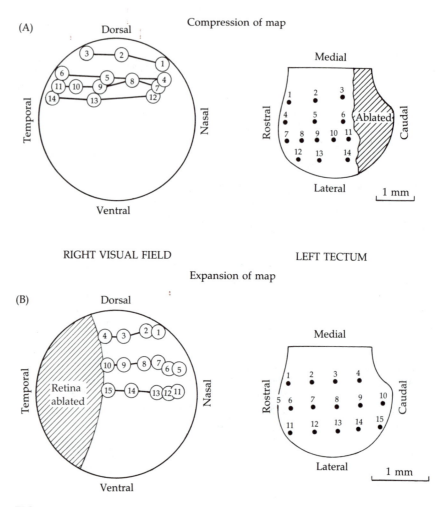

FIGURE 4. *Size disparity experiments in the retinotectal system. (A) Compression of the retinotectal map. The retinotectal projection was mapped in a goldfish several months after excision of the caudal half of the tectum and interruption of the contralateral optic nerve (the retinal axons decussate completely; see Figure 1). Numbers in the right visual field indicate the location of the stimulus that caused maximal activation of the corresponding point on the tectum (cf. Figure 1). (B) Expansion of the retinotectal map in a goldfish. Many months after cutting the optic nerve and removing about half the retina, the residual fibers project in an orderly manner across the entire tectum. The uniform compression or expansion of the retinotectal projection in these experiments is incompatible with absolute matching of retinal and tectal cells. (A after Yoon, 1971; B after Schmidt et al., 1978.)*

1978), perhaps explaining the apparent discrepancy with Sperry's observations, which were made relatively soon after the initial lesion.

A second class of experiments that belied a rigid matching of retinal and tectal markers involved the surgical creation of "compound" eyes. For instance, an eye comprising two nasal (or two temporal) halves was implanted in a tadpole and the retinotectal map tested in maturity (Gaze

Roger Wolcott Sperry (b. 1913)

Roger Sperry was born in Hartford, Connecticut. He graduated from Oberlin College in 1935 as an English major and obtained his Ph.D. from the University of Chicago in 1941, where he was a graduate student in the zoology department under P. A. Weiss (see Box A). After several years of postdoctoral research at Harvard with Karl Lashley and a subsequent stint at the Yerkes Laboratory of Primate Biology, he returned to the University of Chicago in 1946 as a member of the anatomy department. In 1952 he was named chief of the developmental neurology branch at the National Institutes of Health, and in 1954 became the Hixon professor of psychobiology at the California Institute of Technology, where he has remained.

Sperry's scientific work can be divided into two major parts. Beginning with his graduate work and lasting through the early 1960s, his major concern was the basis of specificity in the nervous system. His indoctrination began during his years with Weiss and Lashley, who, in quite different ways, argued that neural function transcended selective connections between presynaptic and postsynaptic cells. Unsatisfied with this notion, Sperry carried out a series of experiments that raised doubts about this interpretation. In the early 1940s he turned his attention to the retinotectal system; this work led him to the conclusion that nerve cells recognize one another by virtue of complementary surface labels. His steadfast promotion of chemoaffinity resurrected this important idea. Under the circumstances, this achievement was quite remarkable. As V. Hamburger put it, "I know of nobody else who has disposed of the cherished ideas of both his doctoral and postdoctoral sponsor, both at that time acknowledged leaders in their fields" (Hamburger, 1979, p. 5).

The second line of investigation that Sperry pursued (cited as his major contribution when he was awarded the Nobel prize for physiology and medicine in 1981) was his work on communication between the two hemispheres of the primate brain. Sperry's so-called split-brain studies in man and monkeys established that when pathways between the two hemispheres are interrupted by surgical section of the corpus callosum, the two halves of the brain are capable of functioning independently. This conclusion was largely established by ingenious behavioral tests on patients who had undergone this surgery because of intractable epilepsy. Information given the right hemisphere of a right-handed person cannot be verbalized after callosal section and is in this sense unconscious. Nonetheless, such patients are "aware" of the information. Even though mute, the nondominant hemisphere has considerable cognitive ability. These results are among the most interesting in human neurology and are nicely summarized in Sperry's *Harvey Lectures* in 1968 (see also Sperry, 1982).

Sperry's ability to carry out two such different, yet successful programs of research is a testament to his genius for picking questions of fundamental interest and performing decisive experiments.

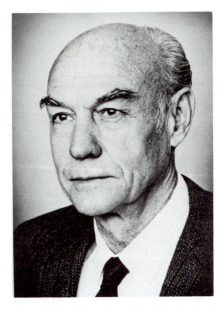

Roger W. Sperry. (Courtesy of V. Hamburger.)

et al., 1963, 1965). If retinotectal markers were unique, then both halves of the compound eye would have projected to only half the tectum. In fact, axons from such compound eyes innervated the entire tectum, although here again axons showed some initial predilection for the appropriate region of the tectum (Gaze and Straznicky, 1980; Straznicky et al., 1981).

A third class of experiments involved an analysis of the disposition of retinal projections during normal development. These developmental studies showed that the retinotectal connections initially formed are not permanent but represent a continually shifting set, as might be predicted from the continually changing size and spatial relationship of the retina and tectum (Chung et al., 1974; Gaze et al., 1974, 1979; Meyer, 1978; Reh and Constantine-Paton, 1984a; see also Fujisawa et al., 1984). This flexibility is especially apparent in goldfish, in which ganglion cells are continually added to the retinal periphery at the rate of some 50 per day throughout life (Johns, 1977; Easter et al., 1981). Whereas the newborn neurons in the retina form a ring, new tectal cells are generated in a crescent-shaped area on the caudal side of the tectum (Meyer, 1978; Raymond and Easter, 1983). In spite of the topological dissimilarity of the retinal and tectal growth zones, the map in older animals is just as orderly as in younger ones. It is difficult to imagine how this could occur without continual rearrangement of retinotectal connections (Easter, 1983; Easter et al., 1984; Stuermer and Easter, 1984; Easter and Stuermer, 1984).

In the aggregate, these experiments refute the idea that retinal axons are rigidly matched to corresponding tectal cells. However, the general idea that retinal axons have selective affinities for their target cells is, if anything, strengthened by this work. Whatever the experimental perturbation, orderly (if sometimes different) maps are established, apparently as a result of relative preferences.

ATTEMPTS TO DEFINE THE MOLECULAR BASIS OF CHEMOAFFINITY

Evidence for some form of intercellular recognition in the retinotectal system has stimulated a broad effort to discover the molecular basis of this apparent selectivity. The approach to this problem has, in general, relied on assays of cell adhesion or immunological techniques.

Intercellular adhesion as a measure of cell recognition

Because chemoaffinity cannot be assessed directly, a common approach to this problem has been to study adhesion between cells dissociated from various parts of the embryonic nervous system (Figure 5) (Frazier and Glaser, 1979; Gottlieb and Glaser, 1980). The assumption here is that recognition is mediated by complementary adhesive molecules (Roth, 1968; Roth et al., 1971). This work is predicated on the classic studies of J. F. K. Holtfreter (see Chapter 4), who showed that cells

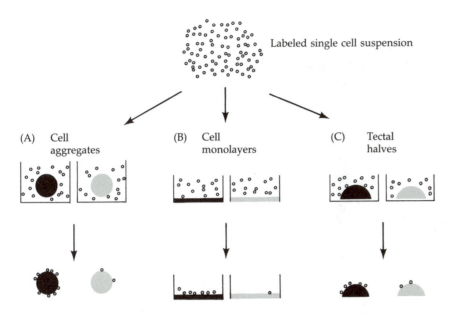

FIGURE 5. *Diagram of in vitro adhesive assays for retinotectal specificity. A suspension of dissociated cells is prepared from the tissue to be tested and labeled with a radioactive isotope or in some other way. The relative adhesivity of the cell suspension can then be measured by monitoring adherence to cell aggregates (A), to cell monolayers (B), or to pieces of intact tectal tissue (C). Subsequent measurements of the amount of radioactivity bound to the test surface gives a measure of adhesivity. (After Roth and Marchase, 1976.)*

from different tissues prefer to aggregate with each other when given a choice (e.g., liver cells prefer liver cells to kidney cells, and so on). Holtfreter's discovery of tissue-specific aggregation led to the finding that cells dissociated from particular regions of the brain also tend to aggregate preferentially with one another (Roth, 1968; Roth et al., 1971; Garber and Moscona, 1972a,b).

When different areas of the retina are tested for adhesivity, another aspect of histiotypic aggregation is observed: cells dissociated from the ventral retina adhere preferentially to dorsal tectal cells, whereas dorsal retinal cells prefer ventral tectal cells; moreover, growing retinal axons can discriminate membranes of one tectal region from those of another (Figure 6) (Barbera et al., 1973; Barbera, 1975; Balsamo et al., 1976; Gottlieb et al., 1976; Halfter et al., 1981; Kerns-Viets and Bonhoeffer, 1984). Such preferential adhesion has now been demonstrated in a variety of in vitro situations and has been shown to vary as a function of developmental age (Gottlieb et al., 1974; Gottlieb and Arington, 1979; Halfter et al., 1981; Bonhoeffer and Huf, 1980, 1982). What makes these results particularly intriguing is that the pattern of adhesive preferences tends to parallel the normal topography of the retinotectal projection.

So far, attempts to define the molecules involved in the preferential adhesion of retinal and tectal cells have been frustrated. Some specific

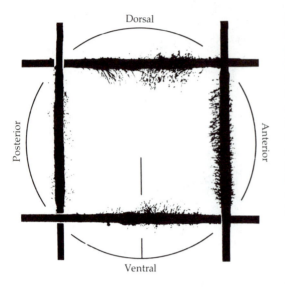

Dorsal

Posterior

Anterior

Ventral

FIGURE 6. *Preferential adhesion of embryonic chick retinal neurites to tectal membranes as a function of position. Strips from different portions of the retina (dorsal, ventral, anterior, or posterior) from a 6-day-old chick embryo were cultured for 30 hours. A suspension of tectal membranes was then added, and after an additional 2 hours the unattached membranes were washed off. These composite photomicrographs suggest that more binding has occurred to neurites extending from relatively anterior retinal cells than to neurites from relatively posterior retinal cells. The preparation has been stained with Sudan black; vertical line indicates the position of the choroid fissure. (From Halfter et al., 1981.)*

suggestions have been put forward, but none have evolved very far. D. I. Gottlieb, L. Glaser, and their colleagues found that an extract of embryonic chick neural retina inhibits the reaggregation of retinal cells in rotating culture (Merrell et al., 1975; Gottlieb and Glaser, 1980). This raised the possibility that the agent of this effect might provide some insight into the basis of recognition in the retinotectal system. However, the molecule that is probably responsible for inhibiting retinal reaggregation, a 10,000-dalton protein called ligatin, is widely distributed and serves as a "baseplate" for the attachment of other surface molecules (Jakoi and Marchase, 1979; Marchase et al., 1981). Evidently, ligatin is not itself an adhesion molecule.

A related hypothesis about the molecular mechanism of retinotectal recognition was based on ideas put forward by S. Roseman in the early 1970s (Roseman, 1970; Roth et al., 1971). Roseman's suggestion was that complex carbohydrates on cell surfaces might interact with one another in highly specific ways by means of glycosyltransferases. According to this view, glycosyltransferases might cause specific intercellular recognition by binding to complementary oligosaccharide acceptors. Some support for this notion was provided by the demonstration of cell-surface glycosyltransferases (Roth et al., 1971) and by an apparent gradient of ganglioside binding activity on the surface of chick tectum (Marchase, 1977; see also Balsamo and Lilien, 1975). Attempts to isolate the relevant molecules were unsuccessful, however, and interest in this particular possibility gradually waned. The disappointment with efforts to define the molecular basis of retinotectal adhesivity was summed up by one wag in this field, who, in referring to Roth's attempts to isolate the gradient molecule, asked: "What hath Roth got?"

Immunological attempts to identify molecules involved in intercellular recognition

The application of immunological techniques to neurobiology, particularly the monoclonal antibody method (see Box C), has offered another means of exploring the molecular basis of chemoaffinity. A particular advantage of the immunological approach is that antibodies to a molecule of interest can be introduced into a developing animal to establish the biological role of a putative agent.

Perhaps the most intriguing use of monoclonal antibodies in the context of chemoaffinity has been the demonstration of a molecule in chick retina that is distributed in a dorsal–ventral gradient (Figure 7) (Trisler et al., 1981). Monoclonal antibodies to homogenized chick retina were screened by applying them to intact retinas and observing the intensity and distribution of binding by a second labeled antibody to mouse immunoglobulins (see Box C). In this way, M. Nirenberg and his colleagues found an antibody directed against a molecule they called

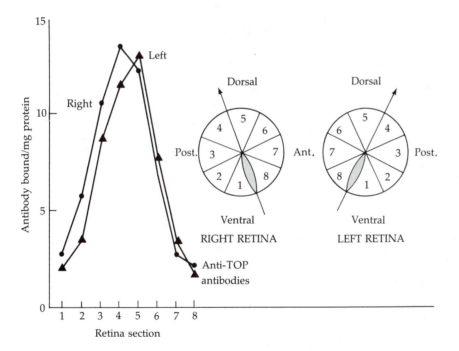

FIGURE 7. *Gradient of TOP molecules in the developing chick retina. Retinas were cut into pie slices at 14 days of incubation, as shown in the diagrams on the right (the shaded area is the choroid fissure, which served as a reference point). The slices were then dissociated and incubated with a solution of radioactively labeled TOP antibody. The numbers within each slice correspond to the numbers on the abscissa of the graph (left). About 35 times more antigen was detected in the dorsal retina than in the ventral retina. (After Trisler et al., 1981.)*

BOX
C

Monoclonal Antibodies

Every decade or two, a new technique changes the way people study a subject. A case in point for neurobiology is the discovery of the monoclonal antibody method by G. Köhler and C. Milstein at the MRC laboratory in Cambridge, England, in 1975.

Of course, an immunological approach to problems in developmental neurobiology was used to advantage before the advent of "monoclonals": consider, for example, the work of S. Cohen and R. Levi-Montalcini on nerve growth factor antiserum (Chapter 7). The traditional method of raising an antiserum, however, has several disadvantages. One disadvantage is the need for a relatively pure antigen at the outset. A second disadvantage is that the serum produced by immunizing a rabbit or some other experimental animal contains a variety of antibodies; the antibody of interest can be obtained only after laborious purification procedures, and then only in small amounts. A third problem is the variability of the immune response of different animals.

These problems were solved when Milstein and Köhler discovered that mouse myeloma cells can be fused with lymphocytes to produce an immortal line of antigen-secreting cells, which can then be raised in large quantities. The principles of the technique are simple. A mouse is immunized by injecting an antigen of interest (relevant examples are homogenized leech ganglia or chick retinas). The mouse will then produce a variety of antibodies, each of which is the product of a different clone of antibody-producing cells (the B lymphocytes). After a suitable period, these cells can be harvested from the spleen of the immunized mouse. Under ordinary circumstances, the antibody-producing cells could not be carried in culture because lymphocytes do not normally grow in vitro. This dilemma was solved when Milstein and Köhler found that lymphocytes can be fused with myeloma cells by using polyethylene glycol. Successful fusion results in hybrid myeloma–lymphocyte cells which grow well in culture and can be maintained indefinitely. The range of antibody-producing cells harvested in this way is initially very large. One therefore needs an assay of some sort to select from this population the clones of cells producing antibodies relevant to the question of interest. This selection is usually done by culturing individual cells in microwells and assessing large numbers of such wells, usually by examining antibody binding to the neurons being studied. Appropriate clones are then selected and carried in culture, stored for later use, grown in mass culture, or injected into an

TOP (for its peculiar topographical distribution), which bound some 35 times more avidly to dorsal retina than to ventral retina. A molecule with this distribution could, in principle, provide information about retinal position. The antigen is a glycoprotein that varies in concentration continually across one dimension of the retina (in parallel with the choroid fissure) but not across the other. Light microscopical studies showed anti-TOP binding to be most intense in the portions of the retina with the highest density of neurons, a result suggesting association with neuronal membranes.

Whether TOP is actually important in retinotectal specificity has not yet been established; this could be explored by treating developing animal to produce tumors secreting large amounts of the desired antibody.

Some of the advantages of this approach are obvious (Milstein, 1980). First, the method gets around a long-standing immunological problem: when an immunized animal producing a useful serum died, the researcher had to start all over again. Second, large amounts of an antibody are helpful in both research and clinical applications. Not only can large amounts of antibody be made for passive immunization, but new immune therapies can be tried at relatively little cost. Third, and perhaps most important for neurobiology, from a relatively impure preparation investigators can identify antibodies of interest simply by the use of an adequate assay. For example, antibodies to neuronal cell surface components can be quickly selected by a fluorescence binding assay without any purification of the membrane constituents that may ultimately be studied (see figure). Alternatively, one can start with a relatively specific material and make large quantities of antibody, which can then be used to identify the time of appearance and distribution of the antigen, as in the case of CAM (see text). Given the extraordinary effort presently being devoted to the making of monoclonal antibodies to various components of the nervous system, many useful findings can be expected (see, for example, Barnstable, 1980; McKay et al., 1983). This technique is especially important in developmental neurobiology, where conventional physiological and biochemical methods are, for a variety of reasons, often difficult to apply. Certainly the monoclonal an-

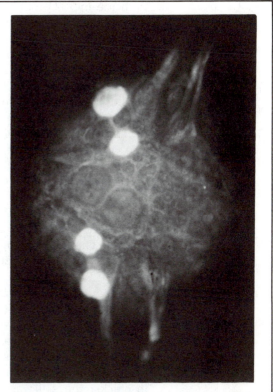

A leech ganglion stained with a monoclonal antibody and rhodamine-labeled second antibody; the monoclonal antibody, derived by injecting a mouse with homogenized leech ganglia, selectively stains four neurons. (From Zipser and McKay, 1981.)

tibody technique provides a powerful means of attacking the biochemical basis of cell recognition in the nervous system.

chicks with antibodies to TOP and evaluating the subsequent integrity and specificity of the retinotectal connections. For the time being, the importance of this work is the demonstration that differences in the concentration of membrane-bound molecules present in small quantities (perhaps 10^3–10^5 molecules/cell) can be revealed by immunological methods and that some of these molecules are distributed in a pattern consistent with encoding information about cell position.

Another class of molecules that have been identified by immunological means and may be important in recognition are the cell adhesion molecules (CAMs) discovered by G. M. Edelman and his co-workers (Edelman, 1983). Edelman, who won the Nobel prize in physiology and medicine in 1973 for studies on the structure of antibodies, used his immunological expertise to isolate and characterize a cell-surface glycoprotein from chick retina. His approach was to raise in the rabbit polyclonal antibodies to chick retinal cells, using inhibition of retinal cell aggregation as an assay. Eventually, Edelman and his colleagues found an antibody that blocked cell adhesion. By testing various fractions of neural extracts for their ability to neutralize this blocking effect, Edelman was able to partially purify the antigen that mediated retinal cell adhesion. Using this partially purified protein as an immunogen in turn, these workers then produced an even more potent antiserum, which they used to further purify what is now called N-CAM (neural cell adhesion molecule) (Thiery et al., 1977; Edelman, 1983). Neural cell adhesion molecule is a sialoglycoprotein that seems to be an integral part of the cell membrane and may constitute as much as 1 percent of the surface protein. The protein moiety has a molecular weight of about 120,000. The mechanism of adhesion mediated by CAM is thought to be dimer formation between CAM molecules on adjacent cells (Edelman, 1983).

Using a monoclonal antibody to N-CAM, Edelman's group showed that the molecule is restricted to the nervous system and is found on the surfaces of all nerve cells as well as on muscle cells and several other tissues. Neural cell adhesion molecule shows a great deal of microheterogeneity in its sugar moiety; and it is peculiar in losing much of its sialic acid content as development proceeds (Rothbard et al., 1982). In chicks, the sialic acid content of N-CAM is about 26 percent by

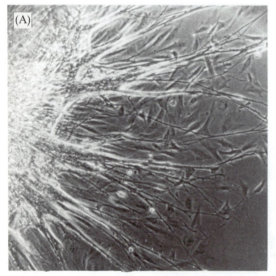

FIGURE 8. *Effects of anti-N-CAM on neurite fasciculation. (A) Fascicles of neurites emerging from an explanted chick dorsal root ganglion in culture for 24 hours. (B) A similar culture grown in the presence of* *anti-N-CAM. Normally neurites tend to fasciculate; in the presence of antibody, the outgrowth is more disordered. (From Rutishauser et al., 1978.)*

weight, whereas sialic acid constitutes only 9 percent of the molecule in full-grown chickens.

Monovalent antibody fragments against N-CAM reduce the diameter of the neurite fascicles that typically radiate from cultured explants of dorsal root ganglia (Figure 8) (Rutishauser et al., 1978). Edelman and his colleagues have suggested that this effect represents interference with the normal mechanism by which neurites adhere to one another. Furthermore, anti-N-CAM disrupts the histiotypic pattern of retinal cell aggregation that normally occurs in culture (Buskirk et al., 1980) and appears to have some effects on retinal axon outgrowth when injected into the developing eye of the chick (Thanos et al., 1984). Finally, a mutant mouse (*staggerer*), which shows gross disorganization in several regions of the central nervous system, fails to show the usual change in sialic acid content of N-CAM during maturation (Edelman and Chuong, 1982).

The upshot of all this is the suspicion that N-CAM may be important in early neural development and, more specifically, that it may be involved in neuronal recognition. Even if N-CAM turns out to be only a general glue, it will still be a molecule to reckon with in understanding events that involve nerve cell movement and the making and breaking of synaptic connections (see also Chapters 1 and 4).

ALTERNATIVES TO THE CHEMOAFFINITY HYPOTHESIS

Part of the appeal of chemoaffinity as the basis of cell–cell recognition in neural development is the paucity of attractive alternatives. Nonetheless, a number of other explanations have been suggested.

The resonance hypothesis

The dominant view before Sperry's work on the retinotectal system was Weiss' theory that neuromuscular specificity comes about by functional matching. In Weiss' scheme, specificity had no anatomical correlate; rather, axons were thought to ramify indiscriminately, stimulating appropriate muscles by virtue of particular patterns of activity (Weiss, 1924, 1928; see also DeSilva and Ellis, 1934). Because the general idea was that individual muscles picked out the appropriate pattern of activity in much the same way that a taut string vibrates sympathetically to a tone of a certain frequency, this idea was referred to as the "resonance hypothesis."

This early formulation of Weiss' hypothesis was soon disproved by the discovery that action potentials in nerves are not directed indiscriminately to all muscles during movement but only to the muscles that are active (Wiersma, 1931). Although these and other findings invalidated the simplest conception of resonance (see Harris, 1980, 1984; Landmesser and O'Donovan, 1984), the analogy is not without its uses. For example, the sympathetic and parasympathetic axons that innervate smooth muscles often release their transmitters at some distance from the target cells. Whether or not a particular postsynaptic cell responds depends on the presence of receptors for the respective neurotransmitters. In this sense, sympathetic and parasympathetic target cells in the same location are "tuned" to their innervation and are differentially active in the presence of the same neural signals. Perhaps Weiss would find some vindication in this for the ideas he put forward in the 1920s.

When the resonance hypothesis was disproved, Weiss modified his views but continued to maintain that specificity might come about by a transformation of connections made more or less haphazardly during early development (Weiss, 1936, 1941a, 1965). The gist of his revised theory was that targets modulate the central connectivity of motor neurons that innervate them more or less by chance. Because muscles were thought to dictate central wiring, this scheme was called "myotypic specification." This theory was discredited by Sperry's demonstration that axons grow to a particular place and that the connections made on the parent neurons are not reorganized following contact with an "inappropriate" target. In spite of this, retrograde modulation of neuronal connections remains a plausible idea (see for example, Frank and Westerfield, 1982).

The contact guidance hypothesis

In the 1930s and 1940s, Weiss carried out further experiments that led him to suggest yet another mechanism of specificity. In tissue culture, axons pay close attention to mechanical features in their environment, for example, lines of tension in a plasma clot or scratches on the surface of a culture dish (Weiss, 1934, 1939, 1941b, 1945). Based on these observations, Weiss proposed that axons might arrive at their destination without any chemical recognition cues at all, a theory that still has some proponents (Horder and Martin, 1979; see also Chapter 5). The contact guidance hypothesis contends that axons simply maintain their neighbor relationships on the way to their target, where they then connect appropriately because of continued alignment. Although this mechanical scenario is most unlikely as a general explanation of patterned connections, maintenance of neighbor relationships is probably important in some instances. There is, for example, an obvious ordering of axons in the optic nerve and tract of some lower vertebrates (Scholes, 1979, 1982; Fujisawa et al., 1981). On the other hand, retention of neighbor relationships between axons is not a sufficient explanation for retinotectal specificity. Whatever their arrangement enroute, as optic nerve axons approach the tectum their arrangement is completely reorganized (Scholes, 1979, 1982); moreover, retinal axons arising from the same region of the retina in mammals stray rather widely among other axons in the optic nerve (Horton et al., 1979; Williams and Rakic, 1984). Even in lower vertebrates, the final pattern of connectivity in the tectum after optic nerve regeneration is apparently attained only through a certain amount of local trial and error (Figure 9) (Fujisawa, 1981a; Fujisawa et al., 1982).

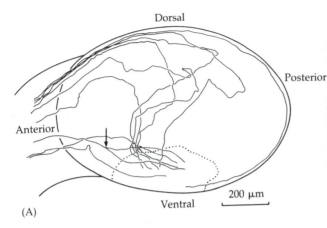

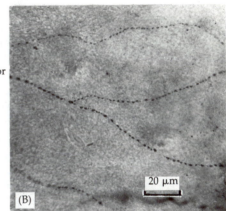

FIGURE 9. *Accurate retinotectal reconnection does not depend on retention of neighbor relationships. (A) Camera lucida drawing of the paths of horseradish per-oxidase-filled retinal fibers several months after inter-ruption of the contralateral optic nerve in an adult newt. The label was injected into the dorsal retina. Although* all the fibers appear to terminate in the appropriate region of the ventral tectum (dotted outline), many axons reach their destination by a devious route. (B) *Photomicrograph of the HRP-labeled fiber indicated by the arrow in A. (After Fujisawa, 1981a.)*

The target labeling hypothesis

Another alternative that would undercut the usual interpretation of chemoaffinity is that tectal cells, when contacted by retinal axons, are altered in a more or less permanent way. This idea has been put forward by J. T. Schmidt (1978) and is based on a series of difficult experiments involving serial reinnervation of the optic tectum. Schmidt found that retinal axons will reinnervate an inappropriate region of the tectum if that region has been innervated earlier by the same axons. This suggests that retinal axons somehow change the properties of the cells they contact. Some caution in interpreting these experiments is probably warranted because of their technical complexity. Nonetheless, the idea of a posteriori specification cannot be ruled out. An unfortunate aspect of this hypothesis is that it implies different rules for establishing appropriate connections in regeneration and in development. Indeed, if this idea were correct, then the bulk of the work on the retinotectal system (which is predicated on reinnervation) would be largely irrelevant to neural development.

Other theories of retinotectal specificity

A number of additional theories that have appeared might be regarded as degraded models of Sperry's original view, that is, theories that require some kind of biochemical labeling, but with less order and exclusivity than Sperry supposed. In one such scheme—the arrow model—tectal cells are not specified in any absolute way but are distinguished only by local information about relative position (Hope et al., 1976). In this conception, information about polarity across the tectum causes fiber alignment, giving the appearance of more detailed affinities between cells than actually exists. Another model along these lines compares retinotectal specificity to a trading situation between tea salesmen from India and buyers in Britain (von der Marlsburg and Willshaw, 1977). In this scenario, it is imagined that marker molecules are continually synthesized by a small number of cells in the presynaptic population. These molecules are then transferred from presynaptic axons to postsynaptic cells at a rate proportional to the synaptic interaction between them. The authors suggest that this mechanism would result in a kind of self-organization based again on information about relative position.

Although such models may explain certain aspects of retinotectal specificity, they suffer from a number of drawbacks. First, the many underlying assumptions are not easily understood or tested. Second, the models are vague enough so that new experimental results can be accommodated by minor tinkering. In consequence, they have relatively little predictive power and provide no clear indication of what a biochemist might actually look for in the retina or tectum.

CONCLUSIONS

As in the peripheral nervous system, specificity in the retinotectal system does not appear to be based on complementary molecules that act as locks and keys; rather the recognition that presumably guides axons and governs selective synaptogenesis seems based on biases that change the probability of interactions between cells without influencing the absolute limits of connectivity. In the retinotectal system, this conclusion is supported by the outcome of size disparity experiments, experiments using compound eyes, and observations that indicate shifting connections during development and optic nerve regeneration.

In spite of a great deal of debate over the years, the idea that cell surface molecules mediate recognition remains an attractive explanation of many aspects of patterned connections. It is clear, however, that surface recognition molecules provide a relatively weak force that modulates the development of connectivity rather than dictating it. Attempts to establish the biochemical basis of such recognition are still at an early stage, but there seems no reason why they should not ultimately succeed. One should hasten to emphasize, however, that surface recognition is only one of a number of mechanisms that lead to patterned innervation (specificity); specific responses to trophic factors, competition for trophic support, and the modulatory effects of neural activity on target cells are examples of other influences that play a major part in the establishment of neural connections. Thus, although important, the biochemical identity of surface recognition molecules is not really the Holy Grail. Ironically, it is not the inadequacy of biochemical methodology that impedes this quest but uncertainty about what recognitional molecules actually do in normal development.

Rearrangement of Developing Neuronal Connections

INTRODUCTION

During development, neurons and their targets establish qualitatively appropriate synaptic connections: each nerve cell must contact particular postsynaptic cells, avoiding other potential synaptic partners that are in some sense incorrect (Chapters 10 and 11). Neural function, however, also depends on precise quantitative relationships between nerve cells: each axon innervates an appropriate *number* of target cells, and each target cell is innervated by an appropriate *number* of axons. The variation in divergence and convergence in different regions of the nervous system is immense. For example, some nerve cells are innervated by a single axon, which makes such a powerful connection that an action potential in the presynaptic neuron invariably drives the postsynaptic cell to threshold. At the other extreme are neurons innervated by many thousands of axons, each one of which exerts only a miniscule postsynaptic influence; in these cases the effects of many converging axons must sum to fire the postsynaptic cell. The functional importance of these different patterns implies that quantitative as well as qualitative regulation is a central theme of neural development.

In general, the quantitative apportionment of innervation during development occurs by a gradual, competitive rearrangement of initial connections. This conclusion derives from evidence in several regions of the nervous system.

SYNAPTIC REARRANGEMENT IN DIFFERENT PARTS OF THE DEVELOPING NERVOUS SYSTEM

Synaptic rearrangement in skeletal muscle

Considerable insight into the way in which quantitative accuracy is achieved has been provided by studies of developing neuromuscular junctions. In the early part of this century, anatomists noted the difference in appearance of the neuromuscular junction in neonatal muscle and in mature muscle (Figure 1) (Tello, 1917; Boeke, 1932). When axons were stained with silver, each adult mammalian muscle fiber appeared to be contacted by a single axon terminal, whereas neonatal fibers

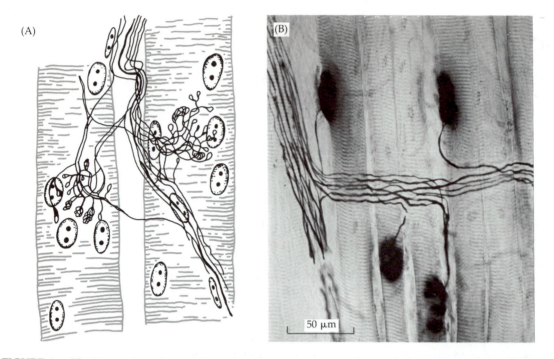

FIGURE 1.   *The innervation of neonatal and mature mammalian muscle fibers. (A) Drawing made by J. Boeke in 1926 of motor nerve endings on two muscle fibers from the tongue of a 4-day-old mouse (silver stain). Each fiber is innervated by endings from several different axons. (B) Photomicrograph of several adult muscle fibers in the rat extensor digitorum longus. Each adult fiber receives innervation from a single axon. The preparation has been impregnated with silver and stained for cholinesterase. ×310. (A from Boeke, 1932; B from Gorio et al., 1983.)*

appeared to be innervated by several different axons. Little attention was paid to this observation until P. A. Redfern (1970) confirmed by electrophysiological means that skeletal muscle fibers in neonatal animals are indeed innervated differently than adult muscle cells are. Rapidly contracting (twitch) skeletal muscle fibers in adult vertebrates are usually innervated by only one axon. Intracellular recordings from individual muscle fibers in neonatal animals, however, indicate a different arrangement. Such recordings characteristically show discrete steps in the postsynaptic potential elicited by gradually increasing the strength of motor nerve stimulation (Figure 2). These multiple steps provide evidence for innervation by several different axons (Redfern, 1970; Bennett and Pettigrew, 1974; Letinsky, 1974; Brown et al., 1976; see also Jansen et al., 1978; Brown et al., 1981; Van Essen, 1982). Morphological, electrophysiological, and pharmacological studies all show that these several synaptic contacts are located at approximately the same place along the fiber length, the eventual site of the mature endplate (Bennett and Pettigrew, 1974, 1976; Brown et al., 1976; Korneliussen and Jansen, 1976; Riley, 1976, 1977a,b, 1981).

The change from the neonatal to the adult pattern of muscle inner-

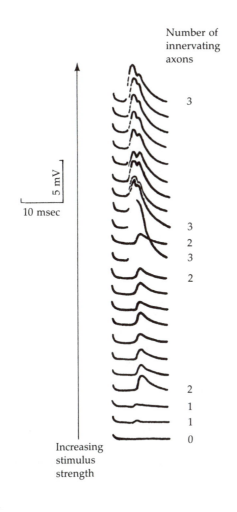

Number of
innervating
axons

3

3
2
3

2

2
1
1
0

5 mV

10 msec

Increasing
stimulus
strength

FIGURE 2. *Intracellular recording from a fiber in the diaphragm of a rat pup, showing multiple innervation of neonatal skeletal muscle fibers. Gradually increasing the strength of motor nerve stimulation (arrow) elicits three different postsynaptic responses; this result indicates innervation by three different axons recruited at slightly different stimulus intensities. Similar experiments in adult animals give only a single postsynaptic response that cannot be fractionated by graded stimulation. The preparation was partially curarized to prevent the endplate potentials from reaching threshold. (After Redfern, 1970.)*

vation implies that some initial neuromuscular synapses must have been removed; thus, this process has been called "synapse elimination." For technical reasons, the time of onset of elimination has been difficult to assess. Synapse elimination does not always progress at the same rate; however, in many mammalian muscles it certainly begins before birth and continues into the first few weeks of postnatal life (Figure 3) (Bixby and Van Essen, 1979; Pockett, 1981; Dennis et al., 1981). In the chick as well, elimination of synaptic contacts begins in ovo and continues after hatching (Bennett and Pettigrew, 1974, 1976). Because there is little evidence of nerve terminal degeneration in neonatal muscles, it seems likely that many of the initial synaptic contacts are withdrawn into the parent axon (Korneliussen and Jansen, 1976; Bixby, 1981; see, however, Rosenthal and Taraskevich, 1977).

Although some motor neurons may die after synapses are made and some new muscle fibers may appear after innervation (Betz et al., 1980; Harris, 1981; Nurcombe et al., 1981; Bennett et al., 1983), in many instances synapse loss occurs without an obvious change in the number

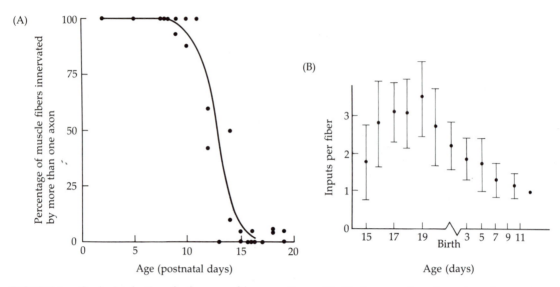

FIGURE 3. *Gradual reduction of polyneuronal inner-* *vation of mammalian muscle fibers. (A) Graph shows* *the percentage of rat soleus fibers innervated by more* *than one axon during early postnatal life. Determina-* *tions were made by intracellular recording, as in Figure* *2; each point represents measurements from at least 20*

fibers. (B) Similar recordings in embryonic rats show *that this process begins several days before birth. Each* *point represents the average response of 30–60 fibers;* *bars show standard deviation. (A after Brown et al.,* *1976; B after Dennis et al., 1981.)*

of innervating neurons or target fibers (Bagust et al., 1973; Brown et al., 1976; Oppenheim and Majors-Willard, 1978). If the number of motor neurons and muscle fibers remains constant, then the number of muscle fibers contacted by each motor axon (the motor unit) must be reduced during early postnatal life. Motor unit size can be measured by esti- mating the percentage of total tension that is developed in a muscle by each axon; such measurements show that there is indeed a several-fold decrease in the average size of motor units during the first few weeks of life (Figure 4) (Bagust et al., 1973; Brown et al., 1976). It should be noted, however, that rearrangement of terminals can also occur in neo- natal muscles with only a modest reduction in motor unit size (Betz et al., 1979).

Most studies of synapse elimination have examined skeletal muscle fibers that are ultimately innervated at a single point along their length; a few studies have also looked at synapse elimination from muscles that are multiply innervated in maturity (Figure 5). Such multiply in- nervated (tonic) muscle fibers in vertebrates are usually contacted at more or less regular intervals by a number of different synaptic endings (Chapter 9). By both electrophysiological and morphological criteria, each endplate site along such fibers in the chick is contacted by several axon terminals early in life, but by only a single axon a few weeks later (Bennett and Pettigrew, 1974, 1976). Thus synapse elimination in muscle appears to be quite general.

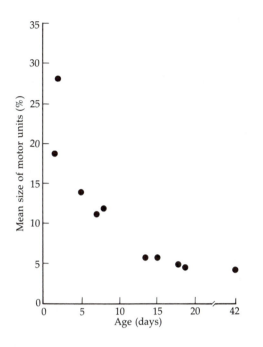

FIGURE 4. *Postnatal reduction in the size of motor units. Unit sizes in the soleus muscle of young rats were measured as the percentage of the total muscle tension elicited by stimulating individual motor axons. The size of motor units estimated in this way gradually decreases during the first few weeks of life. Thus, each motor neuron in the soleus pool innervates more muscle fibers at birth than it does in maturity. Each point represents the average size of units at different ages; in general, smaller units showed less change than large ones. (After Brown et al., 1976.)*

Synaptic rearrangement in the autonomic nervous system

The postnatal elimination of some initial synaptic contacts is not limited to muscle but also occurs when target cells are neurons. The simplest neuronal system in which synapse elimination has been studied is the submandibular ganglion of the rat (Lichtman, 1977, 1980). The cells in this parasympathetic ganglion are similar to skeletal muscle fibers in that most of them are innervated by a single axon in maturity. As in muscle, these ganglion cells at birth are innervated quite differently: each neuron is initially contacted by about five different preganglionic axons (Figure 6). The initial convergence of several different axons onto

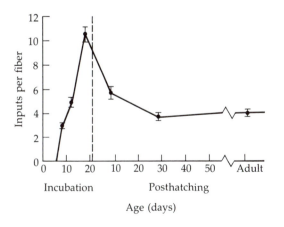

FIGURE 5. *Elimination of axon terminals from the fibers of a tonic muscle. This graph shows a gradual increase and then a decrease in the mean number of axon terminals detected in the vicinity of a recording electrode impaling chick anterior latissimus dorsi muscle fibers during incubation and early life. Unlike mammalian skeletal muscles, these fibers are innervated in maturity by several axons, the terminals of which are distributed along the fiber length. Synapse elimination apparently occurs at each of these sites. Bars indicate standard error of these averages. (After Bennett and Pettigrew, 1974.)*

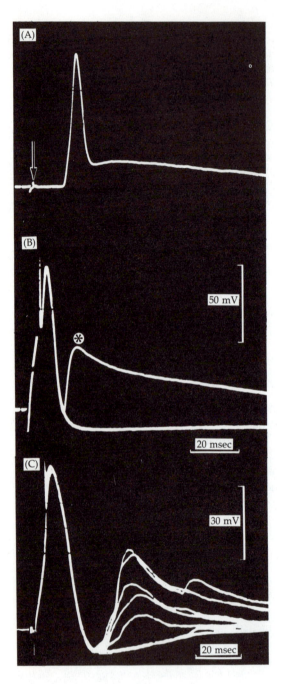

FIGURE 6.   *Electrophysiological evidence of synaptic rearrangement in autonomic ganglia. (A) Intracellular recording from an adult submandibular ganglion cell in the rat; stimulation of the preganglionic nerve (arrow) elicits a suprathreshold synaptic response. (B) When an action potential induced by injecting current through the microelectrode precedes the nerve stimulus, the underlying synaptic potential is revealed (asterisk). Two traces are superimposed. As in adult muscle fibers, graded stimulation usually elicits only a single postsynaptic response that cannot be fractionated. (C) Similar recording from a neonatal ganglion cell shows a number of different steps in the synaptic response, indicating innervation by several different axons (six separate steps could be observed in this neuron). (After Lichtman, 1977.)*

each target cell is reduced to the adult pattern over the first few weeks of postnatal life (Figure 7).

The similarity of this process in muscle and in a simple parasympathetic ganglion raises the question of whether the phenomenon of synapse elimination is restricted to those muscular or neural targets in

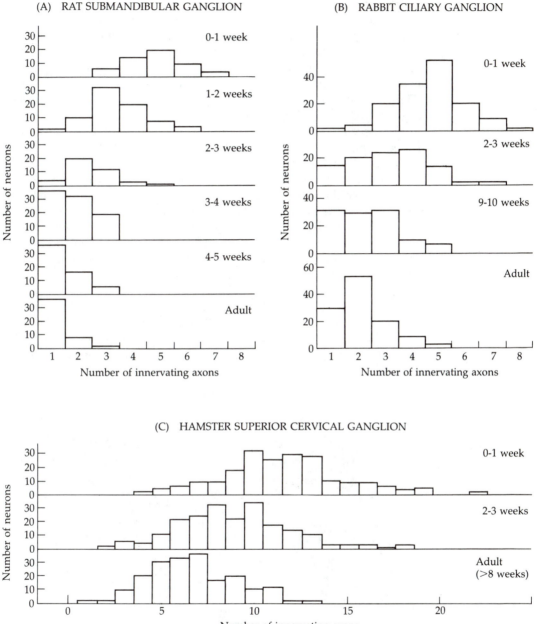

FIGURE 7.   *Postnatal reduction of multiple innervation in autonomic ganglia. Each graph summarizes experiments carried out in a different autonomic ganglion
in which the number of axons innervating the target
neurons at different developmental ages was estimated
electrophysiologically (as in Figure 6): (A) rat submandibular ganglion; (B) rabbit ciliary ganglion; (C) hamster superior cervical ganglion. In each system there is*
*a gradual transition from multiple to either single or
less profound multiple innervation. Note, however, that
this effect is most pronounced in ganglia where the
neurons are ultimately innervated by a single axon (A)
and least pronounced in ganglia in which cells show a
substantial degree of multiple innervation in maturity
(C). (A after Lichtman, 1977; B after Johnson and
Purves, 1981; C after Lichtman and Purves, 1980.)*

which there is ultimately a one-on-one pattern of innervation. At least some classes of neurons that remain multiply innervated in maturity also undergo some degree of synaptic rearrangement in early life. In the hamster superior cervical ganglion, for instance, in which each adult neuron remains innervated by a number of different axons (about six), neonatal ganglion cells are innervated by about twice as many axons (Figure 7) (Lichtman and Purves, 1980). These and other examples suggest that although synaptic rearrangement may occur rather widely in the nervous system, the degree of initial elimination is inversely proportional to the final number of axons that innervate the target cells (cf. Figure 7A, B, C; see also later).

In the autonomic nervous system, as in muscle, it is important to ask whether the populations of innervating cells and target cells are stable during the period of synaptic rearrangement. This has been evaluated in the ciliary ganglion of the rabbit where synapse elimination also occurs in early life (Johnson and Purves, 1981). Even though the number of axons innervating each neuron is reduced by about 50 percent, retrograde labeling of preganglionic neurons with horseradish peroxidase shows that the number of cells innervating the ciliary ganglion (about 40) changes little, if at all, from birth to maturity. Nor does the number of ciliary ganglion cells (about 400) change postnatally. Thus, the number of target cells innervated by each preganglionic axon (the neural unit) must decrease during the postnatal period. This out-

(A) 1 day old

(B) Adult

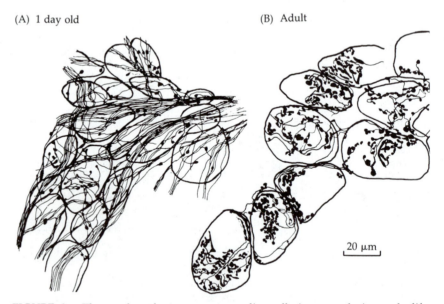

20 μm

FIGURE 8. *The number of synapses on ganglion cells increases during early life. Camera lucida drawings of neurons from the submandibular ganglion of neonatal (A) and adult (B) rats treated with zinc iodide–osmium. This reagent preferentially stains synaptic boutons. The number of boutons on neurons increases during the period of synapse elimination, a fact confirmed in this and other autonomic ganglia by electron microscopy. (After Lichtman, 1977.)*

come is similar to the reduction of motor unit size evident in many developing muscles.

There is, however, one important feature of synaptic rearrangement in autonomic ganglia that appears to be different from muscle: the number of synapses actually *increases* during the period when some inputs are being eliminated (Figure 8). Thus, more synaptic contacts are present on ganglion cells at the end of the first few weeks of life than are present at birth (Lichtman, 1977; Smolen and Raisman, 1979; Johnson and Purves, 1981; Rubin, 1985c). Indeed, this gradual accumulation of synapses during early postnatal life appears to be characteristic of many parts of the nervous system (although synaptic density may later decline; Chapter 9). Thus, the phrase "synapse elimination" is actually a misnomer because the overall number of synaptic contacts on target cells increases during the period when some initial synapses are lost. On the face of it, the innervation of muscle provides an exception to this rule: if each mature muscle fiber is innervated by a single synapse in maturity and if several different axons innervate each fiber at birth, surely there must be a net loss of synapses (see Figure 10). Although commonly referred to as "a synapse," the vertebrate neuromuscular junction often comprises a number of individual synaptic boutons (Figure 9). Because the size and complexity of the terminal

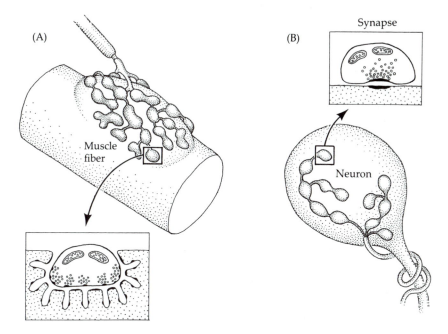

FIGURE 9. *Comparison of the innervation of muscle fibers and neurons. Schematic drawing of the arrangement of synaptic boutons on a snake skeletal muscle fiber (A) and a parasympathetic neuron in the frog heart (B). The implication of this comparison is that the innervation of an endplate by an axon is similar to the innervation of an entire neuronal cell body. In each case a single axon deploys a number of synaptic boutons on a surface area of roughly equivalent size. (After Kuffler and Yoshikami, 1975.)*

arborization within each endplate increases postnatally (Nystrom, 1968; Davey and Bennett, 1982), additional synaptic boutons are evidently elaborated on muscle fibers, just as they are on the surface of autonomic ganglion cells (and other neurons) during this period.

Thus, a general rule for targets where the cells are ultimately innervated strongly by one or a few inputs may be that each innervating axon initially establishes a relatively small number of synapses on a relatively large number of target cells. As development proceeds, these initial synaptic contacts are rearranged and additional synapses are formed so that more and more synaptic endings are established by each axon on fewer and fewer postsynaptic cells (Figure 10).

Synaptic rearrangement in the central nervous system

Early rearrangements of synaptic connections have also been described in several parts of the central nervous system. Perhaps the region that provides the closest analogy to events in the peripheral nervous system is the avian auditory system, in which some neurons are also innervated by one or a few axons in maturity (Jackson and Parks, 1982). Each neuron in the nucleus magnocellularis of chick embryos at 13 days of incubation is innervated by about four different axons from the cochlear nerve (Figure 11). Shortly after hatching, however, these cells are in-

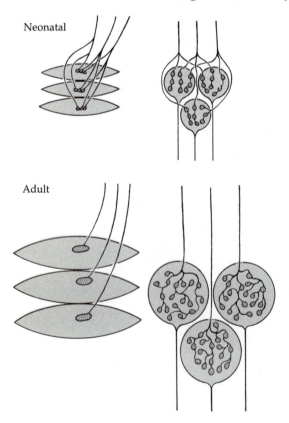

FIGURE 10. *Summary diagram of synapse elimination during the initial innervation of skeletal muscle fibers (left) and ganglion cells that lack dendrites (right). In newborn mammals, both muscle fibers and ganglion cells are innervated by several different axons. In adult animals, however, each of these cells is generally innervated by a single axon. If the number of presynaptic and postsynaptic cells remains constant postnatally, each innervating axon must innervate fewer target cells. At the same time, more and more synapses are elaborated by each axon on a progressively smaller number of target cells. This focusing of innervation is apparently the basic feature of the gradual rearrangement of synapses in these relatively simple systems where the end result is strong innervation of target cells by one or a few axons. (After Purves and Lichtman, 1978.)*

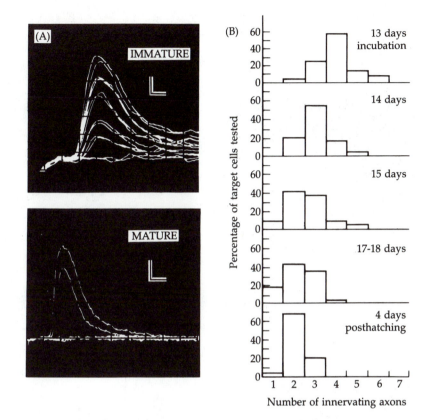

FIGURE 11. *Synapse elimination in the developing avian cochlear nucleus. (A) Intra-cellular recordings from nucleus magnocellularis neurons during increasingly intense stimulation of the cochlear nerve. As in the autonomic system and muscle, some inputs to individual target cells in this brain stem nucleus are lost during development (cf. Figures 2 and 6); recording at top is from a chick embryo at 13 days of incubation; recording below is from a chick 4 days after hatching. Calibration bars correspond to 2 mV, 2 msec above and 5 mV, 2 msec below. (B) Histograms showing the proportion of target neurons receiving different numbers of inputs as a function of age (cf. Figure 7). (After Jackson and Parks, 1982.)*

nervated by an average of only two different axons. This decline is accompanied by a decrease in the number of preterminal branches arising from each innervating axon.

Another example that parallels events in the periphery is the inner-vation of Purkinje cells by climbing fibers in the cerebellum of newborn rats. Although mature Purkinje cells are innervated by many thousands of axons, each of these neurons is contacted by only a single climbing fiber (Figure 12). This one-on-one relationship of climbing fibers to Purkinje cells is apparent both from the anatomy and the electrophys-iology of the adult rat cerebellum. As in muscle or some autonomic ganglia, intracellular recordings from Purkinje cells reveal unitary climb-ing fiber responses that cannot be fractionated by grading the strength

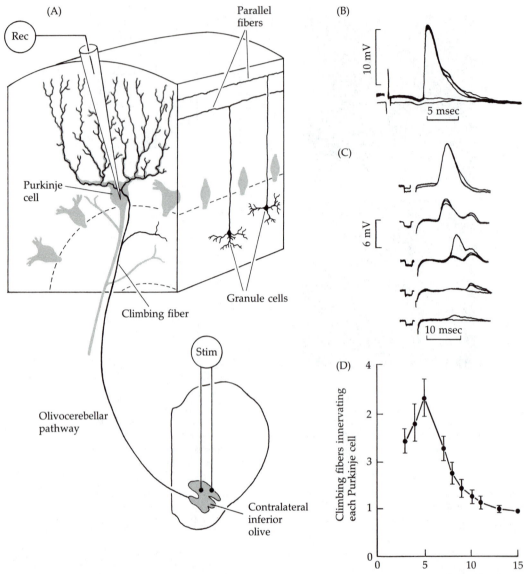

FIGURE 12. *Innervation of cerebellar Purkinje cells by climbing fibers in neonatal and adult mammals. (A) In the mature mammalian cerebellum, each Purkinje cell is innervated by a single climbing fiber. This drawing shows the general arrangement of this system and the method of testing Purkinje cell innervation electrophysiologically. The climbing fibers arise in the contralateral inferior olive and reach the cerebellum via the olivocerebellar pathway; these fibers can be stimulated by electrodes in the inferior olive. At the same time, Purkinje cells can be impaled with a microelectrode. (B) Increasingly intense stimulation of the contralateral olive elicits an all-or-nothing response in individual Purkinje cells,* much the same as in muscle fibers or some classes of adult ganglion cells (cf. Figures 2 and 6). Several traces are superimposed. (C) At birth, however, each Purkinje cell is innervated by several different climbing fibers; as the strength of stimulation is increased (from bottom), additional inputs are recruited. (D) The average number of climbing fibers innervating each cerebellar Purkinje cell in the rat decreases gradually as the animal matures. Each point represents the average of several determinations; bars show 95 percent confidence limits. (A,B after Eccles, 1966; C,D after Mariani and Changeux, 1981.)*

of stimulation (Eccles et al., 1966). However, similar intracellular recordings at birth present a different picture. In newborn rats, complex synaptic responses suggest that each Purkinje cell is innervated by several different climbing fibers; evidently, all but one of these inputs are lost over the first few weeks of postnatal life (Crepel et al., 1976, 1980; Mariani and Changeux, 1980, 1981).

The most interesting example of synaptic rearrangement in the central nervous system occurs in the developing visual cortex. In adult cats and in some species of monkey, neurons in the primary visual cortex are segregated into columns dominated alternately by the right or the left eye (Figures 13 and 14) (Wiesel and Hubel, 1963b, 1965; Hubel and Wiesel, 1965; Rakic, 1977; Hubel et al., 1977; LeVay et al., 1978; Shatz and Stryker, 1978). These columns can be observed in a number of ways. One approach is to make electrophysiological recordings along microelectrode tracks oriented tangentially to the cortical surface. Another is to inject a tracer such as radioactive proline into one eye. The label is transported transsynaptically from the eye through the lateral geniculate to the visual cortex; the pattern of tracer in the cortex is then observed by autoradiography (Figure 14). The importance of ocular dominance columns in the present context is that at birth (and in late embryonic life) there is considerable overlap of the cortical innervation arising from the right and the left eyes (Figure 15) (Rakic, 1976, 1977; Hubel et al., 1977).

Electrophysiological studies have confirmed this relatively unsegregated arrangement at birth. In the adult monkey, most cortical neurons in layer IV (where geniculate afferents terminate) are dominated by innervation from either the left or the right eye. At birth, on the other hand, many of these neurons are binocularly driven (Hubel et al., 1977; LeVay et al., 1978). Evidently, cortical inputs are gradually segregated into alternating columns by synaptic rearrangement.

Segregative phenomena of this sort are apparently widespread in the developing brain. For instance, inputs are gradually segregated into upper and lower cortical layers in the olfactory cortex of developing mammals (Schwob and Price, 1984). Another example is the lateral geniculate nucleus; retinal afferents from both eyes are initially distributed throughout the nucleus but are eventually restricted to appropriate laminae (Rakic, 1977; Shatz, 1983). Segregation can also be induced between afferents that would not normally encounter one another. Thus, if optic nerve fibers from the two eyes of lower vertebrates are forced to innervate the same side of the tectum, the two sets of inputs tend to segregate into discrete patches (Levine and Jacobson, 1975; Meyer, 1976; Meyer and Sperry, 1976; Schmidt, 1978). A striking example of induced segregation occurs following implantation of an extra eye (Constantine-Paton and Law, 1978; Law and Constantine-Paton, 1981; see also Law and Constantine-Paton, 1982). In the frog, axons from the two retinas normally decussate completely so that the left eye projects to the right tectum, and vice versa. Thus, the projections from each eye are not mixed at this level under normal circumstances. If,

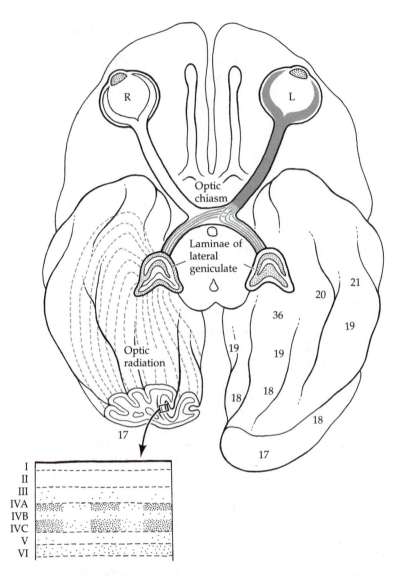

FIGURE 13. *Diagram illustrating the major visual pathways in the rhesus monkey. About half the axons originating from the retinal ganglion cells in each eye cross at the optic chiasm and project to three laminae of the lateral geniculate. The rest of the axons remain ipsilateral and project to the three other layers of the geniculate; thus, inputs from the two eyes remain separate at this level. The principal neurons of the lateral geniculate project in turn to the primary visual cortex (area 17), via the optic radiation, and terminate in sublayers IVA and IVC, as shown in the blowup of a section through this cortical region. During development inputs from the two eyes gradually segregate into ocular dominance columns (see Figure 14). The numbers 18, 19, 20, 21, and 36 indicate other cortical areas concerned with vision. (After Rakic, 1977.)*

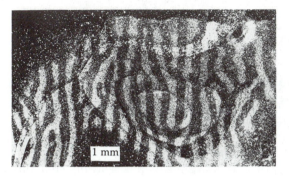

FIGURE 14. *Ocular dominance columns in the monkey striate cortex. This figure shows an autoradiograph of what amounts to a surface view of the striate cortex of an adult monkey; the contralateral eye had been injected with radioactive proline 2 weeks before. This picture was made by cutting deeper and deeper parallel sections through layer IVC and then superimposing them to produce this composite view (cf. Figure 13). A striking array of zebra stripes representing ocular dominance columns is apparent when the silver grains in the exposed film are illuminated by a dark-field condenser. (After Hubel et al., 1977.)*

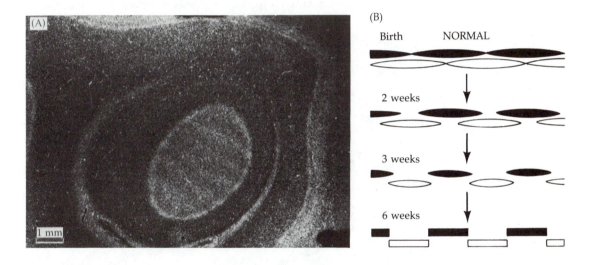

FIGURE 15. *The development of ocular dominance columns in layer IVC of the monkey visual cortex. (A) Autoradiograph of the striate cortex after injection of radioactive label into one eye at birth shows a pattern very different from that seen in the adult (cf. Figure 14). Although a faint periodic pattern is apparent in the newborn, the geniculate terminals related to each eye evidently ramify throughout layer IVC (and IVA) of the primary visual cortex. View is the same as Figure 14. (B) Diagram of the development of columns. The filled symbols represent the terminations of geniculate afferents from one eye, and the open symbols terminations from the other eye. The width of the lines indicates the approximate density of afferent terminals. Although there is already some periodic variation in density at birth (see A), terminal distributions from the two eyes overlap extensively. Inputs from the two eyes compete with one another such that the weaker input at any point declines while the stronger input is fortified. The result is a progressive segregation as the nondominant terminals retract completely from the columns dominated by the other eye. For the purposes of this drawing it was assumed that the retraction process takes about 6 weeks; the exact time course is not clear. Why competition between inputs from the two eyes produces an array of stripes is not known. (From Hubel et al., 1977.)*

however, a third eye is implanted into a tadpole so that axons from two different eyes grow into the same tectum, then ocular dominance columns develop (Figure 16).

Other rearrangements in the central nervous system

Using tracer techniques, neuroanatomists have described a number of additional projections that become more restricted during development. Whether these rearrangements involve changes in synaptic connections is not yet known. For instance, studies using retrograde and anterograde tracers show that projections across the corpus callosum are more diffuse in young animals than in adults (Innocenti et al., 1977; Ivy et al., 1979; Innocenti, 1981, 1982; O'Leary et al., 1981; Ivy and Killackey, 1981). Moreover, many neurons that project to the opposite hemisphere at birth do not do so in maturity (Figure 17). In certain parts of the parietal cortex, for example, ipsilateral cortical projections are main-

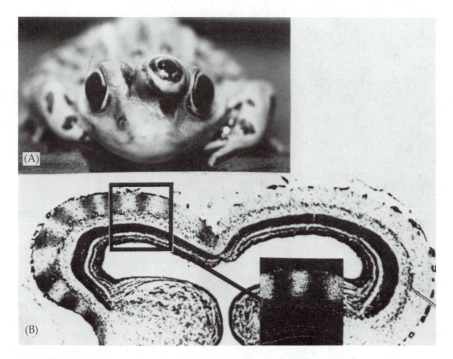

FIGURE 16. *Segregation of ocular inputs following implantation of a supernumerary eye. (A) This three-eyed frog (Rana pipiens) was created by implanting a donor eye into a tadpole before metamorphosis. Normally, retinal axons decussate nearly completely in the frog; therefore inputs from the two eyes are always separate. Because the axons of the implanted eye must go to one tectum or the other, this procedure forces projections from two different eyes to interact. (B) Autoradiograph of the optic tectum of a full-grown, three-eyed frog after injection of tritiated proline into the normal eye. Inset shows a dark-field enlargement. Ocular dominance columns strikingly similar to those in monkeys are apparent (cf. Figures 13 and 14). (From Constantine-Paton and Law, 1978.)*

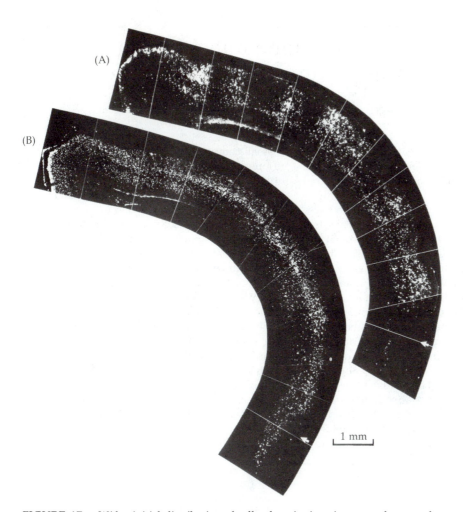

FIGURE 17. *Wider initial distribution of callosal projections in neonatal mammals. (A) Fluorescence photomicrograph of rat cortex after a series of True blue injections into the contralateral hemisphere on postnatal day 17; the animal was sacrificed 4 days later. The labeled cell bodies form characteristic clusters. (B) Similar injections on day 2 followed by a 19-day survival period (True blue has the quality of persisting in cells for many weeks). The retrogradely labeled cells are now more widespread, and no clustering is apparent. Evidently, some neurons that project across the corpus callosum at birth no longer do so several weeks later (cf. A and B). This restriction is not a result of cell death because neurons labeled early in life can still be seen after the projection has contracted (B). Arrows indicate the rhinal sulcus. (From O'Leary et al., 1981.)*

tained during development, but contralateral projections are lost (Ivy and Killackey, 1981, 1982). A related example is the presence of a substantial ipsilateral retinal projection to the tectum in birds and mammals, a projection that largely disappears during development (Land and Lund, 1979; O'Leary et al., 1983). Finally, many neurons from the occipital cortex project to the pyramidal tract in newborn but not in

Elimination of Some Initial Inputs Is Not a Universal Feature of Neural Development

Although many synaptic rearrangements in the developing nervous system reflect a decrease in the degree of initial convergence, this is not always the case.

Perhaps the most thoroughly studied synaptic interaction in the central nervous system is the muscle afferent innervation of spinal motor neurons. In adult animals, HRP labeling of both presynaptic and postsynaptic elements in the spinal cord shows a pattern of innervation that seems quite different from that seen in autonomic ganglia; each Ia axon makes only a small number of synaptic boutons (about 5–10) on each motor neuron it innervates. Each motor neuron, however, is innervated by many Ia axons (see Chapter 10). In contrast, autonomic neurons are innervated by relatively few axons, each of which makes a relatively large number of synaptic boutons. In accord with this different anatomical picture, the electrophysiological effect of each afferent on spinal motor neurons is small compared to the average postsynaptic response elicited in ganglion cells by activation of individual presynaptic axons.

This different adult pattern is reflected in a different developmental sequence. Thus there is little or no decrease in the convergence of Ia afferents onto spinal motor neurons as each Ia axon innervates the entire pool (Chapter 10; see also Lichtman and Frank, 1984). Indeed, even in autonomic ganglia, *some* target neurons are innervated by about as many axons at birth as in maturity (Hume and Purves, 1981).

These observations make two points. First, one should probably avoid facile generalizations about decreased convergence as a universal mechanism in the development of innervation. Second, those situations in which decreasing convergence is most evident are regions of the nervous system where target cells acquire extraordinarily powerful inputs from one or a very few axons.

adult rats (Stanfield et al., 1982). Evidently these sorts of restrictions are the result of terminal retraction rather than of cell death (Innocenti, 1981; O'Leary et al., 1981; Stanfield et al., 1982; see, however, O'Leary et al., 1984). Wider initial ramifications may also be characteristic of the development of the central nervous system in some invertebrates (see, for example, Goodman and Spitzer, 1981; Wallace, 1984).

In summary, a wide variety of rearrangements have been described in the developing central nervous system. These fall into at least three different categories:

1. Rearrangements that, like events in muscle and autonomic ganglia, reflect a decrease in the convergence of axons onto target cells. Examples are the nucleus magnocellularis and the development of climbing fiber innervation to Purkinje cells.

2. Rearrangements that involve the segregation of inputs across target cell populations. The preeminent example is the development of ocular dominance columns.

3. Rearrangements that involve the loss of a projection to a target population as development proceeds. The best example is the changing pattern of callosal projections in mammals. Unlike the other two categories, it is not clear whether synaptic change is involved here.

MECHANISMS UNDERLYING THE
REARRANGEMENT OF SYNAPTIC CONNECTIONS

Synaptic rearrangement appears to be based on competition

Although a number of mechanisms are probably involved in the rearrangements of synaptic connections that occur so widely in early life, competition between different axons innervating the same target cell is certainly a salient feature of the process: terminals are withdrawn from a target cell because in some sense other terminals have been more successful. Several lines of evidence support this view. When motor unit size is measured in rat lumbrical muscles deprived of all but a single axon, the remaining motor unit fails to decrease in size (Betz et al., 1980). This persistence of abnormally large motor units after neonatal denervation is perhaps the most direct evidence for competition in synaptic rearrangements. In some other developing muscles, however, there is also evidence for an intrinsic tendency for axons to withdraw a portion of their initial arborization. For instance, if a substantial fraction of the innervation to rat soleus muscle is removed at birth, an appreciable reduction of motor unit size still occurs (Brown et al., 1976; Thompson and Jansen, 1977).

| BOX B | # The Relationship of Synaptic Rearrangement to Error Correction |

It seems unlikely that a major function of synapse elimination is to remove qualitatively inappropriate connections. Indeed, because the earliest connections formed by presynaptic neurons on vertebrate muscle fibers, ganglion cells, and spinal motor neurons are for the most part correct, relatively few errors are ever present (Landmesser, 1980; Lichtman and Purves, 1980; Frank and Westerfield, 1983; Rubin, 1985c; see also Chapters 5 and 6). Furthermore, in muscle and autonomic ganglia, an axon that loses contacts with one target cell retains synapses with other nearby cells the functions of which are presumably the same; it is difficult to see how one set of connections in a muscle or a functionally homogeneous parasympathetic ganglion is in some qualitative sense more appropriate than any other. On the other hand, synapse elimination in some muscles and autonomic ganglia *is* weakly influenced by the segmental origin of the innervating axons (Lichtman and Purves, 1980; Miyata and Yoshioka, 1980; Brown and Booth, 1983a,b; Bennett and Lavidis, 1984; see also Gordon and Van Essen, 1983, Thompson, 1983a). To the extent that qualitative criteria influence innervation (Chapters 10 and 11), they will also influence synaptic rearrangement.

A further argument for competition is simply the end result of rearrangement in muscle, in some autonomic ganglia, and in the cerebellum. It is difficult to imagine how a process that did not involve competition could produce the one-on-one relationship observed between these target cells and their innervation. If the withdrawal of axons were simply random, then some target cells would be expected to receive no innervation, whereas others should end up with more than one axon supplying them.

The object of competition during synaptic rearrangement is probably trophic support

If competition is a central feature of synaptic rearrangement, what do axons compete for? Although there is no certain answer to this question, a strong circumstantial case can be made for the involvement of trophic factors produced by the target cells (Chapter 7). To reiterate, trophic interactions between target cells and the neurons that innervate them are a basic feature of neural development. Thus, the death of many neurons in early embryonic life apparently results from failure to obtain trophic support from peripheral targets (Chapter 6). In at least two parts of the nervous system there is good evidence that this trophic support is provided by a specific protein—nerve growth factor—produced by target cells. It is attractive to suppose that axon terminals also compete for target-produced factors during the synaptic rearrangements that usually follow the period of cell death (Purves, 1977). In this view, the number of target cells innervated by each axon is regulated in large measure by the requirement of the presynaptic cell for a particular level of trophic support. Because axons often reorganize their initial connections to innervate a smaller number of target cells, presynaptic neurons may receive more trophic support by innervating a few cells strongly than many cells weakly.

Trophic support is somehow linked to neural activity

In spite of the appeal of this argument, the scenario in which target cells supply limited amounts of trophic molecules to competing presynaptic cells does not entirely account for what is observed. As noted earlier, in some regions of the nervous system the number of synaptic boutons actually increases during the period of interaxonal competition in early life. Therefore, trophic support must be available for a larger number of synaptic connections than is initially present; what seems to be lacking is support for connections arising from many *different* axons contacting the same target cell. Moreover, the idea of competition for a limited supply of trophic factor in the local environment of nerve terminals does not explain the restricted innervation of particular target cells in both muscle and ganglia. If presynaptic axons simply required a threshold level of trophic factor, there would be no reason for an axon to innervate strongly a few target cells while completely ignoring neigh-

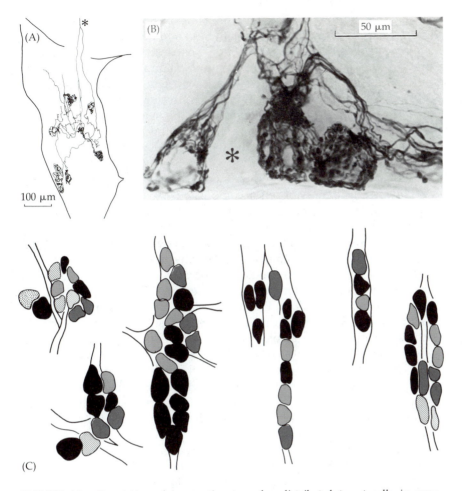

FIGURE 18. *Restriction of innervation to a few distributed target cells in some autonomic ganglia. (A) Camera lucida drawing of the arborization of a single preganglionic axon in the rabbit ciliary ganglion after intracellular axon injection of horseradish peroxidase (HRP). Individual axons ramify widely in the ganglion but make dense clusters of synaptic boutons on a small number of distributed ganglion cells. (B) Photomicrograph of a portion of the arborization of a single HRP-labeled preganglionic axon in the rabbit ciliary ganglion. The three heavily innervated cell bodies abut numerous other cells that receive no innervation from the labeled axon (see also Figure 21). Asterisk indicates a cell not innervated by this axon; it is sandwiched between two heavily innervated neurons. 50-μm section. (C) Camera lucida drawings showing the arrangement of the preganglionic innervation in six different neuronal clusters in adult rat submandibular ganglia (assessed electrophysiologically). Cells innervated exclusively by a particular axon in a cluster (indicated by the same shading) are often interspersed among neurons innervated by different axons. In each of these examples, axons capture particular cells rather than territories. (A after Hume and Purves, 1983; B from Forehand and Purves, 1984; C after Lichtman, 1980.)*

boring cells of the same type (Figure 18). Axons often seem much more interested in focusing their innervation on a few target neurons than in simply establishing a given number of synapses willy-nilly. It is unlikely that this tendency toward exclusive innervation is based on qualitative differences (i.e., chemoaffinity labels) because in many cases the target cells are functionally (and positionally) equivalent (see Box B).

These considerations all suggest that the synapses that ultimately innervate a muscle cell or neuron are somehow treated as *sets* during the process of innervation. Evidently, all the synaptic boutons arising from one axon are identified during competition as being different from the synaptic boutons arising from a competing axon.

How is this identity of sets accomplished? An obvious property held in common by synaptic boutons arising from a particular axon is their pattern of neural activity. There is, in fact, considerable evidence that synaptic rearrangements are influenced by activity. For example, in both muscle and autonomic ganglia, chronically paralyzing nerves with a local anesthetic (or otherwise decreasing activity) decreases the rate of synapse elimination (Benoit and Changeux, 1975, 1978; Srihari and Vrbová, 1978; Riley, 1978; Thompson et al., 1979; Brown et al., 1982; Caldwell and Ridge, 1983; Jackson, 1983). Conversely, increasing the activity of innervating axons by chronic stimulation speeds up synapse elimination (O'Brien et al., 1978; Thompson, 1983b; see also Maehlen and Njå, 1982). Additional evidence for the influence of neural activity on synaptic rearrangement comes from the development of the visual system. When one eye of a monkey is occluded during the first few weeks of life (or removed prenatally), the normal segregation of ocular dominance columns is dramatically altered (Wiesel and Hubel, 1963, 1965; Rakic, 1981a; see Chapter 14). The columns normally activated by the deprived eye shrink, whereas the columns arising from the non-deprived eye persist. Finally, chronic blockade of visual activity with tetrodotoxin impedes the segregation of ocular dominance columns (Stryker, 1981; Meyer, 1982; see also Archer et al., 1982; Schmidt and Edwards, 1983), whereas direct stimulation of the optic nerves of these animals induces segregation (M. Stryker, personal communication).

The overall *amount* of neural activity may be less important in synaptic rearrangement than the *pattern* of neural activity. When both eyes are occluded (presumably reducing activity equally in both ocular pathways), no shift in ocular dominance is observed (Wiesel and Hubel, 1965). Furthermore, profound changes occur in the developing visual cortex without deprivation when the two eyes are simply made disconjugate by cutting one or more eye muscles (or by occluding the two eyes alternately) (Figure 19) (Hubel and Wiesel, 1965). In these circumstances, each eye receives the same amount of stimulation and at maturity the animals appear to see normally with either eye. Yet recordings from single neurons in the visual cortex of animals with strabismus or alternating occlusion show a marked reduction in the number of binocularly driven cells. These results led D. H. Hubel and T. N. Wiesel (see Box C in Chapter 14) to suggest that asynchronous activity en-

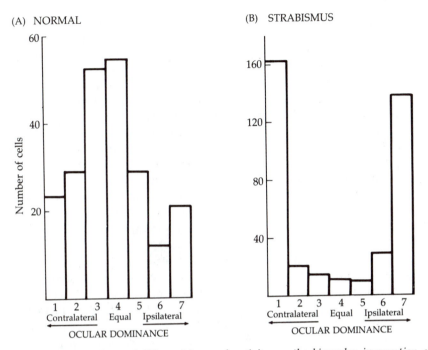

(A) NORMAL

(B) STRABISMUS

FIGURE 19. *Effects of differential neural activity on the binocular innervation of visual cortical cells. (A) Ocular dominance histogram of a large number of cortical neurons in normal adult cats; recordings were made throughout the cortical layers. Each bar in the histogram represents a different level of ocular dominance ranging from complete dominance by the contralateral eye (1) to complete dominance of the ipsilateral eye (7). (B) Ocular dominance in four cats made cross-eyed at birth by cutting some of the extraocular muscles. About 80 percent of cells in normal adult cats are binocularly driven, whereas only about 20 percent of cells in the cross-eyed animals are activated by both eyes. Evidently desynchronizing the activity of inputs from the two eyes stimulates competitive interactions between the two cortical projections so that the target neurons become dominated by one eye or the other. (After Hubel and Wiesel, 1965.)*

hances competition between axons innervating the same cortical neuron, whereas synchronous activity of axons innervating a cell somehow impedes their competitive interaction (Hubel and Wiesel, 1965). A similar result has been described in the developing auditory system (Sanes and Constantine-Paton, 1983).

Hubel and Wiesel's suggestion that asynchronous impulse activity promotes segregation of axon terminals has been useful in a number of ways. For example, this hypothesis provides an attractive explanation of the ocular dominance columns that develop in three-eyed frogs (see Figure 16). Axons from corresponding points on the retinas of the normal and the supernumerary eyes initially project to the same place on the tectum. Under ordinary circumstances, the inputs in a particular region of tectum are active together; the extra eye, however, sees a scene somewhat different from that seen by the normal eye. As a result, the supernumerary axons tend to be out of phase with the corresponding axons of the normal eye. Similarly, when a compound eye consisting of two nasal or temporal retinal halves is implanted in a tadpole in place of a normal eye, the two retinal halves map on the same region of the tectum, presumably because they share the same topographical instructions. As the tadpole matures, however, inputs from the two retinal halves are segregated into alternating strips (Fawcett and Willshaw, 1982; see also Ide et al., 1983). Again the only obvious difference between the two halves is the somewhat different pattern of activity that would arise because corresponding points on the retinal halves view a different scene. In confirmation of this interpretation, blocking normal activity in these sorts of experiments by intraocular injection of tetrodotoxin inhibits the segregation of competing inputs (Meyer, 1982; Reh and Constantine-Paton, 1984b).

In general, attempts to explain the effect of activity in a more detailed way have made use of the idea that terminals are in some sense reinforced when they are active at the same time as the target cell. The notion that coincident activity is important in the formation of neural connections can be traced to D. O. Hebb's book, *The Organization of Behavior*, written in 1949. Hebb suggested an explanation of learning, which states "when an axon of cell A is near enough to excite a cell B and repeatedly and persistently takes part in firing it, some growth or metabolic change takes place in one or both cells such that A's efficiency, as one of the cells firing B, is increased." Since Hebb's formulation, this basic idea has been elaborated in several contexts. The late D. Marr (1969) used a variant of Hebb's postulate to explain learning in the cerebellum. In a theoretical paper, Marr suggested that synchronous impulse activity might explain how the cerebellum gradually modifies movements commanded by the cerebral cortex. In 1973 G. S. Stent outlined a specific mechanism for Hebb's postulate. Stent was impressed on the one hand by Hubel and Wiesel's experiments, which showed that binocularly driven cortical neurons tend to become monocular when the input from both eyes is desynchronized, and on the other hand by T. Lømo and J. Rosenthal's experiments at the neuromuscular junction, which showed that postsynaptic activity blocks denervation supersensitivity (Chapter 8). Putting these observations together, Stent suggested that receptors tend to be eliminated from the postsynaptic membrane by the transient reversals of membrane potential that occur when transmitter release triggers an impulse in the postsynaptic cell. Because the reversal potential for transmitter action is less polarized than the peak of the action potential, Stent surmised that receptors would be more protected in the vicinity of a synapse than away from it during synchronous presynaptic and postsynaptic activity. Conversely, during asynchronous activity, such protection would not occur. The proposal, then, was that simultaneous activity stabilized postsynaptic receptors.

J.-P. Changeux and his collaborators have argued that appropriate neuronal connections are stabilized by patterns of neuronal activity in yet another way (Changeux, 1972; Changeux et al., 1973; Changeux and Danchin, 1976; Changeux and Mikoshiba, 1978). The mechanism envisaged by Changeux involves conversion of receptors from a labile to a stable state. This is suggested to occur "when both an anteriograde factor liberated by the nerve terminal during activity and 'internal coupling factor' are present above a critical concentration and within a given lapse of time on the two faces of the sub-synaptic membrane" (Changeux and Danchin, 1976). This hypothetical stabilization involves a covalent modification of the receptor molecule (e.g., phosphorylation), which is supposed to protect it against proteolysis (Changeux and Danchin, 1976; Gouze et al., 1983). The gist of this view, then, is a biochemical interaction between an anterograde chemical signal and a retrograde signal that reinforces simultaneously active presynaptic and postsynaptic elements by receptor stabilization.

A different idea is that release and uptake of the trophic factors for which axons evidently compete occurs most effectively when the presynaptic and postsynaptic cells are active together (Purves and Lichtman, 1980; Lichtman and Purves, 1981). This idea is predicated on presynaptic reward rather than on stabilization of postsynaptic receptors. The core of this theory is that trophic factor is released by active postsynaptic cells in proportion to depolarization and can only be taken up by a simultaneously active terminal. The greater the postsynaptic activity generated by an excitatory synaptic bouton (or a set of synaptic boutons), the greater the trophic reward. Accordingly, a given number of boutons that are simultaneously active on the same postsynaptic cell will get a larger share of positive reinforcement than will the same number of asynchronously active boutons. This mechanism might explain a number of peculiar features of innervation, such as the apparent ability of presynaptic axons to resolve individual target cells (see Figure 18). Because all of the synaptic terminals arising from a particular axon are linked by their necessarily synchronous activity, a strongly innervated target cell would progressively encourage the establishment of additional terminals by that axon; weaker innervation by the same axon on a neighboring cell might be withdrawn by way of compensation. The protection from competition afforded by synchronous activity might also be explained in this way. If axons were activated together, then the positive feedback provided by trophic support would not distinguish between them. Immunity to competition on this basis might account for the fact that some neural pathways show little evidence of focused innervation or of the elimination of some initial inputs (see Box A).

Whatever the ultimate merits of these various propositions prove to be, most neurobiologists who think about these problems would probably agree that the phenomenon of competition demands that activity play a special role that involves timing and not simply overall amount.

Synaptic rearrangement and target cell shape

Some target cells in maturity are innervated by a single axon, as in the case of muscle fibers or some autonomic neurons, whereas others are innervated by literally thousands of axons, as is the case for many classes of cells in the central nervous system. This wide range of convergence raises a fundamental question: Why does elimination of inputs sometimes continue until only one axon remains in contact with a target cell, whereas in other instances multiple innervation persists? Part of the answer may be mitigation of competition by synchronous activity of presynaptic axons (see the preceding section); another part of the answer apparently has to do with the shape of the postsynaptic cell.

In autonomic ganglia, an obvious difference between cells that are singly innervated and neurons that remain multiply innervated is their geometry. Thus, mature neurons in the submandibular ganglion (which are singly innervated) lack dendrites altogether, whereas neurons in the mammalian superior cervical ganglion (which are multiply innervated) have a number of different dendrites (Purves, 1975; Njå and Purves, 1977a; Lichtman, 1977).

The relation between target cell shape and number of inputs has been explored in greatest detail in the rabbit ciliary ganglion in which the cells display both a range of geometries and a range of inputs (Johnson and Purves, 1981, 1983). Those ciliary ganglion cells that in maturity are innervated by a single axon usually lack dendrites altogether (as do submandibular ganglion cells). Conversely, ciliary ganglion cells innervated in maturity by more than one axon have geometries that increase in complexity in proportion to the number of innervating axons (Figure 20) (Purves and Hume, 1981). A similar relationship has been described in sympathetic ganglia (Purves and Lichtman, 1983). All this suggests a fundamental relationship between the number of inputs a neuron receives and its shape.

This correlation between geometry and inputs is not apparent early in development. Even though all rabbit ciliary ganglion cells are multiply innervated at birth (see Figure 7), their geometry shows the same range of complexity as seen in the adult: some cells lack dendrites altogether, other cells have modest dendritic arborizations and still others have arborizations as complex as the dendritic trees in mature ganglia (Figure 20) (Hume and Purves, 1981). Apparently the confinement of an initial set of inputs to a limited postsynaptic surface (the cell body) forces a resolution in which synaptic contacts from only one axon can survive. Conversely, the presence of dendrites at an early stage somehow allows innervation by a number of different axons to persist. In the rabbit ciliary ganglion, studies of the distribution of innervation suggest that this immunity is conferred because the presence of dendrites allows inputs from different axons to become segregated to some degree (Figure 21) (Forehand and Purves, 1984). The distribution of inputs on dendritic arbors presumably diminishes the competitive axonal interactions that would occur if the inputs were confined to the

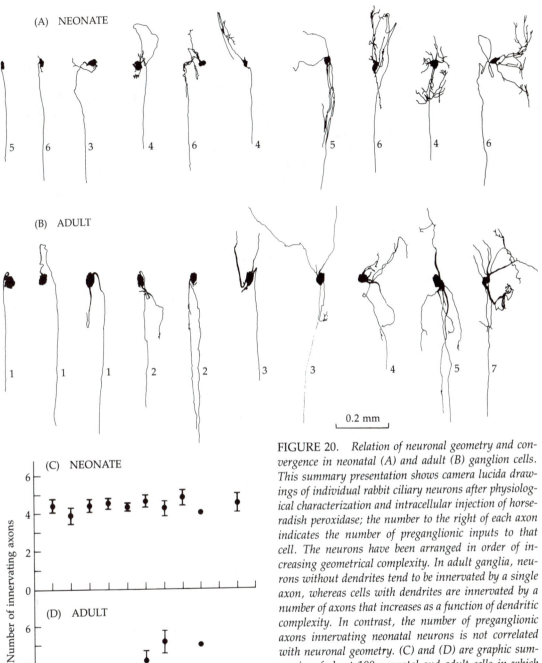

(A) NEONATE

5 6 3 4 6 4 5 6 4 6

(B) ADULT

1 1 1 2 2 3 3 4 5 7

0.2 mm

(C) NEONATE

(D) ADULT

Number of innervating axons

Number of primary dendrites

FIGURE 20.   *Relation of neuronal geometry and convergence in neonatal (A) and adult (B) ganglion cells. This summary presentation shows camera lucida drawings of individual rabbit ciliary neurons after physiological characterization and intracellular injection of horseradish peroxidase; the number to the right of each axon indicates the number of preganglionic inputs to that cell. The neurons have been arranged in order of increasing geometrical complexity. In adult ganglia, neurons without dendrites tend to be innervated by a single axon, whereas cells with dendrites are innervated by a number of axons that increases as a function of dendritic complexity. In contrast, the number of preganglionic axons innervating neonatal neurons is not correlated with neuronal geometry. (C) and (D) are graphic summaries of about 100 neonatal and adult cells in which the number of primary dendrites was used as a simple measure of ganglion cell complexity. Bars indicate standard errors. A strong correlation between geometry and inputs is evident in adults but not in neonates. Evidently, the presence of dendrites mitigates the competitive elimination of some initial inputs. (After Purves and Hume, 1981; Hume and Purves, 1981.)*

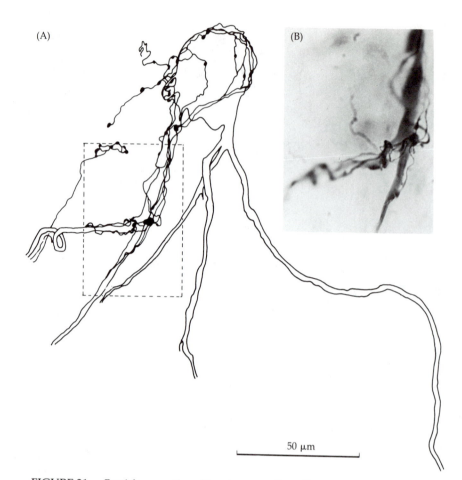

(A)

(B)

50 μm

FIGURE 21. *Partial segregation of inputs on ganglion cells with dendrites. (A) Camera lucida drawing of the apportionment of a single HRP-labeled preganglionic axon on a labeled rabbit ciliary ganglion cell (50-μm section). The presynaptic axon is related to only one of the several dendrites arising from the ganglion cell. (B) Photomicrograph of the boxed region in A. The restriction of the terminals of particular axons to a portion of the postsynaptic surface suggests that spatial separation of competing inputs is important in the maintenance of multiple innervation on these neurons. (From Forehand and Purves, 1984.)*

limited arena of the target cell body (Hume and Purves, 1981, 1983; Purves, 1983; Forehand and Purves, 1984).

Muscle fibers may also retain multiple innervation by increasing the postsynaptic surface available for innervation, albeit in a somewhat different way. Multiple innervation is characteristic of slow (tonic) fibers, on which synaptic sites occur at intervals along the fiber length (Ginsborg and MacKay, 1960; Gordon et al., 1974; Bennett and Pettigrew, 1976). Larger twitch muscle fibers also have two or even three endplates distributed in a proportional way along the fiber length, as if observing a rule of minimum separation (Figure 22) (Nudell and Grinnell, 1983; see also Chapter 9). Evidently, it is not the distance between endplates that is important but the distance between sites of innervation *on a particular cell*; thus, endplates can be virtually contiguous if they are on two adjacent muscle fibers, whereas along an individual muscle fiber they are usually separated by some minimum distance. Experiments on the reinnervation of muscle fibers also indicate a rule of minimum separation; when axons from two different nerves are introduced to a denervated muscle, endplates seldom persist on the same fiber closer than about a millimeter from one another (Kuffler et al., 1977; Grinnell et al., 1979).

The distribution of multiple innervation on muscle fibers, together with the observation that multiple innervation persists on neurons with dendrites, indicates that the arrangement of potentially competing inputs on the surface of postsynaptic cells is another important determinant of the final pattern of innervation. In spite of this general conclusion, comparison of muscle fibers and nerve cells is, in this respect, difficult. A muscle fiber innervated at a solitary endplate site appears to be analogous to a neuron without dendrites: in both cases the innervated surface is sharply limited and all of the synaptic boutons must ultimately be derived from a single axon (note that the axon is analogous to the extrajunctional membrane of a muscle fiber; see Figure 9). Although the rules that govern the single innervation at such sites (endplates or adendritic cell bodies) are not yet understood, it seems likely they will be much the same for nerve cells and muscle cells. The addition of dendrites to nerve cells, which allows multiple innervation to persist, has no obvious analogy in muscle and presumably introduces a new set of rules.

A general rule may be that to achieve multiple innervation, competitive interactions between axons innervating the same target cell must be reduced; conversely, to achieve potent innervation from a given axon (in the limit, innervation derived solely from one axon), competition between axons must be relatively intense. Varying postsynaptic geometry is apparently one way of modulating this intensity.

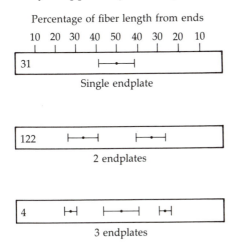

FIGURE 22. *Distribution of multiple endplate sites on twitch muscle fibers. This graph summarizes the average endplate position ($\pm$ the standard deviation) as a percentage of the total length of toad pectoralis fibers innervated by one, two, or three motor nerve terminals. Fibers innervated at a single site tend to have an endplate in the midregion of the fiber; fibers innervated at multiple sites tend to have endplates that are separated by at least 20 percent of the fiber length (1–2 mm). These latter fibers were in general larger than the singly innervated fibers. Numbers in bars indicate sample size. (After Nudell and Grinnell, 1983.)*

Synaptic rearrangements in early life occur in many parts of the nervous system. Although the diversity of these phenomena in muscle, autonomic ganglia, and the central nervous system make any simple summation difficult, in many instances these gradual rearrangements seem aimed at achieving an appropriate degree of convergence and divergence. During this process, individual target cells become innervated by the right number of axons (and synapses), and axons form neural units of an appropriate size and distribution.

The force driving many of these synaptic reorganizations is evidently competition between axons for trophic support. Just as neurons compete for survival (Chapter 6), so, in a more subtle way, do their terminals vie with one another for local maintenance. More specifically, the object of competition is probably a trophic factor supplied by the target cell, although the arguments for this idea remain largely circumstantial.

At least three influences modulate competition between axon terminals in the course of development: the availability of specific trophic agents to which different classes of axons respond, the level and temporal pattern of neural activity among competing axons, and the geometrical complexity of the target cells. The immense range of convergence, synaptic strength, and neural unit configuration in the nervous system is probably generated by varying the proportions of these several influences.

Maintenance and Modifiability of Synapses

INTRODUCTION

The ability of higher animals to modify their behavior as a result of experience (to learn) implies that the nervous system changes continually throughout life. It is thus difficult to define the point at which neural development ends (if indeed it ever does). Most neurobiologists presume (reasonably enough) that synapses are the most likely site for changes underlying learning. Thus, a great deal of attention has been paid to the ways in which mature synapses may be modified. In this chapter we consider two general ideas about synaptic change: (1) that synaptic connections are made and broken throughout life, and (2) that the efficacy of individual synapses is modified. The relative importance of these strategies for altering behavior is not yet clear.

MODIFICATION OF SYNAPTIC CONNECTIONS

Several lines of evidence indicate that the pattern of connectivity achieved during development is a balance between forces that induce synapse formation and forces that promote synapse withdrawal. Support for this view comes, on the one hand, from observations that indicate that neurons can continue to form new synaptic connections throughout life, and, on the other hand, from the observation that neurons also can relinquish synaptic connections. The implication of these facts is that synaptic connections, once formed, must be actively maintained.

Sprouting of axon terminals and the formation of novel synaptic connections

Evidence for the persistent ability of axon terminals to form new connections comes mainly from studies of axonal sprouting. Sprouting is defined as the ability of intact nerves to respond to any one of several stimuli by forming new terminal branches and, in many cases, new synaptic contacts.

The most thoroughly studied stimulus for axonal sprouting is partial denervation of target tissues (Figures 1–3). If a portion of the innervation

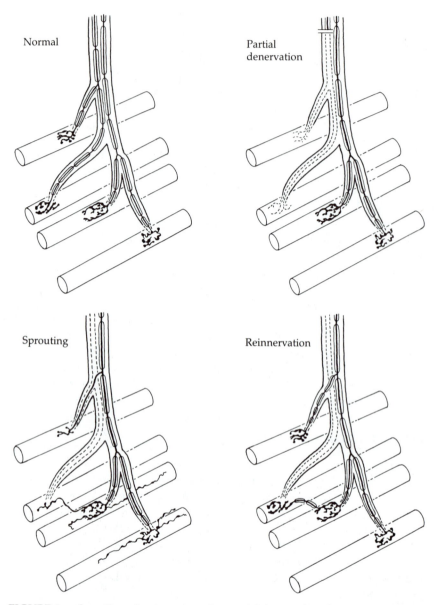

FIGURE 1. *Sprouting of motor axons after partial denervation of mammalian skeletal muscle. Several days after cutting part of a motor nerve, sprouts emerge from intact endings (and nodes of Ranvier) and appear to seek out endplate sites on the denervated muscle fibers. One to two months later, the sprouts that have found denervated endplates are retained, whereas unsuccessful sprouts disappear. (From Brown et al., 1981.)*

to a neural target is destroyed, the remaining axon terminals will proliferate and often will form new synapses with the denervated target cells. This sequence of events has been observed for the motor innervation of skeletal muscle (Edds, 1953; Brown et al., 1981b), preganglionic innervation of autonomic ganglia (Murray and Thompson, 1957; Court-

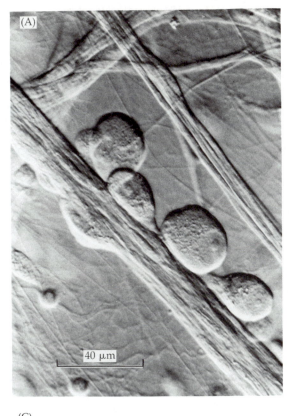

(A)

40 μm

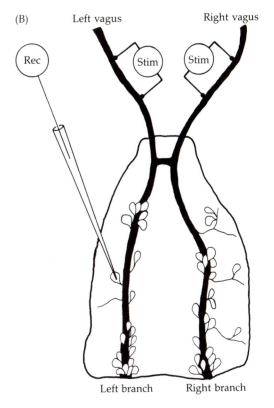

(B)

Left vagus

Right vagus

Rec

Stim

Stim

Left branch

Right branch

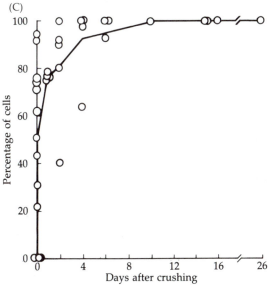

(C)

Percentage of cells

Days after crushing

FIGURE 2. *Sprouting after partial denervation of parasympathetic neurons in the frog heart. (A) Photomicrograph of parasympathetic ganglion cells in the atrial septum (Nomarski optics). (B) Diagram of the interatrial septum and the arrangement of ganglion cells along the branches of the two vagus nerves. The ganglion can be partially denervated by interrupting one of the vagus nerves near its exit from the skull. (C) Innervation of ganglion cells at various times after crushing the left vagus nerve; innervation of neurons was determined by intracellular recording during nerve stimulation as shown in B. Whereas about half the cells in normal ganglia are innervated by the right vagus nerve, within a month after cutting the left nerve virtually all of the cells become innervated by the remaining (intact) nerve. Each symbol represents impalements of 20–30 cells. (A from Roper and Ko, 1978; B,C after Courtney and Roper, 1976.)*

ney and Roper, 1976; Roper and Ko, 1978; Maehlen and Njå, 1981), sensory projections within the spinal cord (Liu and Chambers, 1958), and axonal projections within the brain (Raisman, 1969; Raisman and Field, 1973; Cotman and Nadler, 1978; Tsukahara, 1981; Cotman et al.,

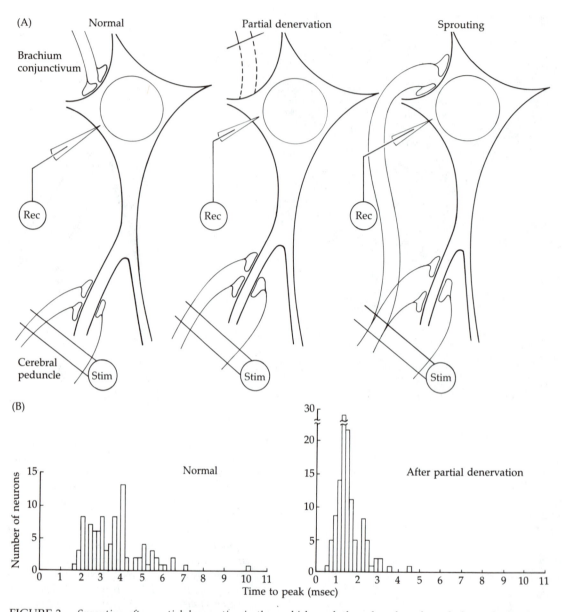

FIGURE 3. *Sprouting after partial denervation in the central nervous system. (A) Because the central nervous system is more complex than muscle or peripheral ganglia, the evidence for sprouting is necessarily less direct. This figure shows the approach to the problem taken by R. Tsukahara and his colleagues in the mammalian brain stem. In these experiments, cells of the red nucleus were partially denervated by cutting the brachium conjunctivum. Within a few weeks fibers from the cerebrum, which reach the red nucleus through the cerebral peduncle, apparently sprout and form new synapses. (B) The evidence for sprouting is that the time to peak of peduncular postsynaptic potentials recorded with an intracellular microelectrode decreases substantially during this period, thereby suggesting that inputs from these fibers (which normally innervate dendritic processes) have sprouted to innervate the cell body as well. (After Tsukahara, 1978.)*

1981). Sprouting of sensory innervation in skin also occurs in response to partial denervation, although synaptic connections are of course not involved in this instance (Diamond and Jackson, 1980; Blackshaw et al., 1982).

Partial denervation is not the only way to induce renewed growth of axon terminals and new synaptic connections: in muscles, sprouting also occurs when neuromuscular transmission is interrupted. Muscles can be paralyzed by local injection of strong neuromuscular blocking agents such as botulinum toxin or α-bungarotoxin (Duchen and Strich, 1968; Holland and Brown, 1980). In these experiments, motor nerve sprouting is apparent within a few days of introducing these irreversible blockers (Figure 4). Similarly, sprouting occurs when muscles are paralyzed by chronic local nerve block (Brown and Ironton, 1977). In this case, neuromuscular block is achieved by a silastic cuff impregnated with tetrodotoxin applied to the motor nerve for several days. This local anesthetic impedes the transmission of nerve impulses but has no ob-

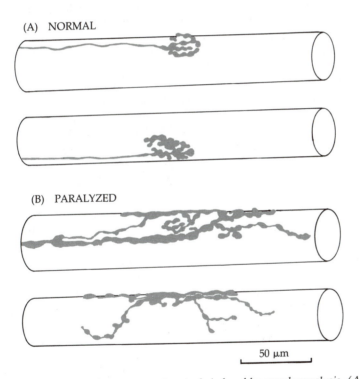

(A) NORMAL

(B) PARALYZED

50 μm

FIGURE 4. *Sprouting of motor nerve terminals induced by muscle paralysis. (A) Two normal endplates in a mouse soleus muscle stained with the zinc iodide–osmium technique. (B) Two endplates from a muscle treated for 7 days with daily local injections of the neuromuscular blocking agent α-bungarotoxin; the presynaptic terminals show extensive sprouting (cf. Figure 1). Tracings were made from the original photomicrograph for the sake of clarity. (After Holland and Brown, 1980.)*

vious effect on axonal transport. When the blocked motor nerve terminals are evaluated anatomically with the zinc iodide–osmium method, they are found to be more complex and longer than the terminals in control muscles.

Still another stimulus to motor neuron sprouting is irritation of the muscle fiber surface by one of a variety of exogenous agents ranging from egg albumin to pieces of dead nerve or even a fine thread applied to the muscle surface (Hoffman, 1951; Jones and Vrbová, 1974). These peculiar findings suggest that agents that induce local inflammation, including the products of nerve degeneration, also stimulate sprouting. Confirmation of this comes from the observation that when the sensory nerves to muscles are caused to degenerate by dorsal root transection— a procedure that can be done without compromising the integrity or function of the corresponding motor nerve—sprouting of motor nerve terminals is apparent (Brown et al., 1978).

Finally, sprouting of a given cutaneous nerve can be induced by blocking axoplasmic transport in the nerves innervating adjacent skin (Aguilar et al., 1973; Diamond et al., 1976). In these experiments, rather than blocking nerve conduction with local anesthetic, axoplasmic transport is blocked with colchicine (Figure 5). Sprouting of cutaneous nerves into the territory of the treated nerve indicates that some aspect of intact axoplasmic transport is needed to maintain a balance between neighboring cutaneous fields. J. Diamond and his collaborators have interpreted this effect as a response to loss of an inhibitory agent secreted by the colchicine-treated nerve; in the normal course of events this agent is supposed to neutralize a sprouting factor secreted by the skin (Diamond et al., 1976). In this view, then, the balance of cutaneous fields is maintained by a mutual inhibition of adjacent nerves mediated through the target. A somewhat different interpretation of this result is that interference with axoplasmic transport prevents the uptake of a target-secreted agent that would then become available to adjacent nerves and cause them to sprout.

How can such a wide spectrum of sprouting stimuli be explained? One possibility is that the common denominator of sprouting is a trophic agent supplied by postsynaptic cells. The gist of this idea is that when target cells are denervated they continue to secrete (or perhaps even increase their secretion of) a trophic agent normally produced to *maintain* innervation (Purves, 1977; see also Brown et al., 1981). Whereas this agent would normally be taken up (or its secretion inhibited) by the full complement of innervating axons, following partial denervation an excess of the agent becomes available and remaining intact axons therefore sprout. This notion is consistent with what is known of the trophic dependence of sympathetic and sensory nerve terminals on nerve growth factor. For example, nerve growth factor acts locally on neurites to regulate their growth and retraction (Chapter 7). Moreover, NGF-secreting targets, when implanted into the anterior chamber of the eye, cause sprouting of sympathetic postganglionic fibers in the iris (Olson and Malmfors, 1970). It is not difficult to imagine, therefore,

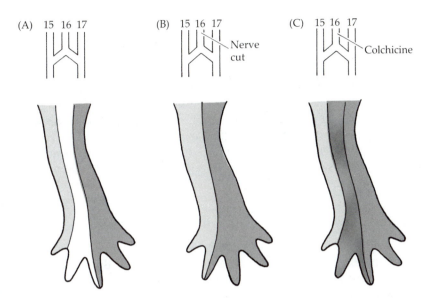

FIGURE 5. *Sprouting of cutaneous nerves in the salamander hind limb after pharmacological blockade of axoplasmic transport. (A) Control limb showing the typical arrangement of cutaneous innervation by spinal nerves 15, 16, and 17 determined electrophysiologically; the territories supplied by spinal nerves 15 and 17 do not normally meet. (B) An experimental limb in which nerve 16 was cut several weeks earlier; the territories innervated by nerves 15 and 17 have expanded to innervate the territory usually supplied by nerve 16. (C) Experimental limb in which nerve 16 was treated with colchicine to block axoplasmic transport; the grey area indicates expansion of the territory supplied by 15 and 17, as in B. Note, however, that nerve 16 remains intact. (After Diamond et al., 1976.)*

that target-derived agents similar in function to NGF but operating in other parts of the nervous system cause the sprouting that follows partial denervation (see, for example, Gurney, 1984). By extension from what is known about NGF, the stimulating effects of postsynaptic paralysis and of blocked axonal transport might arise from a net increase in the amount of available trophic factor due to the increased secretion and/or decreased uptake of a putative chemical signal.

Even if a superabundance of trophic factor is the major cause of nerve sprouting, other more subtle influences are almost certainly involved. For example, Diamond and his co-workers have found that sensory axons in the cutaneous nerves of rats and salamanders sprout more vigorously within their own dermatomes than they do in adjacent ones (Diamond et al., 1976; Jackson and Diamond, 1980; MacIntyre and Diamond, 1981; Diamond, 1982). This finding suggests that sprouting is also influenced by appropriate position. A further observation is that terminals subserving different sensory modalities sprout independently. Thus, in leech skin, sensory terminals sprout only if their homologues are removed (Blackshaw et al., 1982); this result implies that different sensory modalities are sensitive to different sprouting factors (see also

Kramer and Kuwada, 1983). Finally, G. E. Schneider (1973) has shown that removing some of an axon's branches causes reactive sprouting in the rest of its arborization, a phenomenon referred to as the "pruning effect." For instance, if the retinal projection to the upper layers of the superior colliculus is destroyed in newborn hamsters, abnormal retinal projections are subsequently found at a number of sites in the brain. In general, the greater the destruction of the normal projection, the more extensive the abnormal projection (Schneider, 1973). This observation suggests that, in addition to exogenous sprouting stimuli, neurons also respond to intrinsic signals, which impel them to extend arbors of a particular size (see also Chapter 12).

Retraction of synaptic connections in the adult nervous system

Another quite different body of evidence indicates that terminal arborizations are also capable of contracting in maturity, thus providing additional support for the idea that synaptic connections must be actively maintained. Since the work of G. H. Acheson and his collaborators in the 1940s, it has been known that cutting the axon of a nerve cell causes a reduction in the efficacy of synaptic transmission onto the injured cell (Figure 6) (Acheson et al., 1942). A number of studies have shown that this involves retraction of terminal arborizations. For example, if the axons linking sympathetic ganglion cells and their peripheral targets are interrupted, most of the synaptic contacts made on ganglion cells by preganglionic axons are withdrawn (Figure 7) (Matthews and Nelson, 1975; Purves, 1975, 1976; see also Purves and Njå, 1978). When ganglion cell axons regenerate, the preganglionic contacts on the ganglion cells are restored. When, on the other hand, peripheral regeneration is prevented (by chronic ligation, for example), then the synapses normally present on ganglion cells are not reestablished (Purves, 1975). This retrograde influence of axon interruption on the synapses contacting the injured neurons is not limited to sympathetic

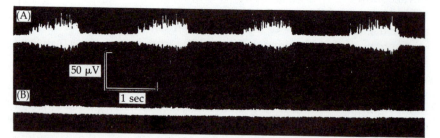

FIGURE 6.   *Depression of respiratory discharge recorded from the proximal portion of a cat phrenic nerve after section close to the diaphragm 15 days earlier. (A) Discharge recorded from the normal phrenic nerve. (B) Discharge from the proximal stump of the cut phrenic nerve. These records provided the first evidence of depressed transmission onto neurons after interruption of their connections to targets. (From Acheson et al., 1942.)*

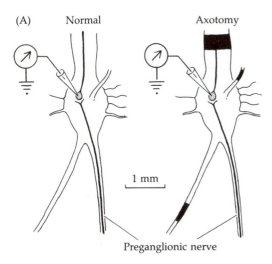

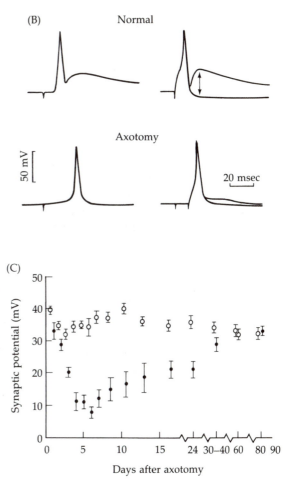

FIGURE 7. *Loss of preganglionic synapses after post-ganglionic axotomy. (A) Diagram of normal guinea pig superior cervical ganglion (left) and an experimental ganglion (right) in which the three major postganglionic nerves were crushed. (B) Intracellular recordings from a normal neuron (upper two records) and from a neuron 6 days after axotomy (lower two records). The synaptic potential (indicated by the arrow) is measured in the refractory period of an action potential that is elicited directly by current injection. The response is markedly reduced after postganglionic axon interruption. (C) Time course of the development of, and recovery from, synaptic depression after axotomy. Filled circles represent the average amplitudes of synaptic responses after postganglionic axotomy; open circles are responses from control neurons in contralateral ganglia. Recovery corresponds with the approximate time course of axon regeneration to peripheral targets. Bars show standard errors of determinations in 5–28 neurons. (After Purves, 1975.)*

ganglion cells. Synapse loss after axotomy also occurs in parasympathetic ganglia (Brenner and Johnson, 1976), in the spinal cord (Downman et al., 1953; Eccles et al., 1958; Kuno and Llinás, 1970; Mendell et al., 1976), and in brain stem nuclei (Blinzinger and Kreutzberg, 1968; Sumner and Sutherland, 1973; Watson, 1974; Sumner, 1975, 1976). Thus, at least for nerve cells with axons that can be cut easily (i.e., those that send their axons over substantial distances), the loss of synapses from the surfaces of the injured neurons after axon interruption appears to be a general rule.

The mechanism of synapse loss after axotomy seems to be based on a signal that reaches the cell by retrograde transport. When axoplasmic transport in sympathetic axons is interrupted by colchicine application, synapse loss and the other phenomena that follow the surgical interruption of axons are still seen (Pilar and Landmesser, 1972; Watson, 1974; Purves, 1976). Because axon section requires the nerve cell to regenerate its distal part whereas colchicine leaves axons intact, this experiment distinguishes between the effects of injury as such and the interruption of a peripherally derived message.

Further experiments in mammalian sympathetic ganglia suggest that the retrograde signal may involve nerve growth factor. Thus, when exogenous nerve growth factor is supplied locally to sympathetic ganglion cells following axotomy, many of the synapses that would otherwise have been lost are spared (Njå and Purves, 1978a; see also Schäfer et al., 1983). Conversely, when adult animals are treated for several days with a course of antiserum to nerve growth factor, substantial synapse loss from the surfaces of sympathetic ganglion cells is induced, even though their axons have not been cut. Because nerve growth factor is peripherally acquired by sympathetic neurons and retrogradely transported to sympathetic ganglia (Chapter 7), these experiments argue that a component of the signal operating between the periphery and the ganglion cells is this protein or a second messenger induced by it.

One explanation of these observations is that when a neuron's connection with its target is interrupted, a cascade effect is initiated: in response to the disappearance of a peripheral signal such as NGF, the ability of the injured neuron to attract and maintain its own innervation (perhaps by the secretion of a second trophic factor) is temporarily inhibited. When peripheral connectivity is restored, normal signaling is resumed and synapses are regained.

In this respect the loss of synapses after axotomy may be closely related to sprouting; indeed, these two processes may be two sides of the same coin. Increasing the availability of the signals underlying synaptic maintenance induces axon terminals to proliferate and establish new synaptic connections, whereas a reduction or loss of these signals causes retraction of axon terminals. This view postulates the persistence in the adult nervous system of the trophic dependencies that are obvious at early developmental stages.

Balance between sprouting and retraction

Observations on the retraction of synaptic fields during the reinnervation of targets provide direct evidence for a balance between the forces of synaptogenesis and retraction. The fate of sprouts competing with regenerating axons in mammalian autonomic ganglia was investigated by L. Guth and J. J. Bernstein (1961; see also Murray and Thompson, 1957) and more recently by J. Maehlen and A. Njå (1981; 1984). In Guth and Bernstein's work, the upper thoracic ventral roots supplying about 90 percent of the innervation to the superior cervical ganglion were crushed and allowed to regenerate. Six weeks later the remaining lower thoracic segments activated an abnormally wide spectrum of end organ responses, indicating extensive sprouting. Six months after this operation, however, the usual end organ responses to ventral root stimulation had been largely restored (see Chapter 10). Thus, most of the synapses formed by sprouting were suppressed or displaced by the regenerating axons. Maehlen and Njå carried out a more detailed study after partial denervation using intracellular recording. They confirmed that the sprouted connections are displaced when the ganglion is reinnervated (Maehlen and Njå, 1984).

Displacement of terminal sprouts during regeneration has also been described in a parasympathetic ganglion in the frog heart. This preparation is particularly convenient for such studies because the ganglion is innervated by both vagus nerves (see Figure 2); thus partial denervation and sprouting can be induced by cutting one of the nerves (Roper, 1976). S. Roper and C.-P. Ko (1978) found that as the cut vagal fibers regenerated, the proportion of ganglion cells that were innervated by sprouts from the intact nerve declined. A further experiment in this same preparation was carried out by P. B. Sargent and M. J. Dennis (1977). The atrium was chronically denervated by resecting both vagus nerves, a procedure that induces the formation of collateral connections between ganglion cells. Such intrinsic connections do not normally occur in this ganglion, although they are present in some other autonomic ganglia. On regeneration of the vagus nerves, the synapses formed between the denervated neurons were progressively lost (Sargent and Dennis, 1981). A similar retraction of sprouts occurs during reinnervation of muscle (Chapter 10; see also McArdle, 1975; Gorio et al., 1983). Such displacements of synapses during regeneration probably represent the competitive redress of an imbalance in the synaptic fields of the sprouted and regenerating fibers.

The fact that the terminal arborizations of axons can either extend or contract throughout life argues that the forces that promote synapse formation and the forces that induce synapse withdrawal are normally poised in a delicate balance.

Normal modification of synaptic connections

If the number of synaptic connections finally attained represents a balance between sprouting and retraction, to what degree is this equilibrium dynamic? The possibility that synapses turn over continually at some steady level in the absence of any experimental manipulation has been raised several times over the years (see, for example, Barker and Ip, 1966; Tuffery, 1971), but this idea has not been widely accepted. As techniques have improved, however, evidence for normal turnover has gradually grown. At the neuromuscular junction some turnover at the level of individual neuromuscular junctions almost certainly occurs (Figure 8) (Wernig et al., 1980a,b, 1981; Mallart et al., 1980; Cardasis and Padykula, 1981; Haimann et al., 1981; Anzil et al., 1984; Bieser and Wernig, 1984; Wernig et al., 1984; see also Pumplin, 1983). In the main, this work has taken advantage of anatomical methods that highlight the detailed geometry of presynaptic and postsynaptic elements in relation to one another. The presynaptic terminal is demonstrated with a silver stain; the postsynaptic element is usually outlined by staining junctional cholinesterase. Using these methods, presynaptic terminals unopposed by a postsynaptic specialization are often seen; this configuration is taken to represent a recently formed nerve sprout that has not yet had time to induce a corresponding postsynaptic specialization. Conversely, postsynaptic specializations unopposed by presynaptic terminals are often found. These configurations are interpreted as sites

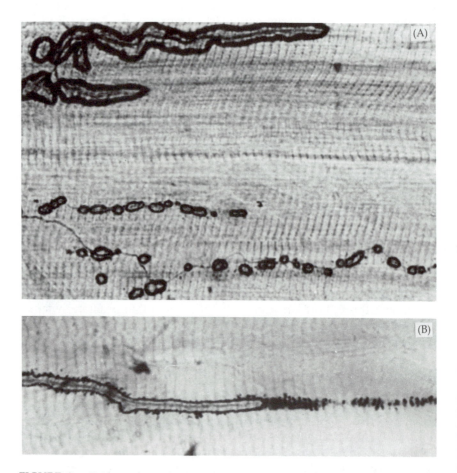

FIGURE 8. *Evidence for synaptic turnover at neuromuscular junctions in normal frogs. (A) Usually, as on the upper fiber, cholinesterase stain completely outlines nerve terminals at the endplates of cutaneous pectoris muscle cells (the nerve is stained by silver impregnation). The presynaptic axon innervating the lower fiber, however, is not opposed by postsynaptic cholinesterase deposits at every point along its course. This discrepancy suggests that portions of this nerve terminal have recently sprouted to occupy this region. (B) At this junction a portion of the postsynaptic specialization (transverse lines of cholinesterase reaction product) lacks a corresponding nerve ending. The presence of postsynaptic cholinesterase unopposed by a corresponding presynaptic terminal suggests that the nerve ending has recently withdrawn from this site. (Courtesy of A. Wernig.)*

recently vacated by regressing nerve terminals at which the postsynaptic specialization has not yet been lost. Because both configurations are evident in normal, adult muscle (Figure 8), these observations argue for some degree of normal synaptic turnover. In accord with this idea, electrophysiological variation in transmission along normal synapses suggests the retraction or extension of portions of the terminal (Haimann et al., 1981; Anzil et al., 1984; Beiser and Wernig, 1984).

Evidence from other parts of the nervous system also argues for some normal synaptic turnover. Degenerating and regenerating autonomic nerve endings have been observed in the ciliary muscle of monkeys (Townes-Anderson and Raviola, 1978) and in other smooth muscles. Fluorescent endings in the human uterus, for example, disappear nearly entirely during pregnancy but gradually return postpartum (Owman, 1981). Finally, some observations suggest that synaptic turnover occurs in the central nervous system. C. Sotelo and S. L. Palay (1971) have described abnormal presynaptic nerve endings in the vestibular system of the rat; these endings contain giant mitochondria, concentric laminar arrays of cisternae, and have decreased numbers of synaptic vesicles. Growth cone-like structures were sometimes seen extending from such terminals. These features are consistent with degenerating and regenerating synapses.

In spite of these various observations, considerable uncertainty about normal turnover will persist until the inferences gleaned from static images can be verified by direct observation.

Modification of synaptic connections in old age

No older person doubts that age alters neural function. Memory loss, diminished speed of reflexes, and other more subtle changes in mentation are almost certainly based in part on modifications of neuronal connections that occur with aging. The most obvious objective finding in the aging nervous system is a progressive decline in neuronal numbers (Ellis, 1920; Brody, 1955; Vijayashankar and Brody, 1979). Other effects are changes in the arrangement and complexity of dendritic arborizations (Figure 9) (Scheibel et al., 1975, 1976, 1977; Hinds and McNelly, 1977; Vaughan, 1977; Mervis, 1978; Weiss and Pysh, 1978; Buell and Coleman, 1979, 1981; Connor et al., 1980) and a net loss of synaptic contacts on surviving neurons in at least some regions (Geinisman, 1979, 1981). Morphological changes also occur at individual terminals. Thus, neuromuscular junctions in senescent rodents show more terminal branching and a greater number of terminal boutons (Figure 10) (Pestronk et al., 1980; Smith and Rosenheimer, 1982; Fahim et al., 1983; Banker et al., 1983; see also Courtney and Steinbach, 1981; Fahim and Robbins, 1982). In spite of this increased complexity, aged neuromuscular junctions are more easily depressed, contain fewer synaptic vesicles, and are less capable of sprouting (Smith, 1979; Fahim and Robbins, 1982; see also Kelly and Robbins, 1983).

Some of these changes in the senescent nervous system may rep-

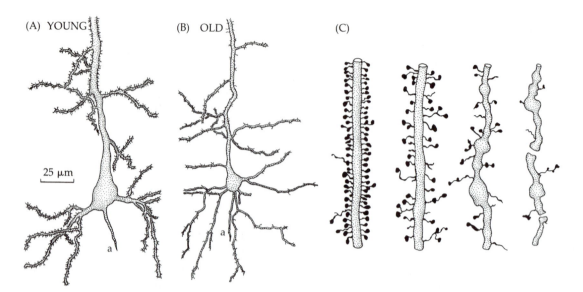

FIGURE 9. *Changes in neuronal structure with age. (A) Camera lucida drawing of a Golgi-impregnated, layer V pyramidal cell from area 17 of a 3-month-old rat. (B) Similar neuron from a 34-month-old (senile) rat. Neurons from this region of senescent animals are generally smaller and have diminished numbers of syn-* *aptic spines. a, Axon. (C) Progressive changes (left to right) in the detailed appearance of cortical dendrites in aging humans. Based on Golgi impregnations; drawn at ×1250. (A,B after Peters and Vaughan, 1981; C after Scheibel, 1982.)*

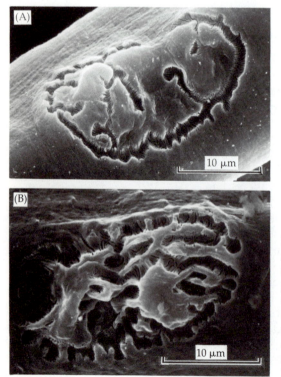

FIGURE 10. *Changes in the structure of the mammalian neuromuscular junction with age. (A) Scanning electron micrograph of motor endplate on mouse muscle fiber from a normal adult (7 months old). The motor nerve terminal has been removed from the muscle surface by enzyme treatment to reveal the underlying endplate structure. (B) Endplate from a 29-month-old mouse; the endplates in aged animals were typically more complex than endplates in younger animals. (From Fahim et al., 1983.)*

resent further adjustments in the equilibrium that is established during development and maintained throughout most of adult life.

MODIFICATION OF SYNAPTIC EFFICACY

In addition to regulation of the numbers of synaptic contacts mediating various neural circuits, neural connections can also be modified by altering the functional characteristics of existing synapses. It is this aspect of synaptic modification that has attracted most attention as a possible basis for learning.

Changes with use at individual nerve–muscle synapses

An important question explored by B. Katz and his colleagues in the 1950s was how synaptic function changed with use at the neuromuscular junction (Katz, 1969; see Box A). When action potentials in a motor neuron follow each other within a few hundred milliseconds, succeeding impulses produce a progressively larger postsynaptic response (Figure 11A). This effect, called facilitation, is the result of an increase in the amount of transmitter released in response to succeeding action potentials (Del Castillo and Katz, 1954). When the number of acetylcholine packets liberated by each nerve impulse is reduced by lowering the calcium:magnesium ratio, the number of quanta released can be counted directly. Katz and his colleagues found that the facilitated response had a larger quantal content than the initial postsynaptic potential. The increased transmitter release is probably the result of an accumulation of calcium in the presynaptic terminal during repetitive stimulation. Katz and R. Miledi (1968) corroborated the importance of calcium by local application of calcium ions to the neuromuscular junction in a calcium-deficient bath. They found that unless calcium was present at the time of the first impulse, the second postsynaptic response was not facilitated (see also Zucker, 1982).

When action potentials occur in a train over a period of a few minutes, a further aspect of synaptic change with use is evident. Although the first few impulses are facilitated, the synaptic response eventually begins to decrease in amplitude and can become very small (Figure 11B) (Del Castillo and Katz, 1954). This phenomenon, called depression, is also a presynaptic effect and has the interesting property of wearing off very slowly. Although the exact mechanism of depression is unclear, it probably represents an actual (or effective) depletion of synaptic vesicles at release sites.

When repetitive activation of the neuromuscular junction ceases, still another phenomenon is revealed: post-tetanic potentiation (Figure 12) (Hutter, 1952; Del Castillo and Katz, 1954). As this phrase implies, within a short time after a train of impulses (a "tetanus"), the release of transmitter is actually increased beyond normal. The effect is again presynaptic, i.e., the quantal content of the post-tetanic response is increased (Del Castillo and Katz, 1954; Liley, 1956); in fact, the effect

FIGURE 11. *Changes in the efficacy of synaptic transmission induced by repetitive activity at chemical synapses. (A) At many synapses, when one action potential closely follows another, the second postsynaptic response is enhanced. This is called facilitation. In this example, facilitation is shown at the crayfish neuromuscular junction; during repetitive stimulation of the excitatory axon supplying the muscle, the amplitude of the response grows progressively in a frequency-dependent manner. (B) With longer periods of repetitive firing, depression occurs. This graph shows the magnitude of depression, and the slow time course of recovery, at the frog neuromuscular junction following 4 minutes of stimulation at 5 Hz (shaded bar on abscissa). (A after Dudel and Kuffler, 1961; B after Del Castillo and Katz, 1954.)*

(A) FACILITATION

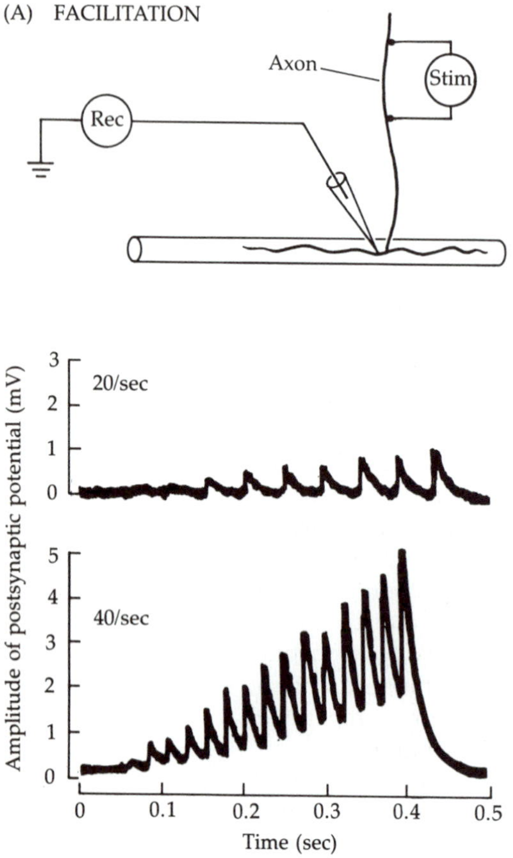

(B) DEPRESSION

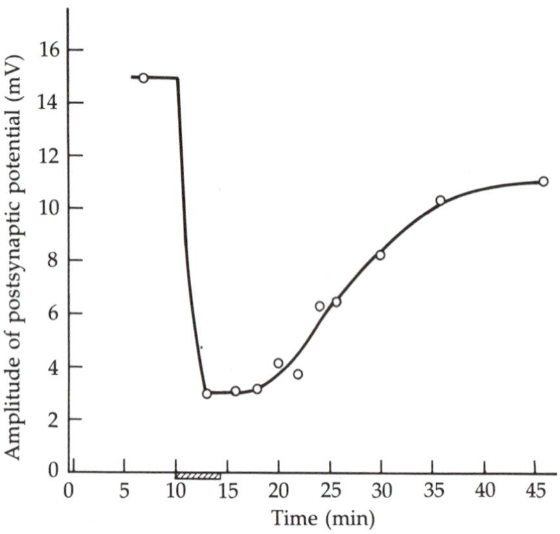

builds up during repetitive activation but is obscured by the superimposed depression (Magleby, 1973). Post-tetanic potentiation also depends in part on calcium and, in this respect, presumably involves either an increase in the availability of intracellular free calcium or in the availability of releasable vesicles in the presynaptic terminal (Rosenthal, 1969; Weinreich, 1971). Sodium ions, however, are also involved in post-tetanic potentiation at the neuromuscular junction; thus depolarization in the absence of Na^+ entry does not produce a normal degree of potentiation (Rahamimoff et al., 1980; Lev-Tov and Rahamimoff, 1980).

Although different classes of chemical synapses show differences in their functional response to use, the phenomena of facilitation, depression, and post-tetanic potentiation are commonly observed. In spite of the considerable gap between the time course of these relatively brief changes with use and the time course of the acquisition (or loss) of learned behavior, these functional changes provide reasonable grounds for exploring changes in the efficacy of individual synapses as a potential basis of learning. It should be emphasized, however, that the behavioral significance of facilitation, depression, or post-tetanic potentiation in most situations in which they have been studied is entirely unclear. The importance of these phenomena in the present context is that they have provided the basis for interpretation of more recent work aimed at establishing directly the nature of synaptic change in reflex pathways subserving a behavior that is modified for long periods.

Modification of central synaptic function in invertebrates

In the 1950s and 1960s, a number of neurobiologists were attracted by the idea of studying synaptic modification in relatively simple invertebrate nervous systems. The rationale behind this approach is indeed appealing (Krasne, 1976; Kandel, 1976). The neural basis for even the simplest reflex in a mammal (or other vertebrates) involves hundreds or thousands of cells that are often inaccessible and difficult to keep alive in isolation for any significant length of time. Invertebrates, on the other hand, have vastly simpler nervous systems in which one or a few readily identified cells often subserve the sensory or motor linkage of a reflex behavior. In the situation provided by such quantitatively simpler nervous systems, one can study directly changes associated with learning.

The animal that has been used to best advantage in this project is the sea hare, *Aplysia californica*. Like many other invertebrates, *Aplysia* has a relatively small nervous system, comprising about 20,000 neurons.

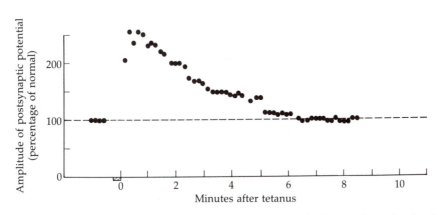

FIGURE 12. *Testing the efficacy of transmission before and after a prolonged train of impulses (a "tetanus") reveals a further modification at many synapses: the response after the train is enhanced. This is called post-tetanic potentiation. In this example, the increase in amplitude of the endplate potential at the rat neuromuscular junction is plotted as a function of time after a train of high-frequency stimuli (200 Hz) for 15 seconds (shaded bar at* t *= 0). (After Liley, 1956.)*

Bernard Katz (b. 1911)

Bernard Katz was born in Leipzig, Germany, where he received his M.D. degree from the University of Leipzig in 1934. Shortly thereafter he emigrated to England, where he studied under A. V. Hill at University College London, receiving his Ph.D. there in 1938. Katz then moved to Australia as a Carnegie Research Fellow to work in J. C. Eccles' laboratory in Sydney. The entry of Japan into the war in 1942 interrupted Katz's research with Eccles (and S. W. Kuffler); from 1942 until 1945 he served as a radar expert with the Royal Air Force in the Pacific. After the war, Katz returned to University College, where he became head of the biophysics department upon A. V. Hill's retirement in 1952, a position he held until 1975.

If Kuffler's style was eclectic (see Box C in Chapter 8), then Katz is surely the counterexample of the scientist who pursues an important problem with undiminished vigor throughout an entire career. Although Katz made outstanding contributions with A. L. Hodgkin and A. F. Huxley to understanding the ionic basis of the action potential, in the late 1940s he turned his attention nearly exclusively to the mechanism of chemical synaptic transmission at the neuromuscular junction. Using this simple preparation he and his colleagues proceeded, over a period of some 30 years, to answer most of the fundamental questions about the physiology of chemical synapses; the answers led to the modern view that transmitter agents are released in quantal packets that correspond to synaptic vesicles. Of particular importance for the present chapter was Katz' proposal and verification of the so-called calcium hypothesis, the view that an influx of calcium into the presynaptic terminal is the link between action potential depolarization and transmitter release (Katz, 1969). Most current theories of synaptic modulation involve regulation of this calcium entry.

The cells are clustered into well-defined ganglia, and within each ganglion many of the cells can be identified from animal to animal because of their large size and distinctive position (see Figure 14). Indeed, some of the nerve cells in *Aplysia* are among the largest neurons known, measuring up to a millimeter in diameter. Work on the neural basis of learning in *Aplysia* has been carried out over a period of about 20 years now by E. R. Kandel and his colleagues, who have focused their attention on the abdominal ganglion of the animal (Kandel, 1979a,b,c). The attractive feature of this ganglion is its role in mediating the central connections of several reflexes.

The reflex that has been studied in most detail is gill withdrawal, a defensive response in which the gill is rapidly retracted when it (or a nearby structure) is touched (Figure 13). The gill withdrawal reflex exhibits a common behavioral modification called habituation, defined as the gradual decrease of a response when it is elicited repeatedly. Habituation presumably allows animals to ignore stimuli that *might* be significant but, in fact, are ongoing and innocuous. As D. H. Hubel

When Katz began to work on the neuro-muscular junction, it was generally accepted that calcium was essential for neuromuscular transmission. In the 1960s Katz and R. Miledi, who succeeded Katz in 1975 as the head of the biophysics department at University College, examined the detailed role of Ca^{2+} in transmitter release. A first step was the demonstration that calcium is needed at the endplate site itself and that it must be present just before the moment of depolarization (Katz and Miledi, 1967a). Katz and Miledi then went on to show that calcium entry is a prerequisite for transmitter release by demonstrating that when the terminal membrane is held at the equilibrium potential for calcium (thereby precluding Ca^{2+} entry), transmitter release fails (Katz and Miledi, 1967b; see also Katz and Miledi, 1969). Subsequently, Miledi (1973) showed that the injection of calcium directly into a nerve terminal enhances transmitter release. An excellent summary of most of these experiments is found in Katz's Sherrington Lectures and the accompanying commentary in 1968 (Katz, 1969). In 1970 Katz received the Nobel prize in physiology and medicine for his work on syn-

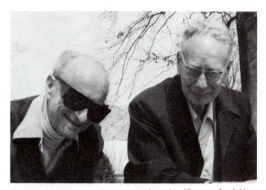

Bernard Katz (right) and Stephen Kuffler at the Missouri Botanical Garden in St. Louis in 1980. (Courtesy of D. A. Johnson.)

aptic transmission. (The award was shared with J. C. Eccles and U. von Euler.)

Although the calcium hypothesis is now taken for granted, there were moments of doubt. Some flavor of the opposition to Katz's views and an example of his consummate ability to demolish false prophets can be found in his review of D. Nachmanson's book, *The Chemical and Molecular Basis of Nerve Activity* (Katz, 1960).

(1979) put it, imagine the problems that would arise if we were constantly aware that our socks were on. Because habituation is a behavioral phenomenon evident at many phylogenetic levels, the neural basis of this response in *Aplysia* might have general relevance.

As a first step, Kandel and his collaborators identified some of the sensory and motor neurons mediating the gill withdrawal reflex by recording intracellularly from identified ganglion cells (Figure 14) (Pinsker et al., 1970; Kupfermann et al., 1970; Castellucci et al., 1978). They then asked whether changes in the efficacy of the relevant synaptic response might provide an explanation of the habituation of gill withdrawal. With repeated stimulation of the gill, they indeed found that some of the synapses mediating the reflex became depressed. Quantal analysis of this response (which is much more difficult in the invertebrate central nervous system than at the neuromuscular junction) showed that the quantal content of some of the synapses between sensory and motor neurons was reduced by successive stimuli (Castellucci and Kandel, 1974; see also Zucker, 1972).

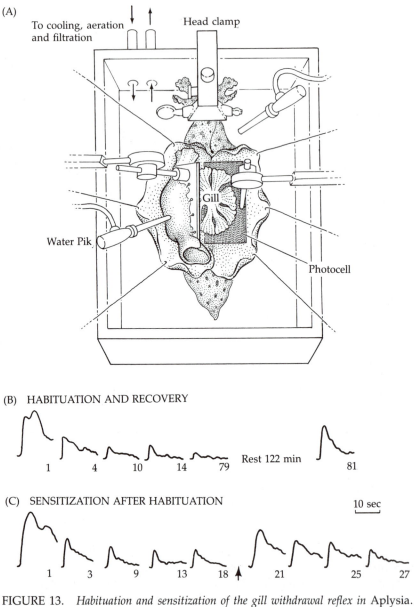

(A)

To cooling, aeration and filtration

Head clamp

Gill

Water Pik

Photocell

(B) HABITUATION AND RECOVERY

1   4   10   14   79   Rest 122 min   81

(C) SENSITIZATION AFTER HABITUATION

10 sec

1   3   9   13   18   21   25   27

FIGURE 13.   *Habituation and sensitization of the gill withdrawal reflex in* Aplysia. *(A) Experimental arrangement for behavioral studies in a restrained, but otherwise intact, animal. The* Aplysia *is immobilized in a small aquarium; reflex withdrawal of the gill in response to jets of water delivered to a nearby structure called the siphon are measured by the amount of light impinging on a photo cell. (B) During some 80 repetitions of the tactile stimulus at 3-minute intervals, the normal response measured in this way is gradually attenuated (numbers below indicate trials). This is called habituation. Complete recovery of the response occurs in about 2 hours. (C) Habituation is again induced by repetition of the stimulus, this time at 1-minute intervals. A strong and prolonged tactile stimulus to the neck region (arrow indicates time of delivery) causes an immediate restitution of the habituated response. This is called sensitization. (After Kandel, 1976.)*

Kandel and his group proposed that habituation arises because of decreased free calcium in the presynaptic ending (Castellucci et al., 1970). In support of this idea, the inward movement of calcium into the cell bodies of the sensory neurons during repeated activation is decreased (Klein et al., 1980). In these experiments, sensory neurons (either in intact ganglia or in isolation) were voltage-clamped under conditions in which membrane currents due to Ca^{2+} could be examined. When the cell body was repeatedly depolarized, the Ca^{2+} current declined in parallel with the postsynaptic response recorded in the motor neuron (see Figure 14). Based on these observations, Kandel and his collaborators concluded that habituation of the gill withdrawal response arises from decreased movement of Ca^{2+} into presynaptic terminals with repeated activity, perhaps as a result of a direct influence of depolarization on Ca^{2+} channels (Klein et al., 1980; Kandel and Schwartz, 1982). There is some uncertainty, however, in inferring events at synaptic endings from cell body recordings. In *Aplysia* and other invertebrates, synaptic connections are made in a central neuropil, which is at some distance from the cell body. Therefore, events studied at the level of the cell soma do not necessarily reflect conditions at the synaptic terminals.

The fact that habituation can last for many days adds considerable interest to this system. V. Castellucci, T. J. Carew, and Kandel (1978) discovered that even a few training sessions could cause habituation (and synaptic depression) that persisted for as long as 3 weeks! Whether the mechanism of this remarkably long-term effect is also based on decreased inward calcium current or on modification of synaptic connections is not yet clear (see Bailey and Chen, 1983).

An equally interesting aspect of the gill withdrawal reflex in *Aplysia* is the rapid restoration of the habituated response by a noxious stimulus to the head of the animal (e.g., an electrical shock) (see Figure 13). This effect depends on a general arousal of the animal and is called sensitization. The phenomenon is particularly intriguing because it is in some ways similar to classical conditioning: activation of one neural pathway enhances reflex action in another. In the isolated abdominal ganglion, a synaptic change that parallels behavioral sensitization can be produced by stimulating the nerve to the abdominal ganglion from the head or neck (Castellucci et al., 1970; see also Kandel and Tauc, 1965). Castellucci and Kandel (1976) have suggested that the basis of sensitization is roughly the opposite of events underlying habituation, i.e. that the behavior is restored by enhancing the quantal content of the synaptic response. Enhanced release of transmitter from sensory terminals during sensitization is postulated to occur because of increased calcium entry (Klein and Kandel, 1978, 1980). The agent of this effect is thought to be the release of serotonin from modulator neurons activated by the noxious stimulus; serotonin in turn increases cyclic AMP levels in the sensory neuron endings. In accord with this scheme, incubation of the abdominal ganglion in serotonin produces an increase in cyclic AMP content with a time course that is similar to the duration of sensitization

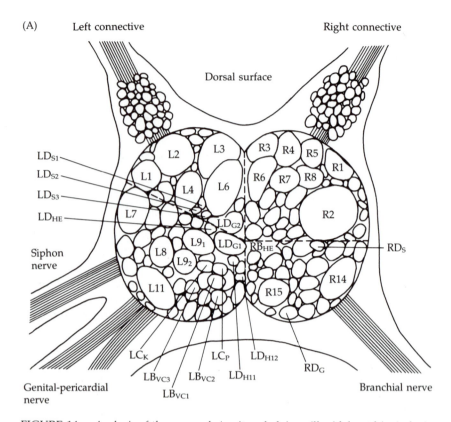

(A) Left connective   Right connective

Dorsal surface

LD_{S1}
LD_{S2}
LD_{S3}
LD_{HE}

Siphon
nerve

Genital-pericardial
nerve

FIGURE 14. *Analysis of the neuronal circuit underlying gill withdrawal in Aplysia. (A) The abdominal ganglion (consisting of about 1500 cells) contains many neurons that can be identified from animal to animal by virtue of their size and position. Some of these are the sensory and motor neurons involved in gill withdrawal. (B) Scheme of the circuit underlying this reflex. The skin of the siphon is thought to be innervated by about 24 sensory neurons, 8 of which are shown here. These make synaptic connections (probably monosynaptic) with six gill motor neurons (L7, . . ., RD_G; see A). A number of interneurons are also involved in the circuit, some of which are shown. (C) Intracellular recording from one of the gill motor neurons (L7), showing a decline in the amplitude of the synaptic response elicited during repetitive stimulation of one of the siphon sensory neurons at 10-second intervals (numbers indicate trial). The similar time course of synaptic depression and behavioral habituation suggests a relationship between these events (cf. Figure 13). (After Kandel, 1979a.)*

(Kandel and Schwartz, 1982). Furthermore, serotonin enhances the synaptic response of some gill motor neurons when it is applied exogenously. Finally, when cyclic AMP is injected into the cell body of the sensory neuron, it enhances the postsynaptic response in a manner similar to the effect that accompanies behavioral sensitization (Brunelli et al., 1976). Kandel and his co-workers have further argued that increased levels of cyclic AMP in the sensory endings activate a protein kinase that phosphorylates and inhibits a K^+ channel, thus prolonging depolarization of the terminal and increasing Ca^{2+} influx (Kandel and

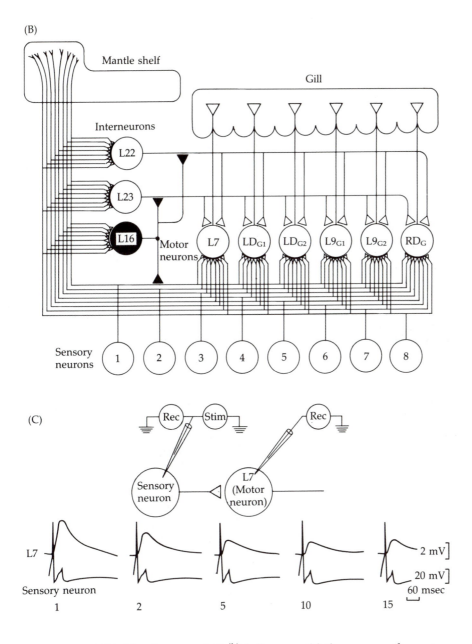

(B)

Mantle shelf

Gill

Interneurons

L22

L23

L16

Motor neurons

L7   LD_{G1}   LD_{G2}   L9_{G1}   L9_{G2}   RD_G

Sensory neurons   1   2   3   4   5   6   7   8

(C)

Rec — Stim   Rec

Sensory neuron   L7 (Motor neuron)

L7

Sensory neuron

1   2   5   10   15

2 mV]
20 mV]
60 msec

Schwartz, 1982). The increased Ca^{2+} influx would then cause the sensory terminals to release more transmitter, leading to restoration of the behavioral response. This general idea is based in part on work by P. Greengard and others that suggests a variety of long-lasting postsynaptic effects involve increases of cyclic nucleotides; this increase in turn influences protein phosphorylation by virtue of its effect on protein kinases (Greengard, 1976, 1981; Nestler and Greengard, 1983). The link between cyclic AMP-dependent protein phosphorylation and synaptic efficacy is supported by two sorts of findings: (1) injection of the sensory

Compensatory Responses to Distorted Perception

Although most successful studies of neural "plasticity" have been carried out in much simpler systems, some remarkable observations have also been made in human subjects. The most interesting examples involve the ability of people to correct for gross distortions that occur when the world is viewed through prisms.

The idea of studying human responses to a distorted visual world dates from the work of G. M. Stratton at the University of California, who, like many early investigators, used himself as a subject (Stratton, 1896–1897). Two other investigators in the 1920s, T. Erismann in Austria and J. J. Gibson in the United States, undertook further experiments of this sort, in which volunteers wore various types of prisms for a period of several weeks (Kohler, 1962). One of the first reports of a dramatic adaptation to a novel visual world came from a subject of Erismann's who wore goggles that transposed left and right. Erismann found that after a few weeks his subject became so adept at maneu-

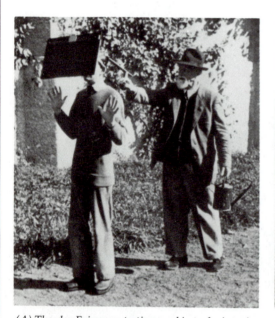

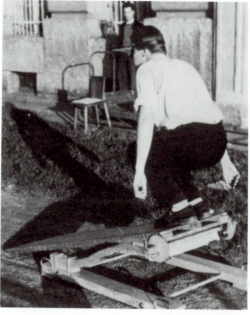

(A) Theodor Erismann testing a subject who is trying to walk forward while looking backward. (B) A sub-ject using a springboard while wearing goggles that transpose up and down. (From Kohler, 1962.)

neuron with a cyclic AMP-dependent protein kinase stimulates transmitter release (Castellucci et al., 1980); and (2) injection of an inhibitor of protein kinase blocks the sensitization response (Castellucci et al., 1982).

This molecular model may provide a basis for exploring some aspects of learning in vertebrates.

vering in his reversed visual world that he could drive his motorcycle through the narrow streets of Innsbruck without difficulty.

I. Kohler extended Erismann's experiments in the 1950s and 1960s (Kohler, 1962). He found that some subjects adapted in a remarkable and rather sudden fashion to the distortions induced by prisms. The mystery of this adaptation was highlighted by what happened when the volunteers removed their goggles; to their consternation, they found that when they first looked at the world without goggles it was distorted in an opposite way to the distortion experienced while wearing the prisms. This effect diminished over several days, and eventually all of the subjects again perceived the world normally.

Kohler also carried out a series of adaptation experiments involving color (Kohler, 1962). In one experiment, he had subjects wear glasses in which each lens was half blue (on the left) and half yellow (on the right). Thus, when the subject looked to the left the world was blue, but when he looked to the right the world was yellow. As in the prism experiments, the subjects became accustomed to this odd effect, and after some time no longer noticed that the world was blue in one direction of gaze and yellow in another.

Another perceptual challenge was acoustical transposition achieved with what was called a "reversing pseudophone" (Young, 1928). These experiments were limited by a number of problems including headaches and the considerable embarrassment that arose from being seen in this device (see figure). According to the author this latter problem was partially relieved by a "large loose-fitting cap." After 3 or 4 days with the pseudophone in place, Young (again his own subject) found that when he looked at objects producing a noise the sound was localized to them, even though the actual

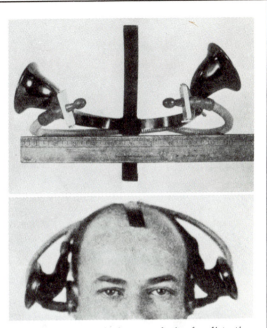

The reversing pseudophone, a device for distorting the aural world by introducing sound originating on the subject's left side into the right ear, and vice versa. (From Young, 1928.)

sounds were being presented in reversed fashion to the two ears.

Based in part on these experiments, a number of workers are currently exploring the basis of long-term adaptation to perceptual distortion in animals such as monkeys, who tolerate wearing goggles for long periods and whose responses can be tested with sophisticated techniques like unit recording (see, for example, Miles and Lisberger, 1982). Although the basis of such long-term adaptations is not yet understood, it is clear that the visuomotor system (and perhaps the auditory system) can cope with remarkable distortions by adjustments made over a period of days to weeks.

Modification of synapses following repetitive activity in the hippocampus

In spite of the obvious difficulties, a number of workers have chosen to investigate synaptic changes with use in parts of the vertebrate nervous system that are more complicated than the neuromuscular

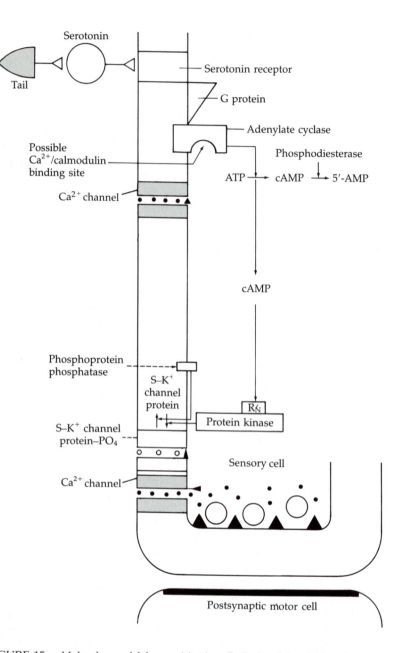

FIGURE 15. *Molecular model for sensitization. E. R. Kandel and his colleagues have suggested that sensitization is mediated by serotonergic interneurons that end on or near sensory terminals. As a result of transmitter (serotonin) release by the sensitizing pathway, the levels of cAMP in the sensory terminals are supposed to increase. This in turn inhibits K^+ channels by protein phosphorylation, reducing the repolarization of the action potential and enhancing Ca^{2+} influx. Increased Ca^{2+} entry then causes more transmitter to be released by sensory terminals when they are reflexly active. (After Kandel et al., 1983.)*

junction. In the 1940s, M. G. Larrabee and D. W. Bronk (1947) described post-tetanic potentiation in mammalian sympathetic ganglia (see also Brown and McAfee, 1982); shortly thereafter, D.P.C. Lloyd (1950) described a similar effect in the monosynaptic reflex pathway in the cat spinal cord. More detailed studies in the early 1970s reported potentiation of synaptic responses in the dentate area of the rabbit hippocampus after stimulation of the pathway that provides excitatory input to this region (the so-called perforant pathway) (Bliss and Lømo, 1973; Bliss and Gardner-Medwin, 1973). This latter effect routinely lasted minutes and, in some animals, could be detected even after a few days (Douglas and Goddard, 1975; Swanson et al., 1982).

Two general approaches have been taken to analyze the basis of potentiation in the hippocampus. G. Lynch and his collaborators have studied the effects of high-frequency stimulation on the structure of synapses in the rat hippocampus (Lee et al., 1980). In these experiments, one group of animals was stimulated repetitively for about a second; a control group received the same total number of action potentials but spread out over a longer period so that potentiation did not occur. The brains were then fixed and the relevant parts of the hippocampus examined electron microscopically. Although most parameters studied showed no significant change, about 30 percent more synaptic contacts were found on the dendritic shafts of the potentiated neurons. A second approach in the hippocampus has been to look for biochemical changes associated with potentiation. Small, but perhaps significant, shifts in the spectrum of phosphorylated proteins extracted from the affected region of the hippocampus have been reported (Swanson et al., 1982).

Although it will be difficult to relate such morphological and biochemical effects to behavior, these observations could conceivably represent alterations in brain structure and chemistry that have something to do with learning.

CONCLUSIONS

Synapses are not immutable in maturity but can change in at least two important ways: (1) the number of synaptic contacts between neurons and their targets can be altered by synaptogenesis and synaptic withdrawal, and (2) the efficacy of existing synapses can be modified by changing the amount of neurotransmitter released with each nerve impulse.

With respect to the first of these points, a great deal of evidence indicates that synaptic connections in adult animals represent a balance between a tendency of axon terminals to sprout and a tendency to withdraw. Whether this equilibrium of synaptic *number* is dynamic in the sense of a continual synaptic turnover is a question of considerable interest. Should synaptic turnover in maturity prove to be a general phenomenon, this fact would have profound implications for the neural basis of behavioral change.

A second way in which synapses can be modified concerns changes in the function of individual synaptic contacts with use or disuse. Interest in this aspect of synaptic malleability stems from the widely held belief that changes in synaptic *function* must account for a large part of our ability to learn and remember, at least in the short term. Although no generally accepted answers are yet available, there is no doubt that synaptic function can change with use at the neuromuscular junction, in the central nervous system of simple animals like *Aplysia* and, indeed, in the mammalian central nervous system. In the case of *Aplysia*, changes in synaptic function have been correlated with behavioral alterations that can be considered simple forms of learning, and a molecular scheme for short-term learning at these synapses has been proposed.

The degree to which learning and memory are based on changes in the number and distribution of synaptic boutons, changes in their individual efficacy, or some combination of these strategies remains an open question.

The Development of Behavior

INTRODUCTION

The reductionist approach of most earlier chapters tends to obscure the fact that the goal of neural development is appropriate behavior. Many of the most valuable contributions to understanding the development of behavior have come from ethologists and psychologists, who have examined this issue without explicit reference to the nervous system and who have often worked without the benefits (or burdens) of modern technology. This difference in style between neurobiologists and ethologists stems quite naturally from the still profound gap between neuronal events and their concerted action to produce behavior. In recent years this distance has gradually narrowed. Perhaps the best example is the present understanding of birdsong; in this and other instances, the psychological concepts of the 1950s and 1960s have begun to be translated into neurobiological terms.

The theme of much work on the development of behavior—as on other aspects of development—is the familiar nature–nurture controversy. By and large, the vehement debates earlier in the century between those who argued that behavior is engendered by experience and those who favored an intrinsic basis for behavior have given way to the more balanced view that the truth lies somewhere in between.

INNATE QUALITY OF MANY BEHAVIORS

Instinctual behavior

The idea that animals already possess a set of behaviors appropriate for a world not yet experienced has always been a difficult notion to accept. However, as the ethologist K. Z. Lorenz pointed out, the preeminence of instinctual responses is obvious to any biologist who studies what animals actually do. Darwin, for instance, cited many examples of inherited behaviors in his argument for natural selection (Darwin, 1859). Darwin was particularly impressed with the elaborate yet stereotyped behavior of insects. A case in point is the *Sphex* wasp (Emerson, 1958). This wasp lays its eggs in a specially constructed burrow and then stings a cricket, which it drags to the threshold. Following an inspection of the burrow's interior, the wasp pulls the cricket in; the paralyzed but still living cricket provides fresh food for the newly hatched grubs. This behavioral sequence appears purposeful and premediated; in fact, it is simply programmed. If the cricket is moved a few centimeters away while the wasp is inspecting the burrow, on emerging the wasp will bring the cricket back to the entrance and repeat the inspection. If the cricket is moved again during the inspection, the routine will be repeated over and over: the wasp never grasps the predicament and has no ability to modify its now useless behavior. An example noted by Darwin is the hammock-building behavior of certain caterpillars. If a caterpillar that has completed its hammock up to the sixth stage of construction is put into a hammock built only to the third stage, the caterpillar will complete the job. "If, however," wrote Darwin, "a caterpillar were taken out of a hammock made to the third stage and put into one finished up to the sixth stage, far from deriving any benefit from this, it was much embarrassed, and in order to complete its hammock seemed forced to start from the third stage, where it has left off, and thus tried to complete the already finished work" (Darwin, 1859).

Darwin could not resist comparing this sequence in the caterpillar to human behavior, adding that this reminded him of a musician who was interrupted in performing a memorized piece and could not complete it without going back to the beginning. Indeed, programmed behavior is commonplace in vertebrates. Perhaps the most thoroughly studied examples occur in young birds (Tinbergen, 1953; Lorenz, 1970).

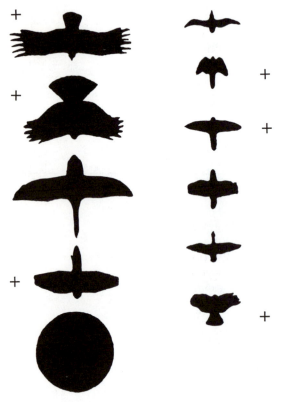

FIGURE 1. *Silhouettes used to study alarm reactions in young birds. The shapes that were similar to the shadow of the bird's natural predators (+) elicited escape responses (crouching, crying, running for cover); silhouettes of songbirds and other innocuous species elicited no obvious response. (After Tinbergen, 1961.)*

Hatchlings arrive in the world with an elaborate set of innate behaviors. First, of course, is the complex behavior that allows the chick to emerge from the egg. Having emerged, a variety of additional behaviors are evident and indicate how much of its early life is preprogrammed. Chicks of precocial species preen, peck, gape their beaks, follow a parent, and carry out a variety of other complex acts almost immediately. In some species, hatchlings automatically crouch down in the nest when a hawk passes overhead but are oblivious to the overflight of an innocuous bird. Lorenz and N. Tinbergen used hand-held silhouettes to explore this phenomenon in naive chicks. "It soon became obvious," wrote Tinbergen, "that . . . the reaction was mainly one to shape. When the model had a short neck so that the head protruded only a little in front of the line of the wings, it released alarm, independent of the exact shape of the dummy" (Figure 1) (Tinbergen, 1961). Evidently even knowledge about predators is built into the nervous system of some animals.

The execution of automatic programs of behavior is obviously not limited to early life or to birds. Lorenz and Tinbergen describe numerous more or less automatic behaviors in adults that, at first glance, seem intelligent. An amusing example in a mature bird is the so-called egg-rolling behavior of the greylag goose. Although to the casual observer the behavior seems purposeful, Lorenz demonstrated that the goose is simply executing a stereotyped sequence (Figure 2).

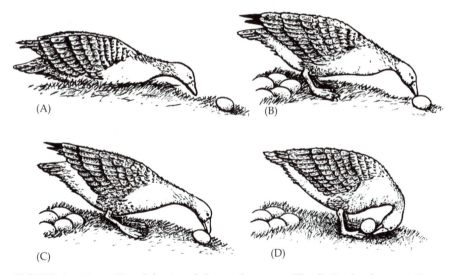

FIGURE 2. *Egg-rolling behavior of the greylag goose. The distinction between "instinctual" behavior and behaviors based on some more intelligent analysis of the situation may be subtle. In this example, the goose appears to react sensibly to the sight of an egg outside the nest by retrieving it with its bill (A–D). When K. Lorenz studied this behavior in detail, however, he found that this elaborate motor action was quite automatic. If by accident the egg rolled away during retrieval, the goose continued to roll the now nonexistent object and settled back onto the nest as if successful. When the egg was spotted anew, the goose, in Lorenz' words, "seems to exhibit amazement at seeing 'yet another' egg outside the nest." (After Lorenz, 1970.)*

The inherent nature of many behaviors is also well-known to animal breeders, who go to some pains to select stock with desirable behavioral qualities that subsequently breed true. "How strongly these domestic instincts are inherited," Darwin pointed out, ". . . is well shown when different breeds of dogs are crossed. Thus it is known that a cross with a bull-dog has affected for many generations the courage and obstinancy of greyhounds; and a cross with a greyhound has given to a whole family of shepherd-dogs a tendency to hunt hares" (Darwin, 1859).

Evidence for the development of complex neural programs in the absence of experience

The observations of ethologists were buttressed by neuroembryologists, who amassed evidence that the neural substrates of reflexive behavior become organized in early embryonic life without benefit of "experience," or indeed sensory information of any sort (see Coghill, 1929).

In general, embryos begin to move at very early stages of development: salamanders move in the intermediate tailbud stage, mouse embryos move at 14 days of gestation, and human embryos at 7½ or 8 weeks. These movements usually begin with flexion of the head, reflecting the cephalocaudal progression of neural maturation (Chapter 1). For the most part, early movements are convulsive, uncoordinated, and cyclical. In 1885 the German physiologist W. Preyer reported that chick embryos begin to move after only 4 days of incubation, even though they do not respond to stimulation until several days later (Preyer, 1885). This lag between motor competence and sensory responsiveness is presumably related to the ventrodorsal gradient of maturation in the spinal cord (Chapter 1). Eighty years later, V. Hamburger and his colleagues confirmed Preyer's work and extended it by asking whether early motor activity is intrinsic to the spinal cord (Hamburger, 1963, 1968; Provine, 1973; Oppenheim, 1982). They found that surgical isolation of the ventral spinal cord in chick embryos produced little or no reduction in hindlimb motility (Hamburger and Balaban, 1963; Hamburger et al., 1965, 1966). Action potentials in the relevant nerves always preceded muscular contraction; moreover, autogenous early activity persisted in the absence of motor responses which might artifactually have caused the appearance of neural activity (Ripley and Provine, 1972; Provine, 1973). Thus, these early movements are apparently caused by intrinsic motor neuron activity.

Embryonic movements show signs of coordination well before peripheral sensory input modulates motor neurons (Figure 3) (Bekoff et al., 1975; Bekoff, 1976; Landmesser and O'Donovan, 1984). Even at the earliest stages, antagonist and synergist muscles tend to be activated differentially with an appropriate phase lag. In accord with this evidence for autonomous development of embryonic motor behavior, when brachial cord segments are transplanted heterotopically to the lumbrosacral region before embryonic movement begins, subsequent leg movements are simultaneous rather than alternating, as if the legs were trying to flap (Narayanan and Hamburger, 1971).

(A)

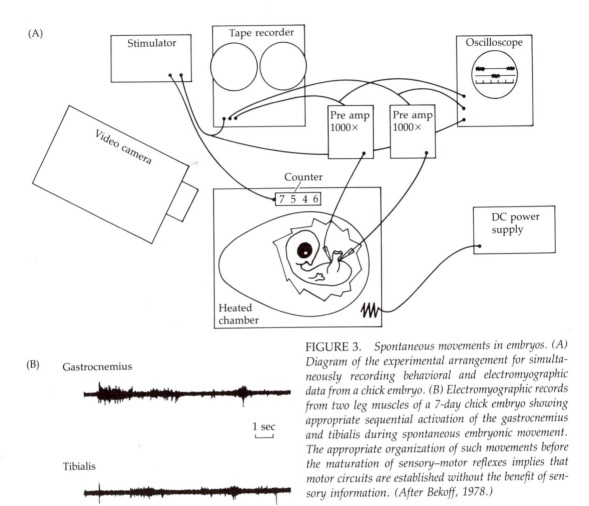

FIGURE 3. *Spontaneous movements in embryos.* (A) *Diagram of the experimental arrangement for simultaneously recording behavioral and electromyographic data from a chick embryo.* (B) *Electromyographic records from two leg muscles of a 7-day chick embryo showing appropriate sequential activation of the gastrocnemius and tibialis during spontaneous embryonic movement. The appropriate organization of such movements before the maturation of sensory–motor reflexes implies that motor circuits are established without the benefit of sensory information.* (After Bekoff, 1978.)

The upshot of these studies is that central patterns of motor organization are present very early. Well-organized activity at such early stages makes an important point: a substantial proportion of neural wiring is established according to rules that have nothing to do with an animal's experience in the sense of receiving interpretable sensory information about the external world. These findings are of course consistent with the expression of complex "instinctual" behaviors at birth; they are also in agreement with the early outgrowth of axons to appropriate targets (Chapter 5) and the establishment of selective synaptic connections as soon as targets are contacted (Chapters 10 and 11).

INFLUENCE OF EXPERIENCE ON THE DEVELOPMENT OF BEHAVIOR

Although the major theme of the preceding section is the importance of intrinsically determined neural circuitry and behavior, ethologists and, more recently, neurobiologists have shown that many behaviors have a malleable component. Imprinting in birds, socialization of primates, and the development of birdsong are good examples of innate behaviors that are modified by postnatal experience to extend and enhance the behavioral repertoire of an animal.

Imprinting

Imprinting was discovered by O. Heinroth (1911), who was interested in the fact that hatchlings of different species do not behave in the same way. Newly hatched ducklings, for example, crouch and then run away when a human attempts to pick them up. Young goslings, on the other hand, are quite different. "Without any display of fear," wrote Heinroth, "they stare calmly at human beings and do not resist handling. If one spends just a little time with them, it is not so easy to get rid of them afterwards. They pipe piteously if left behind and soon follow reliably." (quoted from Lorenz, 1970, p. 125). Thus, if a gosling is exposed to a human being shortly after hatching, subsequent attempts to return the hatchling to its natural parents will be frustrated. "The young gosling shows no inclination to regard the two adults as conspecifics," Heinroth went on, "The gosling runs off, piping, and attaches itself to the first human being that happens to come past; it regards the human being as its parent."

Systematic studies of imprinting in goslings and other species were undertaken by Heinroth's student Lorenz (see Box A). Lorenz and others found that some species of newly hatched birds (the greylag goose is one) will follow the first moving object they see after birth (Figure 4). Although under normal circumstances this object is a goose, imprinting to a variety of less typical "parents" can occur; examples include a passing dog, a moving cardboard box, and in one instance a bouncing football. Evidently it is the mobility of the object that provides the attraction. A second generalization is that imprinting occurs best soon after hatching; the effect wanes after the first day or two of life. Another point is that imprinting in sensory modalities other than vision also occurs; for example, auditory imprinting is common in birds and can even occur to sounds heard in ovo (Oppenheim, 1982). Perhaps the most important generalization is that imprinting seems to be more or less permanent: whatever the young bird imprints to will have a special meaning for it in later life. Another of Lorenz' favorite subjects was the jackdaw. In maturity jackdaws have an elaborate courting behavior, which involves bringing insects and worms to the intended sexual partner. To Lorenz' dismay, one of the jackdaws he had raised showered these attentions on Lorenz himself, attempting to stuff such offerings into Lorenz's ear (Lorenz, 1935).

Effects of early experience on the social behavior of primates

A series of related observations in primates make a good case for the lasting effects of early experience on behavior in higher animals.

In the 1950s H. F. Harlow and his colleagues isolated monkeys within a few hours of birth and raised them in the absence of either natural mothers or a human substitute (Harlow, 1958, 1959; Harlow and Zimmerman, 1959; see also Hinde and Spencer-Booth, 1971). In the best known of these experiments, the baby monkeys had one of two maternal surrogates: a "mother" constructed of a wooden frame covered with wire mesh, which supported a nursing bottle, or a similarly shaped object covered with terry cloth (Figure 5). When presented with this choice, the baby monkeys evidently preferred the terry cloth mother and spent much of their time clinging to it, even if the feeding bottle was with the wire mother. When the babies were placed in a strange environment, the presence of a wire mother had little effect in calming

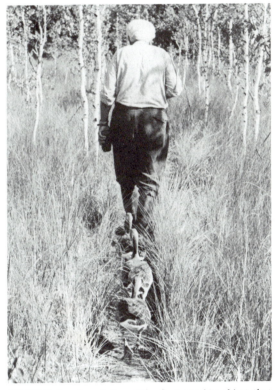

FIGURE 4. *Imprinting. The first moving object that goslings usually see after hatching is their mother; under normal circumstances they have a strong (and useful) inclination to follow her. O. Heinroth and K. Lorenz showed, however, that if the newly hatched birds see a different moving object, they will follow it instead and will persist indefinitely in this maladaptive behavior. They called this abiding impression of parental significance "imprinting." This picture shows Lorenz being trailed by several grown geese, which had been imprinted with his presence shortly after they hatched. (From Nisbett, 1976; photo courtesy of H. Kacher.)*

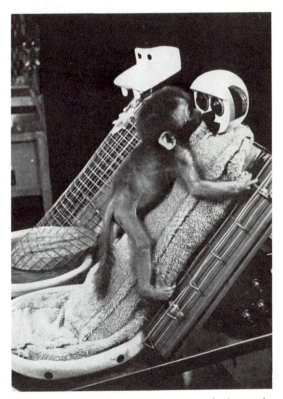

FIGURE 5. *The effects of inadequate mothering on the subsequent social behavior of primates. In studies carried out in the 1950s, H. F. Harlow and his colleagues reared baby monkeys in total isolation or with various maternal surrogates. In this picture, two kinds of surrogates are shown; a wire "mother" on the left and a terry cloth-covered "mother" on the right. Baby monkeys showed a strong preference for the softer mother and spent more time clinging to it even when their nursing bottles were attached to the wire surrogate. Babies raised with surrogates or in isolation showed severe changes in later social behavior. (From Harlow, 1959.)*

Konrad Zacharias Lorenz (b. 1903)

Konrad Lorenz, who is generally considered the founder of ethology, was born in Altenburg, Austria, where his father was an orthopedist. Somewhat unwillingly, he obtained his medical degree from the University of Vienna in 1928, where, until 1935, he was an assistant in the Institute for Anatomy. He went on to obtain a Ph.D. in zoology at the University of Munich in 1936, and was subsequently promoted to lecturer in comparative anatomy and animal psychology at Vienna. In 1941 Lorenz became the head of the department of psychology at Königsberg. Then in 1945 he joined the Max Planck Institute in Büldern, Westphalia, and, in 1961, was appointed director of the Max Planck Institute of Physiology and Behavior at Seewiesen in Bavaria. Finally, in 1973, he became the director of the department of animal sociology at the Institute of Comparative Ethology in the Austrian Academy of Sciences.

In addition to establishing the study of animal behavior as a legitimate field of biology, Lorenz provided evidence that behavior has both innate and acquired components. The idea that much behavior is innate generated considerable controversy; many opponents contended that behavior was primarily a product of learning. Lorenz summed up this battle in the following way:

The fact that the behaviour not only of animals, but of human beings as well, is to a large extent determined by nervous mechanisms evolved in the phylogeny of the species, in other words, by "instinct," was certainly no surprise to any biologically-thinking scientist. It was treated as a matter of course, which, in fact, it is. On the other hand, by emphasizing it and by drawing the sociological and political inferences I seem to have incurred the fanatical hostility of all those doctrinaires whose ideology has tabooed the recognition of this fact. The idealistic and vitalistic philosophers to whom the belief in the absolute freedom of the human will makes the assumption of human instincts intolerable, as well as the behaviouristic psychologists who assert that all human behaviour is learned, all seem to be blaming me for holding opinions which in fact have been public property of biological science since *The Origin of Species* was written (Lorenz, 1970, p. xii).

Lorenz's preeminence is based not only on first rate biology but also on the ability to popularize his ideas. One reason for Lorenz's notable success as a popularizer of animal behavior (several of his books are available on paperback racks) is the ability to extrapolate his findings to human mores.

An example is Lorenz's fascination with the way the greylag gander tries to impress the female. Although this species flies poorly, a courting male often takes to the air over short stretches that would normally be covered by swimming or walking. In addition, the flight is often directed toward an actual or imagined opponent, who is chased off with considerable show. "Demonstrative behaviour in man is extremely similar to that of the Greylag goose," Lorenz wrote. "Even extremely able men talented with powers of self-criticism can, under circumstances involving physical activity (for example when skiing or ice-skating) become considerably more vigorous and dashing when the number of spectators is increased by one attractive girl. In primitive or not quite grown-up men, this is often accompanied—as in the gander described—by attacking or at least molesting weaker pseudo-opponents. The most remarkable fact to be seen from this, however, is that many men perform the dissipation of energy characteristic of demonstrative behaviour with a *machine* if they happen to be riding one. I have repeatedly observed that motor

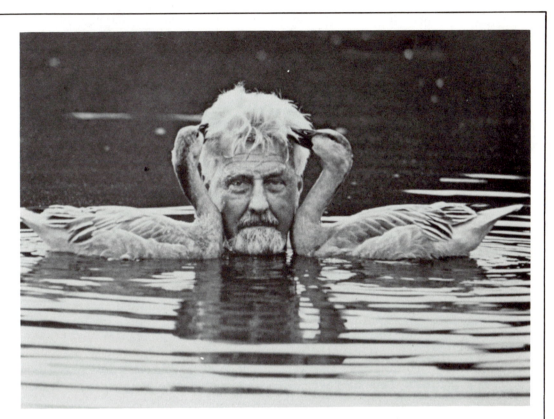

Konrad Lorenz with his geese. (Courtesy of N. Leen and Time-Life Books Inc.)

cyclists in such cases increase the noise-level and energy consumption of their machines by revving and simultaneously adjusting the ignition, without greatly increasing their speed" (Lorenz, 1935). As a popularizer, however, he was joined by less hard-headed colleagues such as D. Morris and R. Ardrey, whose sweeping, if congenial, views were a much greater worry to Lorenz than the easily refuted dogmas of his opponents (see Lorenz, 1970, p. 190).

Among numerous other awards, Lorenz received the Nobel prize for physiology and medicine in 1973 with two other ethologists, N. Tinbergen and K. von Frisch (see Tinbergen, 1969). Although the nervous system per se was never of much concern to Lorenz, his beautifully expressed observations on instinctual behavior provide a major lesson for neurobiologists. Lorenz's colleague Tinbergen summed up the perspective of ethologists and its significance as follows: "Man likes to consider himself a rational being; he not only fails to recognise his instincts, he even scoffs at instincts and considers them inferior. This attitude makes him fall a victim to them much more easily than is necessary. The student of behaviour is struck by the deeper similarity between man and animals; he recognises himself only too often in an animal. Also, he has rather a higher opinion of instincts; for instance, he recognises that they are at the bottom of his subjective experiences. And he has his doubts about the all-controlling power of reason, for he sees its limits too often" (Tinbergen, 1953, p. 239).

them; they showed a variety of disturbed behaviors (crying, rolling on the floor, rocking) that were not mollified by the wire surrogate. However, when the terry cloth mother was placed in the same environment, the baby monkeys clung to it, and many of the signs of distress were said to disappear. Harlow took this to mean that newborn monkeys have a built-in need for maternal care and have at least some idea of what a mother should be like.

The long-term effects of inadequate mothering were apparently profound (Harlow and Harlow, 1973; Ruppenthal et al., 1976); when the deprived monkeys matured they showed obvious and evidently permanent disturbances of social behavior. They often sat and stared for long periods, rocking their bodies for minutes or hours at a time, and developed compulsive habits such as pinching or biting themselves. These effects were most severe in a group of monkeys reared in total isolation, without benefit of even the surrogate mother. Monkeys treated in this way failed to show the usual interest and aggressive response at the approach of a strange human and instead bit or scratched themselves in agitation. Harlow noted the similarity of this kind of behavior to some disturbances of human children.

In accord with Lorenz' observations on birds, the early experiences of primates also had a profound influence on subsequent sexual behavior (Harlow and Harlow, 1973). Males reared in isolation were uninterested in females and were unable to mate. Females reared in isolation could sometimes be mated with a normal male, but the effects of their early experience on mothering were apparently severe. Mothers that had been isolated in early life showed indifference to their own babies and were sometimes overtly aggressive toward them. Interestingly, when these babies grew to maturity, they also showed behavioral anomalies.

The adequacy of mothering is probably not the only aspect of a baby monkey's experience important for its later behavior. In other experiments carried out by Harlow, baby monkeys were raised without mothers but with other young monkeys (Harlow and Harlow, 1973). Monkeys raised with peers developed what was said to be a fairly normal adult pattern of social and sexual behavior. Evidently peer interactions can compensate to some degree for maternal deprivation.

These observations by Harlow and his associates obviously depend on the experimenters' interpretation of what constitutes normal (or abnormal) monkey behavior. Nonetheless, it is difficult to dismiss these studies or their relevance to human development.

Development of birdsong

These ethological studies of birds and monkeys are in accord with a growing body of neurobiological evidence that confirms that experience can modify innate behavior in a more or less permanent way. Particularly instructive is a series of studies on birdsong carried out over the last two to three decades. Rather than conducting explicitly ethological investigations, students of birdsong have begun to look at changes in the relevant parts of the nervous system during maturation in various experimental circumstances. Although one would have little idea where to look for relevant neural changes in a bird during imprinting or in a monkey's brain during maternal deprivation (see, however, Horn, 1981), it is a fairly straightforward matter in the songbird to examine the centers involved in vocal control.

Birdsong consists of a stereotyped set of calls and more complex sounds that constitute a characteristic and well-defined song for each species. In general, males in reproductive condition sing, whereas females do not. The systematic investigation of birdsong began with W. H. Thorpe's work on the chaffinch in the 1950s (Figure 6) (see Thorpe, 1958, 1961, 1963). Using the sonogram (Figure 6A), Thorpe showed that young chaffinches reared in isolation develop a song that, although quite poor, is recognizable as the song of that species. Thus, these birds come into the world with an innate but imperfect idea of what they are to sing; the fully formed song must be learned from conspecifics during a limited (critical) period in early life (Thorpe, 1958).

Thorpe's students (and their students, in turn) have studied a number of other species, greatly extending his initial findings. In zebra finches, for example, song learning is restricted to about the first 80 days after hatching (even though it is not practiced until much later; Immelmann, 1969). Canaries, on the other hand, learn new phrases of song with each successive season and so extend their repertoire (Nottebohm and Nottebohm, 1978). P. Marler and his collaborators showed that song learning has a remarkable degree of specificity (Figure 7). Like chaffinches and zebra finches, male white-crowned sparrows learn song during a defined period in early life. So keen is their preconception of what constitutes a proper song that they will not learn the song of other sparrow species when exposed to it in the laboratory (Marler and Tamura, 1964); even more remarkably, they can learn their species song when it is spliced together on tape with the song of a sympatric species (Marler and Peters, 1977). Thus, these birds recognize the song they are supposed to learn even under confusing and difficult conditions. Evidently vocal learning occurs by modifying vocal output until the auditory feedback generated by the young bird matches a model of species song (Konishi, 1965). All told, these observations amply confirm that the neonatal nervous system already contains detailed information about what behaviors to learn and when to learn them.

Recent work on birdsong has gradually begun to bridge the gap between ethological studies like those of Lorenz and of Harlow and modern cellular neurobiology. Much of the progress in understanding the neurological basis of the ability to sing has been made by F. Nottebohm and his co-workers, who have for a number of years explored the neural correlates of song in chaffinches and canaries (Nottebohm, 1980a). Two aspects of this work are of particular interest. First is the observation that birdsong is lateralized. In canaries and chaffinches, song is produced by modulating the air flow within the syrinx, a spe-

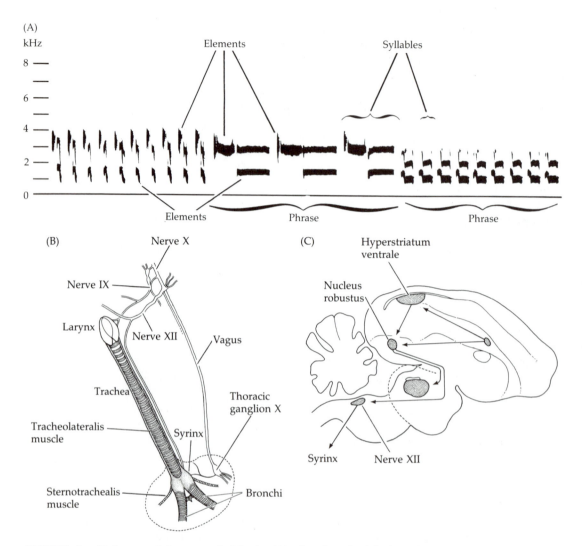

FIGURE 6. *Birdsong and its anatomical basis. (A) Song fragment of a normal adult male canary. Sonograms of this sort allow a detailed study of song during normal development and in a variety of experimental circumstances. (B) Ventral view of the syrinx, trachea, and the related structures involved in birdsong. Song is produced by the syrinx (a specialized organ at the confluence of the two bronchi) as airflow is modulated by the syringeal muscles; the musculature is controlled by a branch of the hypoglossal nerve (XII). (C) Saggital section of the adult male canary brain. Arrows indicate the connections between components of the vocal control pathways. The major stations of the pathway that have been examined in various neurobiological studies are the hyperstriatum ventrale and the nucleus robustus. (A and C after Nottebohm, 1980a; B after Nottebohm, 1971.)*

cialized structure at the confluence of the bronchi and trachea (see Figure 6). The right and left halves of the syrinx have their own muscular apparatus and are innervated, respectively, by the right and left hypoglossal nerves. Thus, each half-syrinx can modulate air flow and produce sound independently. The effects of cutting the left hypoglossal

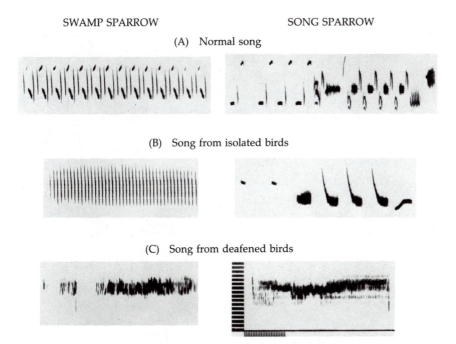

SWAMP SPARROW   SONG SPARROW

(A) Normal song

(B) Song from isolated birds

(C) Song from deafened birds

FIGURE 7. *Development of birdsong. Typical songs of a male swamp sparrow (left) and a song sparrow (right) are shown from normal birds (A), from males reared in isolation (B), and from males deafened in infancy (C). Birds reared in isolation retain some characteristics of the species song, even though the version is much simplified. Evidently normal song has both an innate and a learned component. The innate component, however, must be validated by auditory feedback. Thus, if birds are deafened early in life, the song and its species specificity is severely degraded. (After Marler, 1981.)*

nerve (or destroying its higher control centers) are not the same as the effects of an identical lesion on the right: a left-sided lesion is much more destructive of a bird's ability to sing than a right-sided one (Nottebohm, 1970, 1971, 1977, 1980b; Nottebohm et al., 1976). Thus, birdsong in these species is dominated by left-sided structures, perhaps in the same way that human language is dominated by the speech areas of the left hemisphere. This lateralization can be modulated experimentally. When the left hypoglossal nerve is destroyed in a young male canary, song develops normally but is mediated by right-sided neural structures (Nottebohm et al., 1979). In canaries, which retain the ability to add new songs to their repertoire from season to season, this neural flexibility is not entirely lost in maturity. For example, adult male canaries can re-acquire some song after the destruction of the left-sided brain structures that normally organize singing (Nottebohm et al., 1979).

A second intriguing feature of birdsong is its sexual dimorphism (Konishi and Gurney, 1982). The telencephalic vocal control areas of the songbird brain are much larger in males than in females (Figure 8)

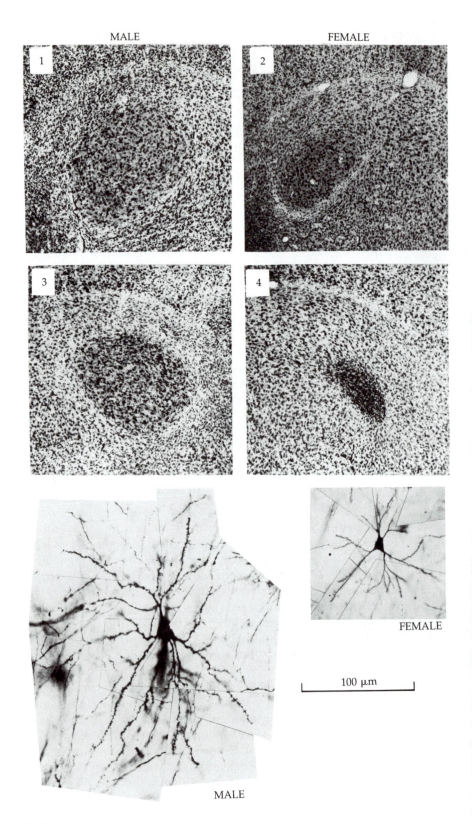

MALE

FEMALE

100 μm

MALE

FEMALE

◄ FIGURE 8. *Sexual dimorphism in the vocal control areas of songbirds. (A) Frontal sections through the nucleus robustus (see Figure 6C) in a male (1) and a female (2) canary; (3) and (4) show the same areas in another songbird, the zebra finch. In both species there is an obvious sexual difference in the size of this brain nucleus. (B) Cellular differences in male and female song nuclei. As far as is known, male and female birds possess the full complement of neuronal types in their song control centers. However, neurons in Golgi preparations from the nucleus robustus of males are typically larger and more complex than the homologous neurons of females. (A from Nottebohm and Arnold, 1976; B from Gurney, 1981.)*

(Nottebohm and Arnold, 1976; Gurney and Konishi, 1980; Konishi and Gurney, 1982). Moreover, these areas are larger in males with more complex song repetoires than in males with simple repetoires (Nottebohm et al., 1981). If testosterone is administered to a developing female, the size of the vocal areas will increase, and song will develop if the treatment is continued (Gurney and Konishi, 1980; Arnold, 1980; Nottebohm, 1980b). Thus testosterone appears to influence both the differentiation of specific brain nuclei and the propensity to sing. Finally, there are demonstrable changes in the size of the telencephalic vocal control nuclei in adult male canaries; these changes parallel the seasonal changes in testosterone levels (Nottebohm, 1981; DeVoogd and Nottebohm, 1981b).

Most of the difference in size between male and female song control nuclei (or between the same nucleus in males from season to season) results from differences in the size and dendritic complexity of the relevant neurons (Gurney and Konishi, 1980; Gurney, 1981; Devoogd and Nottebohm, 1981a,b). Labeling with tritiated thymidine also shows that testosterone treatment induces glial proliferation, and probably some neuronal proliferation, in adult birds (Nottebohm et al., 1981; Goldman and Nottebohm, 1983).

These changes in the brain that occur in parallel with the acquisition of song may provide some insight into mechanisms of learning in the vertebrate central nervous system.

REFINEMENT OF INNATE CONNECTIONS IN THE VISUAL SYSTEM

Among the important conclusions of ethological studies is the idea that various behaviors can only be learned during a restricted (critical) period. Thus, imprinting must occur during the first few days of a hatchling's life, birdsong in some species must be learned during a limited time in the first season, and socialization of monkeys must occur during early life or be forever abnormal. A corollary of these findings is that during these critical periods animals are particularly sensitive to deprivation or "abnormal" experience. In humans with strabismus (in which information from one eye is suppressed by mechanisms that are poorly understood), failure to rectify the problem in infancy by patching the

Neural Correlates of Sexually Dimorphic Behavior in Invertebrates

A number of workers have sought to identify the neural elements underlying stereotyped behaviors in invertebrates. Many of these behaviors, like birdsong, are sexually dimorphic. For instance, the male housefly shows elaborate courtship and chasing behaviors not seen in females. In the region of the brain concerned with chasing behavior, the male fly has two retinotopic columns of neurons and giant "tangential" cells that are not found in the female brain (Strausfeld, 1980; Hausen and Strausfeld, 1980). Because insect sexual behavior is often elicited by a pheromone secreted by the female, a number of studies have focused on the male antennae, the organs of pheromone reception. In the moth, the male antennae are larger than in the female and are specialized for detection and orientation toward the pheromone. In the part of the brain concerned with olfaction, the male has another specialized area (the macroglomerular complex) believed to be responsible for processing the pheromone signal (see figure) (Boeckh et al., 1977; Hildebrand et al., 1980). Projecting into the macroglomerular complex are the dendrites of a set of male-specific neurons that are excited when the antennae are stimulated by the pheromone (Boeckh et al., 1977; Hildebrand et al., 1980; Matsumoto and Hildebrand, 1981).

Sexually dimorphic behavior has also been studied in the fruit fly. During courtship, male fruit flies extend their wings and vibrate them in the direction of females (Bennet-Clark and Ewing, 1970). The neural circuitry underlying

(A)

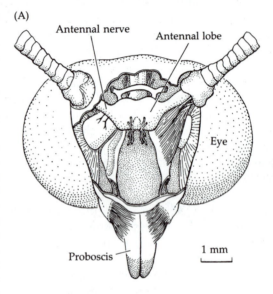

Neuronal correlates of sexually dimorphic behavior in the moth Manduca sexta. *(A) Cut-away view of brain. (B) Cut-away view of the male and female*

other eye or by corrective surgery results in permanent loss of visual acuity. Moreover, injury to language centers in the dominant hemisphere of infants can be compensated by the development of language in the nondominant hemisphere up until the age of 2 or 3 years, but not thereafter. Such anecdotal evidence for critical periods has, in the past 20 years or so, been augmented by detailed studies of the influence of experience on the development of the mammalian visual system; this work has been carried out largely by D. H. Hubel and T. N. Wiesel (see Box C).

this behavior can be dissected using mosaic flies, which are part male and part female (gynandromorphs). Gynandromorphs with a male head and a female thorax extend their wings to females. This indicates, perhaps not surprisingly, that the impetus to begin courtship is in the brain (Hotta and Benzer, 1976; Hall, 1977, 1979; Von Schilcher and Hall, 1979). However, the vibratory wing behavior (called the song) is not well executed unless some male tissue is also present in the thorax. Thus, although the motivation comes from the brain, the wherewithal is in the body. A similar kind of analysis has been carried out in crickets (Stout and Huber, 1972). In the cricket, the male circuitry that generates the familiar courtship song is specified by the same genes as the female circuit that recognizes the song (Hoy and Paul, 1973; Bentley and Hoy, 1974). By analogy, vocal control centers in female birds (see text) may be involved in song recognition.

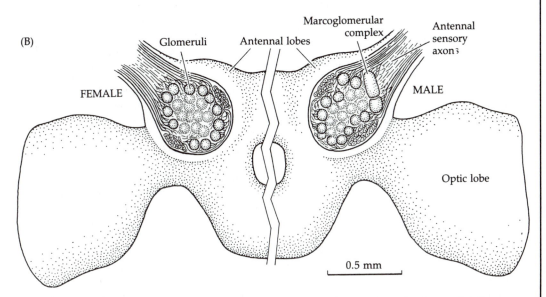

(B)

antennal lobes. Both male and female brains contain specialized regions of neuropil called glomeruli, to which antennal neurons project; the male lobe, however, contains a unique structure called the macroglomerular complex. (After Hildebrand et al., 1980.)

The cat visual system at birth

Studies of adult mammals—the cat, in particular—have demonstrated a hierarchical arrangement of cellular connectivity underlying the initial processing of the information that leads to visual perception (Hubel, 1963; Hubel, 1982b). At the level of the primary visual cortex, inputs driven by corresponding points on the two retinas converge in a retinotopic fashion on cortical neurons in layer IV. These neurons in turn innervate other cells in the layers above and below so that each cortical

BOX

C

David Hunter Hubel (b. 1926) and Torsten Nils Wiesel (b. 1924)

David Hubel was born in Windsor, Ontario. He received both his B.S. (physics, 1947) and his medical degree (1951) from McGill University. Following 3 years of residency training at the Montreal Neurological Institute, he moved to the neurology program at Johns Hopkins in 1954. After a further stint at the Walter Reed Army Institute of Research, he returned to the Wilmer Ophthalmological Institute at Hopkins to work in the laboratory of S. W. Kuffler. There he began a collaboration with Torsten Wiesel that was to last more than 20 years, culminating with the Nobel prize for physiology and medicine in 1981. Wiesel was born in Uppsala, Sweden, and received his medical degree from the Karolinska Institute in Stockholm in 1954. He came to Johns Hopkins in 1955 as a fellow in ophthalmology after a year of assistantship in the department of child psychiatry at the Karolinska Hospital. In 1959 Kuffler persuaded Hubel and Wiesel to accompany him to Harvard Medical School, where they carried out the bulk of their work. In 1983 Wiesel accepted a position at Rockefeller University; Hubel remains at Harvard.

Hubel and Wiesel's work falls into two different, but closely related areas. First was a detailed analysis of the way that retinal information is processed in the mammalian lateral geniculate and cortex. This work depended largely on the development in the 1950s of extracellular tungsten electrodes capable of recording signals from individual neurons in the living mammalian brain. This technique, which Hubel helped develop, is now widely used and has supplanted the electroencephalogram (EEG) as the major tool for brain research.

V. B. Mountcastle, whose work on the somatosensory cortex provided the first evidence of a columnar organization in the mammalian brain (Mountcastle, 1957), was clearly an important influence on the direction of Hubel and Wiesel's early work. A second critical influence, both personally and scientifically, was Kuffler, whose pioneering work on the organization of receptive fields in the retina in 1953 provided the impetus for Hubel and Wiesel's analysis of the organization of the ocular projections to the thalamus and cortex (see Box C in Chapter 8). The major achievement of this aspect of their work was the demonstration that successive relays in the visual pathway systematically transmute visual information into abstractions of the real world. In addition, they showed that the anatomical basis for these abstractions at the cortical level are arrays of repeating cortical entities (hypercolumns) that make up modules; each of these iterated units is capable of a complete analysis of a small portion of visual space. Most current theories of perception rely heavily on Hubel and Wiesel's physiological and anatomical analysis of the visual pathways.

Hubel and Wiesel's second major contribution was an investigation of the effects of visual deprivation on cortical development. These studies have contributed not only to the understanding and prevention of clinical problems such as amblyopia, but to a general understanding of the development of synaptic connections. Armed with a detailed knowledge of how the visual system is organized, Hubel and Wiesel examined the effect on cortical connections of closing one eye in a cat or a monkey at birth. An important result of this work was the definition of a critical period in postnatal life during which connectivity is particularly susceptible to modification (see text). A second result was that the columnar organization of the cortex develops by a process of segregation that involves competition between inputs.

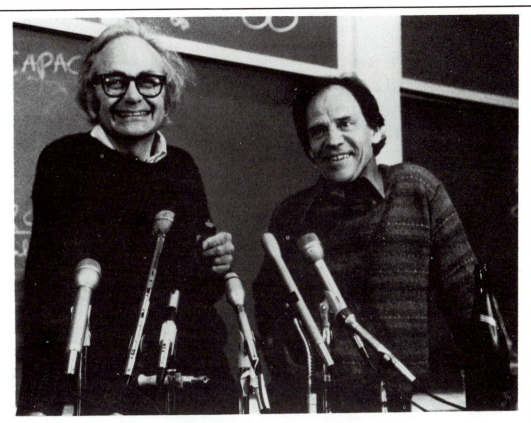

David Hubel (left) and Torsten Wiesel talking to reporters in 1981.

A characteristic of Hubel and Wiesel's work has always been a no-nonsense approach that allowed them to eschew the conventional wisdom and find simple solutions to difficult problems. The following vignette exemplifies their style of thinking: "I remember a momentous occasion," wrote Hubel, "when at Walter Reed, in 1957 or so, I felt pleased enough at finding directionally selective cells in area 17 of a purring cat to drag Bob Galambos down to my lab for a demonstration. Bob was suitably impressed—he always gave wonderful positive feedback and was very tolerant of a stubborn and moody postdoc—but said, 'David, this is fine, but what is the latency of this cell?' Well, I did feel a bit sheepish, to be preoccupied with postgraduate stuff like movement and not to have even established the latency, so I found a strobe light, and quickly found that this cell's latency was 83 msec. That was odd, considering a myelinated pathway a few inches long, and allowing for a delay of about 1 msec per synapse. I took the lesson to heart: that was the first latency I ever measured, and also the last" (Hubel, 1982, p. 367). This scientific style enabled Hubel and Wiesel to ignore K. S. Lashley's conclusion (widely accepted in the 1950s) that cortical function was not localized but depended on holistic mechanisms that might be impossible to analyze. Quite the contrary, Hubel and Wiesel showed that understanding the brain is no different than understanding any other biological problem.

neuron responds to visual stimulation in a specific and restricted way. Thus to activate a given cell the stimulus must fall on the right region of the retina, must have a particular orientation and shape, and must often move in a certain direction at a certain speed and even be a certain color. These restrictions arising from the normal organization of the visual pathway define the "receptive field properties" for each cortical neuron (Figure 9).

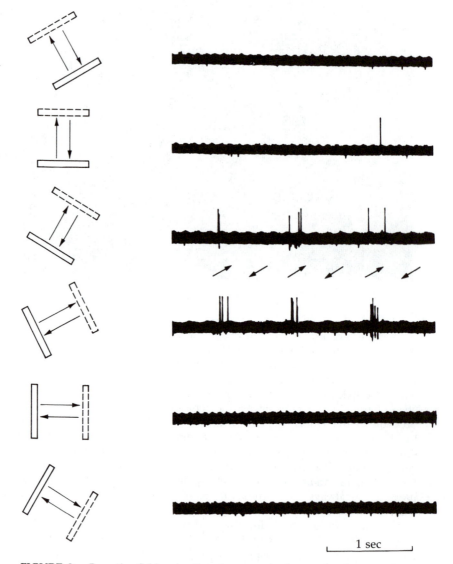

FIGURE 9. *Receptive field properties of neurons in the cat visual cortex. Responses of a single cortical neuron from an adult cat (right) to a moving rectangle of light (left) presented in the region of the visual field in which light excites the cell. The response of this cell was best when the slit was aligned in a particular orientation; note that the cell was also selective for the direction of movement. (From Hubel and Wiesel, 1959.)*

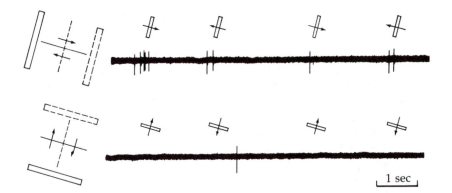

FIGURE 10. *Receptive field properties in kittens. Single-cell response from the cortex of an 8-day-old kitten with no previous visual experience shows orientation selectivity: a stimulus oriented at right angles to the optimal orientation gives no response (cf. Figure 9). The cell responds to both directions of movement (as do some adult neurons), although other neonatal neurons also showed directional selectivity. The specific qualities of the receptive fields of neonatal neurons indicate that much of the cortical circuitry is already established at birth. (After Hubel and Wiesel, 1963.)*

The highly specific receptive fields of neurons in the visual cortex provide a complex but well-understood system in which to study the nature–nurture question in mammals. Because in maturity individual neurons in the primary visual cortex are precisely defined by the stimuli that activate them, one can ask whether the properties of cortical neurons are equally well defined at birth, before the animal has had any visual experience (at least in a loose sense). Although there has been some debate on this issue (Barlow, 1975), most workers are agreed that many receptive field properties are established prior to any experience (Figure 10). To be sure, neonatal neurons are less sharply tuned than their adult counterparts, but the basic wiring that subserves these various aspects of adult responsiveness is largely present at birth (Hubel and Wiesel, 1963). In fact, this general point has already been made in the context of the developing spinal cord (see earlier).

Effects of eye closure

Cats and monkeys reared in darkness, or children with congenital cataracts, have permanent deficits when vision is later tested (Hebb, 1937; Von Senden, 1932; Riesen, 1961). On the face of it, these observations present a paradox. If visual connections are largely established at birth, why does deprivation have such serious effects? The answer is that although many aspects of connectivity depend on intrinsic mechanisms, other aspects of connectivity remain malleable at birth. As a result of further postnatal maturation, experience can influence the final pattern of connections, as Hubel and Wiesel showed in a series of seminal experiments on visual deprivation carried out in the 1960s.

When normal visual experience is abridged experimentally in kittens by occluding one eye for only a few weeks, the arrangement of cortical connections in the adult cat is permanently altered (Wiesel and Hubel, 1963, 1965; Hubel, 1982b; Wiesel, 1982). The most obvious effect of monocular eye closure (achieved by suturing the eyelids) is a sharp decline in the number of cortical neurons that can later be driven by the previously closed eye: following a 3-month period of unilateral eye closure from birth, the proportion of cells that the deprived eye can influence drops from the normal value of about 85 percent to about 7 percent (Figure 11) (Hubel and Wiesel, 1970). These effects are largely permanent: opening the deprived eye for long periods produces only a modest improvement in the number of cortical neurons activated by the previously deprived eye. In accord with these electrophysiological

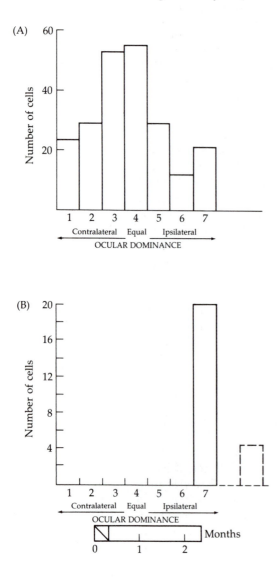

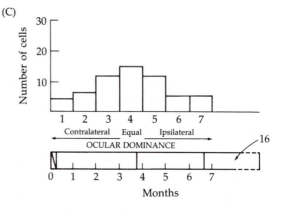

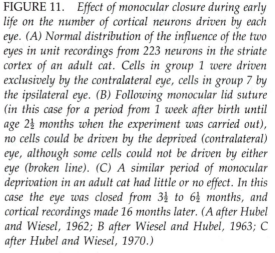

FIGURE 11. *Effect of monocular closure during early life on the number of cortical neurons driven by each eye. (A) Normal distribution of the influence of the two eyes in unit recordings from 223 neurons in the striate cortex of an adult cat. Cells in group 1 were driven exclusively by the contralateral eye, cells in group 7 by the ipsilateral eye. (B) Following monocular lid suture (in this case for a period from 1 week after birth until age 2½ months when the experiment was carried out), no cells could be driven by the deprived (contralateral) eye, although some cells could not be driven by either eye (broken line). (C) A similar period of monocular deprivation in an adult cat had little or no effect. In this case the eye was closed from 3½ to 6½ months, and cortical recordings made 16 months later. (A after Hubel and Wiesel, 1962; B after Wiesel and Hubel, 1963; C after Hubel and Wiesel, 1970.)*

findings, ocular dominance columns fail to segregate normally; the columns activated by the deprived eye are narrower than normal whereas the columns driven by the normal eye are wider (Figure 12; see also Chapter 12). Evidently experience is important in the development of visual connections because it provides a proper balance between competing inputs. When the connections driven by one eye are deprived of normal stimulation, they do not compete effectively with the active inputs from the normal eye and are lost. In the absence of competition, many more of the initial connections of the nondeprived eye persist (Figure 12).

The susceptibility to the effects of eye closure in kittens begins about the fourth week of life, remains high for several weeks, and finally disappears around 3 months of age (Wiesel and Hubel, 1963, 1965; Hubel and Wiesel, 1970). During the period of maximum susceptibility monocular closure for as little as 3–4 days produces an obvious decline in the number of neurons subsequently activated by that eye. On the other hand, monocular closure for over a year in fully grown cats produces no effect (see Figure 11C). A similar phenomenon is apparent in monocularly deprived monkeys, although the period of susceptibility is longer (Hubel et al., 1977).

Critical periods exist for other aspects of connectivity in the visual cortex. For example, over a time span similar (but not identical) to the critical period for monocular deprivation, the tuning of cortical neurons for orientation is also malleable (Daw and Wyatt, 1976; Berman and Daw, 1977). Critical periods for deprivation effects have also been described in other sensory systems (see, for example, Knudsen et al., 1984a,b).

Relevance of deprivation effects to normal development

The deeper significance of such critical periods for sensory deprivation has been assessed in widely discussed (and debated) experiments in which young kittens are raised in various abnormal visual environments. For example, kittens have been raised in a vertically striped environment in order to expose them to a visual world in which everything is oriented the same way (Figure 13) (Blakemore and Cooper, 1970; Hirsch and Spinelli, 1971; Blakemore and Mitchell, 1973; Blakemore, 1974; Barlow, 1974). These experiments are difficult to carry out because the kittens must be kept in the dark except for training periods in the vertical environment. Moreover, for a kitten raised in a vertically striped drum, turning its head or seeing itself might provide other orientation experiences. For these and other reasons this approach has been a controversial one. However, most of the principals seem now agreed that raising an animal in a vertical environment during the critical period does cause important changes in cortical connectivity (see Stryker et al., 1978). The usual result of such an experiment is that an abnormally high percentage of neurons in the primary visual cortex are responsive to vertical stimuli when tested in the adult animal.

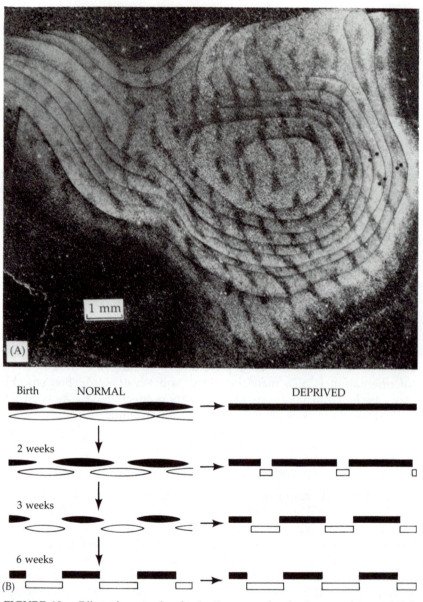

FIGURE 12. *Effect of monocular deprivation on ocular dominance columns. (A) In normal monkeys, ocular dominance columns gradually segregate to give alternating stripes of roughly equal width (see Figure 14 in Chapter 12). This dark-field autoradi-ograph shows a reconstruction of parallel sections through layer IVC of the primary visual cortex of a monkey the right eye of which was deprived by lid suture from 2 weeks of age to 18 months, when the animal was sacrificed. Two weeks before death the normal (left) eye was injected with radiolabeled amino acids. The columns from the nondeprived eye (white stripes) are much wider than normal. (B) Probable explanation of the duration of the critical period. Early deprivation alters competition between the projections from the two eyes because they still overlap widely; deprivation at progressively later times produces less obvious effects because the columns have already segregated. In this scheme, the end of the critical period coincides with the completion of the normal process of segregation. (From Hubel et al., 1977.)*

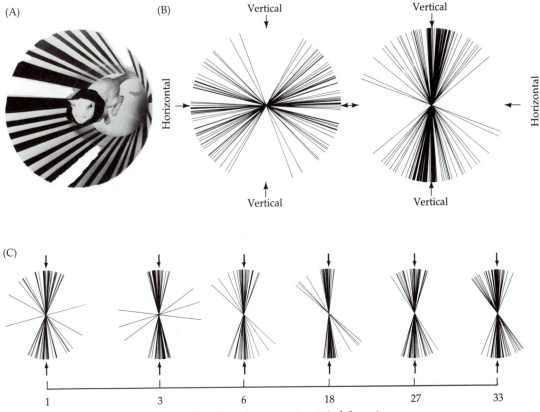

(C)

1	3	6	18	27	33

Duration of exposure to vertical (hours)

FIGURE 13. *Modification of the receptive field properties of visual cortical neurons by altered early experience. (A) Kittens can be raised in rotating drums in which they see only stripes of one orientation. The kittens wear black collars to hide their bodies and stand on a glass plate; except when in the drum for a few hours each day, they are kept in total darkness. (B) These polar histograms show the distribution of the stimulus orientations eliciting optimal responses in 52 neurons from a kitten that had been exposed only to horizontally oriented stimulation (left) and in 72 neurons from a kitten exposed only to vertical stimuli (right). The total visual* experience amounted to about 300 hours over the first 5 months of life (at which time the recordings were made). Each line represents the stimulus orientation eliciting an optimal response in a single neuron (cf. Figures 9 and 10). (C) Responses of kittens reared in darkness and exposed only to vertical stimuli for the number of hours indicated. As in B, each line signifies the optimal orientation for single neuron responses. Evidently, even a few hours of exposure to a particular visual environment can modify cortical connectivity. (A after Blakemore, 1974; B after Blakemore and Cooper, 1970; C after Blakemore and Mitchell, 1973.)*

A variety of experiments based on this paradigm have been carried out with other sorts of limited early visual experience. Thus, cats have been raised in stroboscopically illuminated environments where movement is abolished (Cynader et al., 1973), in environments in which all movement is unidirectional (Pettigrew and Garey, 1974), and in environments in which the visual world consists simply of points of light without any particular shape or orientation (Pettigrew and Freeman, 1973; Van Sluyters and Blakemore, 1973). The outcome of most of these experiments tends to support the idea that the early visual environment has a significant influence on subsequent connectivity (see Stryker et al., 1978).

One reason for the intense interest in these results is the notion that the *purpose* of critical periods is to allow the outside world to influence cortical connectivity. "The final organization of pattern detecting neurons in the visual cortex of a cat," C. Blakemore argues, "is fundamentally determined by the kitten's early visual experience. . . . This mechanism may be adaptive, the feature-detecting apparatus of the visual system being optimally matched to the animal's visual environment" (Blakemore, 1974, p. 105). However, many cells in the neonatal cortex are already organized to respond selectively to orientation at birth (see Figure 10); clearly, visual experience is not a requirement for the *initial* stages of the connectivity that leads to "feature detection." An alternative way of regarding critical periods is that they represent the developmental time when neuronal projections can still compete with one another. This period begins before birth (Rakic, 1977, 1981a) and lasts well into postnatal life (Chapter 12); indeed, some aspects of competition apparently persist indefinitely (Chapter 13). Because neural activity influences these competitive interactions, "experience" (in the sense of postnatal neural activity) will necessarily affect the end result. Whether the influence of experience in this sense is instructive or permissive is another matter. In relatively simple parts of the nervous system such as muscle and autonomic ganglia, it would be foolish to argue that experience instructs the final pattern of innervation (even though neural activity demonstrably plays a role; Chapter 12). On the other hand, in more complex parts of the nervous system, the effect of postnatal experience may generate unique neural circuits. Perhaps the significance of the critical period in the primary visual system lies somewhere between the role of experience in shaping peripheral connections and its role in shaping associational connections.

CONCLUSIONS

A theme that runs throughout this chapter is whether behavior is programmed or is a product of experience. A large body of work generated by ethologists has shown that much animal activity is innate: many behaviors are present at birth and are largely impervious to modification by experience. These same ethologists, however, have also shown that other behaviors are subject to more or less permanent modification: examples are imprinting in some newly hatched birds, socialization in primates, and vocal modification in songbirds. The behavioral programs that impel a gosling to form a lasting attachment to a moving object in the first few hours of life is a product of its development in ovo. On the other hand, whether the object that it follows is the mother goose or a man is clearly a matter of the animal's early exposure. Although the relative contributions of the given and the acquired to the development of behavior will probably be debated for a long time to come, it seems clear enough that many behaviors arise both from what is inherent and what is experienced. Indeed, as work on the developing visual system has shown, where intrinsic influences on neural development stop and experience begins is at best a fine distinction. In relatively simple animals, the portion of behavior engendered by the inherent rules of development seems the larger component of this equation. Even in humans, it would be wrong to imagine that the bulk of behavior is learned as a result of experience. Certainly inherent developmental programs lead to the neural connections that enable most of the functions necessary for survival and reproduction. Consciousness, after all, is only a small corner of our neural universe. Man's view tends to be biased because our minds have no direct access to the myriad neural mechanisms that allow us to function successfully in daily life, mechanisms that certainly are not learned. What we do learn, however, affects us (and other animals) in a profound way. The experiences of a young bird, a young monkey, or a young human have an immense influence on the animal's emotional well being and indeed its biological fitness. The interaction of individual animals and their world continues to shape the nervous system throughout life in ways that could never have been programmed. Modification of the nervous system by experience is thus the last and most subtle developmental strategy.

Principles of (and Some Prejudices About) Neural Development

CHAPTER

15

Authors who have the temerity to call their book "principles" of something should ultimately be called to account. Summarizing neural development has its perils, however. Because so many different factors are involved, syntheses are often more intimidating than helpful (Figure 1). In spite of the difficulty, attempts at distillation are probably useful because ideas that seem attached to particular aspects of development emerge as recurrent themes. In this chapter we have collected some of these ideas and have arranged them in roughly the order of their manifestation during neural development (the order of the book). Although the following points are not principles in any strict sense, they underscore themes that have shaped current thinking about neural development.

1. Neural development, like development generally, depends on genetic and epigenetic influences (Chapters 1 and 2).

Although this statement is certainly hackneyed, the interactive nature of development cannot be overemphasized. Development is not strictly governed by an unalterable plan locked away in the genome; rather, developmental phenomena are initiated by genomic events that depend in turn on epigenetic influences. This means that unraveling the relative contribution of genetic and epigenetic factors to particular developmental events is inevitably frustrated by the fact that genes influence the developmental environment—and that the developmental environment influences the genes (Figure 2).

2. The fate of cells becomes progressively restricted (Chapter 2).

From the perspective of individual cells, development is proliferation and progressive specialization. In general, cytodifferentiation is governed by each cell's genes, its cytoplasm, and the extracellular environment. A great deal of evidence shows that developing cells influence the proliferation and specialization of their neighbors by means of chemical signals (induction). As development proceeds, cells become less susceptible to such extragenetic influences. As a consequence, the fate of many cells becomes increasingly determined.

3. The lineage of specific cell types in many simple animals is largely preordained, whereas in complex animals the fate of individual cells is more flexible (Chapters 2 and 3).

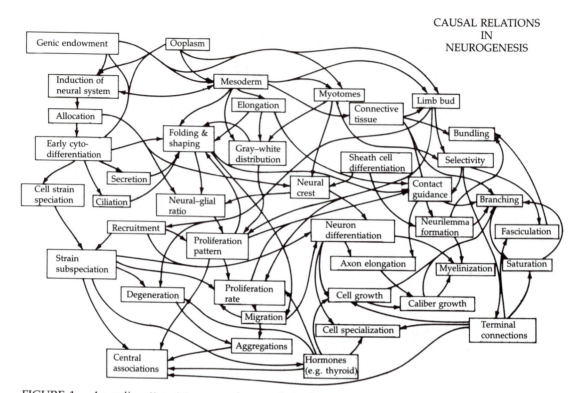

FIGURE 1.   *An earlier attempt to summarize neural development. (After Weiss, 1956).*

In an animal such as the roundworm C. *elegans,* each adult cell is derived from a predictable sequence of divisions of specific precursors. Various experimental manipulations indicate only a limited ability of these cells to compensate for perturbations. In this sense, the fate of every nerve cell in animals of this sort is largely preordained. Studies in other invertebrates (leech, grasshopper) suggest that this dependence of cell fate on lineage may be fairly general at lower phylogenetic levels.

In vertebrates, on the other hand, the relation between lineage and cell fate is less obvious. For example, any ectodermal cell can be induced to form neural tissue by an appropriate signal from underlying mesoderm. Moreover, ablation of relatively large parts of the developing nervous system can be compensated for by regulation of the remaining neural (and nonneural) tissue. This result implies that the fate of individual neurons in vertebrates is not predetermined. In this respect, the strategy of neural development in relatively simple and more complex animals may be different.

4. An important component of the epigenetic influences on differentiation is cell position (Chapter 3).

The importance of cell position is perhaps most obvious in relatively simple systems such as algal chains or insect cuticle, in which differentiation is evidently influenced by absolute position in a gradient across a developing group of cells. In these situations, the mechanism of positional instruction seems akin to induction. In other instances, however, differentiation according to position is more complicated. Regulation within morphogenetic fields during vertebrate development, complete restitution of a severed hydra, or regeneration of an insect limb provide examples of differentiation according to *relative* position.

5. Neuronal precursors, and subsequently neuronal processes, move according to directional cues in their local environment (Chapters 4 and 5).

Neuronal precursors, and somewhat later neuronal processes, move over substantial distances in the embryo to reach appropriate locations. The manner in which this occurs suggests a continual responsiveness to local cues that influence the direction of cell movement. The nature of these cues is not understood, but they almost certainly involve differential adhesion of the leading edge of the moving cell or growth cone to the substrate.

6. As vertebrate neurons mature, they acquire obligatory trophic dependencies (Chapters 6–8).

Whether many of the nerve cells initially generated flourish or succumb in vertebrates depends on the establishment of a relationship with appropriate targets. The present understanding of nerve growth factor and its biological role provides a paradigm for the acquisition of trophic support from targets (Figure 3). In this instance, targets manufacture a protein that is taken up by specific receptors on responsive neurons. The effects of uptake are both general (cell survival) and local (control of terminal arborizations). Innervating neurons in turn sustain many aspects of their target cells; for instance, innervation maintains the integrity and functional properties of muscle cells. The long-term postsynaptic effects of innervation depend on transmitter-induced activity as well as on chemical signals.

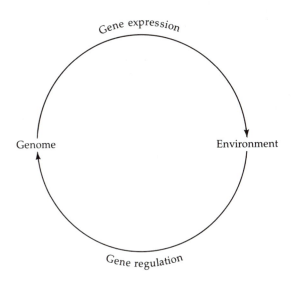

FIGURE 2.   *Genes affect the environment of developing nerve cells, and vice versa.*

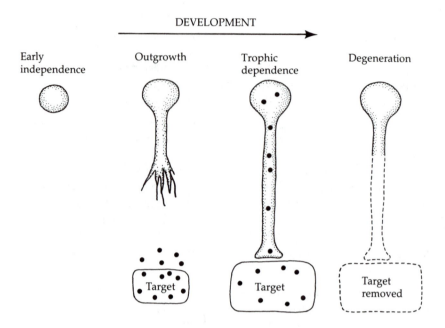

DEVELOPMENT

Early
independence

Outgrowth

Trophic
dependence

Degeneration

Target

Target

Target
removed

FIGURE 3. *Developing neurons acquire trophic dependencies.*

These retrograde and anterograde interactions show that neurons affect the properties of their targets and that targets affect the properties of the nerve cells that innervate them. This kind of interdependence is presumably a means of ensuring that every nerve cell in the adult has a useful function.

7. Vertebrate nerve terminals compete with one another for trophic support (Chapters 6, 7, 9 and 12).

More neurons initially innervate targets than can be trophically supported; as a result, competition occurs. Competition between neurons appears to provide the mainspring of quantitatively appropriate synaptic relationships. Competitive interactions help to regulate the number of nerve cells, the degree of convergence and divergence in neural pathways, and the number of synaptic contacts made between presynaptic and postsynaptic cells. In general, animals with complex nervous systems make extensive use of this sort of feedback and consequent adjustment in establishing neural connections, whereas simple animals seem to depend more heavily on preprogrammed circuitry.

8. The patterns of neuronal connections established during development also depend on recognition between presynaptic and postsynaptic cells (Chapters 9, 10 and 11).

Even competing inputs with the same trophic dependencies express different preferences during synapse formation. Such preferences presumably depend on surface recognition.

Intercellular recognition of this sort is relative rather than absolute.

For example, axons from particular preganglionic neurons are more likely to innervate qualitatively appropriate sympathetic ganglion cells and to make more synapses with them. Less appropriate cells are by no means excluded; they simply receive fewer (and weaker) contacts from the relevant axons. The continuously graded nature of this qualitative accuracy in synapse formation allows an extremely subtle modulation of synaptic connections.

9. Patterns of neural connections are maintained in an equilibrium throughout life (Chapter 13).

Neurons in mature animals can form new synaptic connections or retract existing ones. This implies that the number of synapses maintained between presynaptic and postsynaptic cells represents a balance of two opposing forces: the impetus to sprout and the tendency to withdraw. A lifelong persistence of trophic dependency may explain the continued malleability of neural connections. The sprouting of axon terminals and synapse formation are evidently stimulated by a surfeit of trophic support, whereas synaptic withdrawal is induced by a paucity of trophic support (Figure 4).

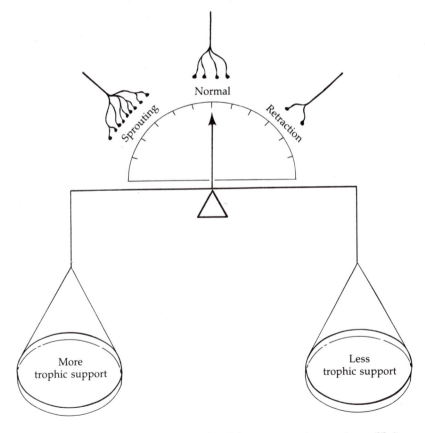

FIGURE 4. *Synaptic connections in the adult nervous system are in equilibrium.*

10. Neural malleability tends to persist in more complex animals (Chapters 13 and 14).

In lower animals, the stereotyped nature of the developmental environment, the brevity of life, and the narrowness of biological purpose may provide little impetus for behavioral flexibility; this is apparently reflected in the largely preprogrammed development of the nervous systems at these levels. Vertebrate neural development, on the other hand, is increasingly susceptible to the influence of experience. Perhaps as a reflection of this, more complex animals prolong developmental processes in the nervous system. Thus, the establishment of patterned neural connections in the primary visual cortex of a cat takes weeks; of a monkey, months; and of a man, years. A rule of thumb seems to be that the more "intelligent" an animal is (i.e., the more complex its nervous system), the more drawn out its neural development, particularly the period during which synaptic connections are malleable.

11. The sphere of influences acting on the nervous system continually enlarges during development (Chapter 14).

At the outset, the epigenetic environment is the milieu provided by the egg cytoplasm. Somewhat later, local cellular interactions (e.g., induction) become important. Later still, neurons send axons to targets that they then influence and are influenced by. Finally, the nervous system, of higher animals at least, is shaped by its experience in the postnatal world (Figure 5). Because each animal's experience is different, persistent neural malleability generates nervous systems that are unique.

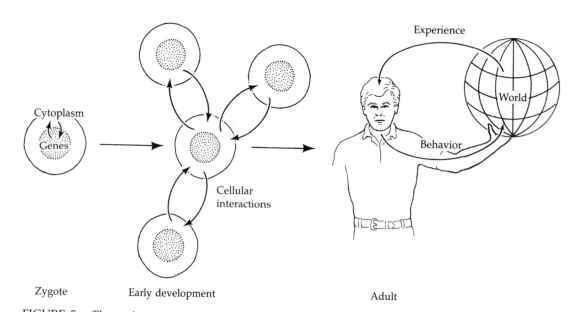

FIGURE 5. *The environment that influences neural development continually enlarges as an animal matures.*

*   *   *

Taken together, these various themes make a further point about neural development. In simpler animals, a relatively small number of elements are connected in a highly stereotyped manner by rigid obedience to genetic instructions and local epigenetic influences. Although no doubt the same fundamental mechanisms of cell biology are involved in the development of the vertebrate nervous system, the strategy of neural development in higher animals has a much more ecological quality: neurons and their synaptic connections behave more like organisms in a biological system than elements in an electrical circuit. What happens to an individual nerve cell cannot be foretold with any exactness because its role in life depends on competitive interactions with peers striving to succeed in the same niche. Exploring this aspect of nerve cell behavior—neuroecology—may provide the best hope of understanding the remarkable properties of the human nervous system.

Acknowledgments

We are greatly indebted to Viktor Hamburger and Josh Sanes who read the manuscript in its entirety and offered numerous valuable criticisms and suggestions. David Bentley, Nigel Daw, Steve Easter, David Gottlieb, Peggy Hollyday, Bob Horvitz, David Hubel, Gene Johnson, Eric Kandel, Peter Lawrence, Rita Levi-Montalcini, Fernando Nottebohm, Cherie Olson, Paul Patterson, Gunther Stent, Wes Thompson, Bob Wilkinson, Tom Woolsey and Bob Zucker gave us valuable advice on specific problems. We are also grateful to Andy Sinauer, Joe Vesely and Laszlo Meszoly for their expert production of the book and to Sue Eads, Margaret McCarthy and Jane Dunford for their patient and intelligent help throughout the preparation of the manuscript. Finally, we wish to thank numerous colleagues who generously provided many of the illustrations.

Glossary

action potential   The electrical signal conducted along axons (or muscle fibers).

adrenergic   Referring to synaptic transmission mediated by the release of norepinephrine.

adult   The mature form of an animal, usually defined by the ability to reproduce.

afferent   An axon that conducts information toward the central nervous system.

Ambystoma   A genus of salamanders with wide mouths and blunt heads. (Because of an error in a classic paper, the spelling *Ambystoma* ultimately replaced the more logical *Amblystoma* at the behest of the International Commission on Zoological Nomenclature.)

ametabolous   A style of insect development that does not involve metamorphosis.

amnion   The innermost membranes around the embryos of reptiles, birds, and mammals.

amniote   A vertebrate that develops in an amnion (i.e., reptiles, birds, and mammals).

amphibian   A cold-blooded vertebrate, the larva of which is aquatic (and breathes by gills), but the adult form of which is usually terrestrial and breathes air (technically, vertebrates of the class Amphibia).

amphioxus   A fishlike chordate of the genus *Branchiostoma* (also called a lancelet).

anamniote   A vertebrate that develops without an amnionic membrane (cyclostomes, fishes, and amphibians).

animal pole   The pole of the egg characterized by abundant cytoplasm and little yolk. This pole defines the region that gives rise to the nervous system (the nervous system was considered an "animal" organ by eighteenth century embryologists).

anlage (plural, **anlagen**)   A German word appropriated by embryologists to signify the embryonic primordium of an organ or embryonic part.

annelid   A segmented worm. Examples are earthworms and leeches (technically, invertebrates of the phylum Annelida).

anterior   Toward the front; sometimes used as a synonym for rostral, and sometimes as a synonym for ventral.

anterograde   A movement or influence acting from the neuronal cell body toward the axonal target.

anuran   An amphibian that lacks a tail as an adult. Examples are frogs and toads.

arthropod   A segmented invertebrate with jointed legs. Examples are insects, spiders, and crustacea (technically, a member of the phylum Arthropoda).

ascidian   Any solitary or colonial tunicate. Examples are the sea squirts (technically, a member of the class Acidiacea).

autonomic nervous system   The part of the nervous system (peripheral and central) concerned with the regulation of smooth muscle, cardiac muscle, and glands.

axolotl   A larval salamander of the genus *Ambystoma* that is sexually mature (usually *A. mexicanum*).

axon   The neuronal process that carries the action potential to a target.

axotomy   Cutting an axon.

basal lamina   A thin layer of extracellular matrix material (primarily collagen, laminin, fibronectin) that surrounds muscle cells and Schwann cells. Also underlies all epithelial sheets.

blastema   A mass of cells from which an organ or body part is formed, either normally or during regeneration.

blastocoele   The cavity of the blastula.

blastomere   A cell produced when the egg undergoes cleavage.

blastula   An early embryo during the stage when the cells are typically arranged to form a hollow sphere.

bouton   A swelling specialized for the release of neurotransmitter that occurs along or at the end of an axon.

caudal   Posterior or "tailward."

central nervous system   The brain and spinal cord of vertebrates (by analogy, the central nerve cord and ganglia of invertebrates).

cerebellum   A large division of the vertebrate brain that is located behind the cerebrum and is concerned with motor coordination, posture, and balance.

cerebrum   The largest part of the brain in man and other mammals, consisting primarily of the two cerebral hemispheres.

chemotaxis   The movement of a cell up (or down) a gradient of a chemical signal.

chemotropism   The growth of a part of a cell (axon, dendrite, filopodium) up (or down) a chemical gradient.

chimera   An experimentally generated embryo (or organ) comprising cells derived from two or more species (or other genetically distinct sources).

cholinergic   Referring to synaptic transmission mediated by the release of acetylcholine.

chordate   A member of the phylum Chordata. These animals are characterized by a notochord, pharyngeal gill slits, and a dorsal nerve cord (includes tunicates, lancelets, and vertebrates).

chorioallantoic membrane   A highly vascular double membrane that surrounds the amnion.

Major taxonomic category	Example (Man)	FIGURE 1. *Taxonomic categories.*

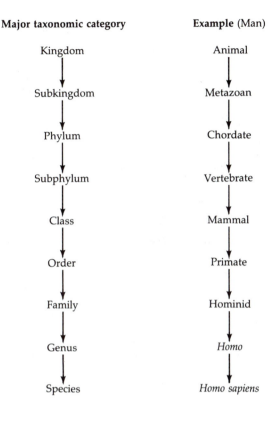

Major taxonomic category	Example (Man)
Kingdom	Animal
Subkingdom	Metazoan
Phylum	Chordate
Subphylum	Vertebrate
Class	Mammal
Order	Primate
Family	Hominid
Genus	*Homo*
Species	*Homo sapiens*

chromosome   Nuclear organelle that bears the genes.

class   A taxonomic category subordinate to phylum; comprises animal orders (see Figure 1).

cleavage   The early cell divisions that subdivide the fertilized egg.

cleavage furrow   A groove formed by division of the egg (or early blastomeres); often coincides with the plane of symmetry (the dorsoventral plane).

clone   All the progeny of a single cell.

compartment   A polyclone in the epidermis of some insects defined by aversion to intermingling with other polyclones across otherwise invisible boundaries.

competence   The ability of an embryonic tissue to respond to an inductive signal.

competition   The struggle among animals, cells, or cell processes for limited resources essential to survival or good health.

contact guidance   The notion that axon outgrowth is directed by mechanical features of the local environment.

contact inhibition   The inhibition of cell movement (or mitosis) that occurs when monolayer cultures divide to the point where cells touch one another.

contralateral   On the opposite side of the body.

convergence   Innervation of a target cell by multiple axons.

coronal   Referring to a plane through the brain that runs parallel to the coronal suture (the mediolateral plane).

corpus callosum   A large collection of axons that unite the two cerebral hemispheres across the midline.

cortex   The outer layers of the cerebral hemispheres and cerebellum, where most of the neurons in the brain are located.

crustacean   Chiefly aquatic arthropod with a hard shell; includes lobsters, crabs, barnacles, and shrimps (technically, a member of the class Crustacea).

cuticle   The outer epidermal layer in insects and other invertebrates. Often used as a synonym for epidermis.

cyclostome   An eel-like aquatic vertebrate characterized by a round, jawless mouth; includes lampreys and hagfishes (technically, a member of the subclass Cyclostomata).

dendrite   A neuronal process, usually branched, that receives synaptic input.

denervation   Removal of the innervation to a target.

depolarization   Reduction of the membrane potential from its resting value toward 0.

dermatome   The area of skin supplied by the sensory axons of a single spinal nerve.

determination   Commitment of a developing cell (or cell group) to a particular fate.

diencephalon   The part of the brain that includes the thalamus and related structures (the portion of the prosencephalon derived from the posterior part of the forebrain vesicle).

differentiation   The progressive specialization of developing cells.

distal   Further away from any point of reference (cf. **proximal**).

divergence   Branching of an axon to innervate multiple target cells.

dorsal   Referring to the back.

dorsal root ganglion (sensory ganglion)   Segmental collections of neurons that mediate sensation in the distribution of each spinal nerve in vertebrates.

ectoderm   The most superficial of the three germ layers (gives rise to the nervous system and epidermis).

efferent   An axon that conducts information away from the central nervous system.

egg   The female gamete.

embryo   The developing organism before birth or hatching.

endoderm   The deepest of the three germ layers (gives rise to the gut and related structures).

endplate   Specialization on skeletal muscle fibers at the site of nerve contact.

ependyma   The epithelial lining of the canal of the spinal cord and the ventricles.

ependymal zone   *See* **ventricular zone.**

epidermis   The outermost layer of the skin; derived from the ectoderm.

epigenetic   Referring to influences on cell development that arise from factors other than genetic instructions.

epithelium   Any continuous layer of cells that covers a surface or lines a cavity.

eukaryote   An organism having cells with nuclei.

explant   A piece of tissue placed in culture.

family   A taxonomic category subordinate to order; comprises genera (see Figure 1).

fasciculation   The aggregation of neuronal processes to form a nerve bundle.

fate map   A diagram of the embryo that indicates the prospective fate of each region.

fetus   The developing mammalian embryo at relatively late stages when the parts of the body are recognizable.

fibrillation   Spontaneous contractile activity of denervated muscle fibers.

field   *See* **morphogenetic field.**

filopodium   Slender protoplasmic projection, arising from the growth cone of an axon or dendrite, that explores the local environment and adheres to a favorable substrate.

forebrain   *See* **prosencephalon.**

galvanotropism   Attraction to a source or sink of electrical current.

gamete   A mature reproductive cell (egg or sperm).

ganglion (plural, **ganglia**)   In vertebrates, a collection of neurons at a particular site outside of the brain and spinal cord; in invertebrates, the stereotyped collections of neurons that make up the "central" nervous system.

gastrula   The early embryo during the period when the three germ layers are formed; follows the blastula stage.

gastrulation   The cell movements (invagination and spreading) that transform the blastula to the gastrula.

gene   A hereditary unit located on the chromosomes; genetic information is carried by linear sequences of nucleotides in DNA that code for corresponding sequences of amino acids.

genome   The complete set of an animal's genes.

genotype   The genetic makeup of an individual.

genus   A taxonomic division that comprises a number of closely related species within a family (see Figure 1).

germ cell   The egg or sperm (or the precursors of these cells).

germ layers   The three primary layers of the developing embryo from which all adult tissues arise (ectoderm, mesoderm, and endoderm).

glia   Supportive cells associated with neurons (astrocytes and oligodendrocytes in the central nervous system, Schwann cells in peripheral nerves, and satellite cells in ganglia).

gradient   A systematic variation of the concentration of a molecule (or some other agent) that influences cell behavior.

gray crescent   A gray-colored cytoplasmic region that appears in some amphibian eggs and identifies the future dorsal side of the embryo.

growth cone   The specialized end of a growing axon (or dendrite) that generates the motive force for elongation.

hemimetabolous   A style of insect metamorphosis characterized by gradual transition of larval stages.

Hensen's node   A cluster of cells in the ectoderm of the avian gastrula that marks the anterior end of the primitive streak (analogous to the dorsal lip of the blastopore in the amphibian gastrula).

hindbrain   *See* **rhombencephalon.**

hippocampus   A deeply infolded portion of the cerebral cortex in higher vertebrates; its function is uncertain. Its discrete and highly organized arrangement has made it a favorite object of neuroanatomical study.

holoblastic   A style of egg cleavage in which the entire egg participates (characteristic of mammalian eggs; cf. **meroblastic**).

holometabolous   A style of insect metamorphosis in which the larva enters a pupal stage, during which it is dramatically transformed into the adult.

homeotic mutant   A mutation that transforms one part of the body into another (e.g., insect antennae into legs).

imaginal disk   Segmentally distributed tissues that occur in some insects; the disks take no part in larval life but generate adult parts at metamorphosis.

imago   The adult form that appears at the final molt of some insects and that was previously encrypted in the imaginal disks of the larva.

induction   The ability of one tissue to influence the fate of nearby cells, presumably by a chemical signal.

instar   A developing insect during the periods between molts.

instinctual behavior   A behavior that is not learned.

instructive   A developmental influence that dictates the fate of a cell rather than simply permitting differentiation to occur.

integration   The summation of excitatory and inhibitory synaptic conductance changes.

interneuron   A neuron that intervenes between sensory and effector neurons.

invertebrate   Any animal without a backbone.

in vitro   Referring to any biological process studied outside of the organism (literally "in glass").

in vivo   Referring to any biological process studied in an intact living organism.

ipsilateral   On the same side of the body.

larva   The postembryonic stage of metamorphosing animals that precedes the transition to the adult form.

learning   The acquisition of novel behavior through experience.

limb bud   The limb rudiment of vertebrate embryos.

mammal   An animal the embyros of which develop in a uterus and the young of which begin to suckle at birth (technically, a member of the class Mammalia).

medial   Located nearer to the midsagittal plane of an animal (the opposite of lateral).

meroblastic   A style of egg division, typical of some fishes, reptiles, and birds, in which cleavage is restricted to one superficial region of the egg (the non-yolky part; cf. **holoblastic**).

mesencephalon   The part of the brain that includes the superior and inferior colliculi, and the aqueduct of Sylvius (derived from the embryonic midbrain vesicle).

mesenchyme   Embryonic connective tissue that is derived largely from the mesoderm and gives rise to blood and lymphatic vessels and to adult connective tissue.

mesoderm   The middle of the three germ layers (gives rise to muscle, connective tissue, skeleton, and other structures).

metamere   *See* **segment.**

metameric   Referring to segmentation.

metamorphosis   The transformation of a larva into an adult form.

metazoan   A multicellular animal (technically, an animal belonging to this subkingdom of the animal kingdom).

midbrain, *see* **mesencephalon.**

modality   A category of function. For example, vision, hearing, and touch are different sensory modalities.

mollusc   An invertebrate usually characterized by a calcareous shell and a soft, unsegmented body. Examples are chitons, snails, squids, octopuses, and bivalves (technically, a member of the phylum Mollusca).

molt   A casting off of feathers, skin, or exoskeleton, which is replaced by new growth.

monoclonal antibody   An antibody molecule raised from a clone of transformed lymphocytes.

morphogen   A molecule presumed to influence morphogenesis.

morphogenesis   The generation of animal form.

morphogenetic field   An embryonic region that can regulate following the ablation of any part of that region.

morphology   The study of the form and structure of organisms; or, more commonly, the form and structure of an animal or animal part.

morula   An early stage in the development of some animals, during which the embryo is a solid mass of cells; precedes formation of the blastula.

mosaic development   Referring to an embryo in which the fate of each early cell is already determined (cf. **regulative development**).

motor neuron   By usage, a nerve cell that innervates skeletal muscle (or the equivalent in invertebrates).

motor unit   The unit formed by a motor neuron and the skeletal muscle fibers it innervates.

myoblast   A developing muscle cell before it fuses with others to form myotubes.

myotome   The part of each somite that contributes to the development of skeletal muscles.

myotube   A developing muscle cell formed by the fusion of myoblasts.

nematode   A roundworm or threadworm (technically, a member of the class Nematoda).

nerve   A collection of axons, usually peripheral, that travel a common route.

neural crest   A group of cells that forms along the dorsum of the neural tube and gives rise to peripheral neurons and glia (among other derivatives).

neural plate   The thickened region of the dorsal ectoderm of a neurula that gives rise to the neural tube.

neural tube The primordium of the brain and spinal cord; derived from the neural ectoderm.

neural unit The collection of target neurons innervated by a single axon.

neurite A neuronal process; used when the process in question could be an axon or a dendrite (e.g., the processes of isolated cells in tissue culture).

neuroblast A dividing cell the progeny of which develop into neurons.

neurogenesis The development of the nervous system.

neuromuscular junction Site of the synapse made by a motor axon on a skeletal muscle fiber.

neuron A nerve cell. Usually defined by the ability to receive and transmit information by means of synaptic connections.

neuropil Regions of the nervous system where axons, dendrites, and synapses are densely intertwined.

neurula The early vertebrate embryo during the stage when the neural tube forms from the neural plate; follows the gastrula stage.

notochord A transient skeletal structure of mesodermal cells underlying the neural plate (and later the neural tube) in vertebrate embryos; may be a permanent structure in other chordates.

nymph The larval stage of a hemimetabolous insect.

ontogeny A synonym for development.

optic tectum The first central station in the visual pathway of many vertebrates (located in the midbrain and analogous to the superior colliculus in mammals).

optic vesicle The evagination of the forebrain vesicle that induces lens formation in the overlying ectoderm.

order A taxonomic category subordinate to class; comprises animal families (see Figure 1).

organizer The part of the dorsal lip of an amphibian gastrula that has the ability to induce a secondary embryo when transplanted ectopically.

parasympathetic nervous system A division of the peripheral autonomic nervous system in vertebrates comprising cholinergic ganglion cells located near target organs (derived from cranial and sacral neural crest).

peripheral nervous system All nerves and neurons outside the central nervous system.

permissive An influence during development that permits differentiation to occur but does not specifically instruct cell fate.

phenotype The visible (or otherwise discernible) characteristics of an animal that arise during development.

phylogeny The evolutionary history of a species (or other taxonomic category).

phylum A major division of the plant or animal kingdom that includes classes having a common ancestry (see Figure 1).

pioneer The first axon that navigates the path to a target.

placode An ectodermal thickening that occurs in vertebrate embryos and gives rise to a sense organ (or sensory ganglion) in the head.

plasticity An overused term that refers to structural or functional changes in the nervous system, usually in the adult.

pluripotent Referring to a cell whose fate is still undecided; the opposite of determined (*see also* **totipotent**).

polarity Referring to a continually graded organization along one of the major embryonic axes.

polyclone A group of cells comprising several clones.

posterior Toward the back; sometimes used as a synonym for caudal and sometimes as a synonym for dorsal.

postsynaptic Referring to the component of a synapse specialized for transmitter reception.

preformation The idea that development represents the growth of miniature but fully formed parts.

presynaptic Referring to the component of a synapse specialized for transmitter release.

primary induction The induction of the neural plate by the underlying mesoderm in amphibian embryos; contrasts with secondary induction (e.g., of the lens).

primate An order of mammals that includes lemurs, tarsiers, marmosets, monkeys, apes, and man (technically, a member of this order).

primitive streak Axial thickening in the ectoderm of the gastrulas of reptiles, birds, and mammals; the mesoderm forms by ingression of cells at this site.

prokaryote An organism the cells of which lack a nucleus and divide by binary fission. Examples are bacteria and blue-green algae.

prosencephalon The part of the brain that includes the diencephalon and telencephalon (derived from the embryonic forebrain vesicle).

prospective fate The anticipated role of a cell (or cell group) and its progeny.

protozoan A unicellular animal (technically, an animal belonging to this subkingdom of the animal kingdom).

proximal Closer to any point of reference (cf. **distal**).

pseudopodium *See* **filopodium.**

pupa The quiescent form of holometabolous insects that precedes the emergence of the adult form.

recapitulation The developmental repetition of phylogeny.

receptive field The peripheral area of the body that activates a sensory neuron.

reflex A stereotyped (involuntary) motor response elicited by a defined stimulus.

regulation The ability of an embryonic anlage to completely compensate for partial ablation.

regulative development Referring to an embryo that regulates; that is, an embryo in which cell fate is flexible (cf. **mosaic development**).

reptile A class of cold-blooded vertebrates that includes snakes, turtles, lizards, crocodilians, and tuatara (technically, a member of the class Reptilia).

resting potential The voltage difference that normally exists across a cell membrane.

retrograde A movement or influence acting from the axon terminal toward the cell body.

rhombencephalon The part of the brain that includes the pons, cerebellum, and medulla (derived from the embryonic hindbrain vesicle).

rostral Anterior or "headward."

sagittal Referring to the anterior–posterior plane of an animal.

Schwann cell The name given the glial cells in peripheral nerves.

segment One of a series of more or less similar anterior–posterior units that make up segmental animals.

segmentation The anterior–posterior division of animals into roughly similar repeating units.

selectivity The ability of an axon to chose appropriately among potential synaptic partners.

self-differentiation The ability of cells or cell groups to differentiate without benefit of induction or other extrinsic influences.

soma A nerve cell body.

somatic cells Referring to the cells of an animal other than its germ cells.

somites Segmentally arranged, blocklike masses of mesoderm that lie alongside the neural tube and give rise to skeletal muscle, vertebrae, and dermis.

species A taxonomic category subordinate to genus; members of a species are defined by extensive similarities, including the ability to interbreed (see Figure 1).

specificity A broad term that refers to the stereotyped outcome of development in the nervous system. Sometimes used as a synonym for selective synapse formation.

sprouting The growth of axon terminals in response to any of a variety of normal or experimental stimuli.

stereotropism Directed axon growth resulting from contact with structural features in the local environment.

supersensitivity An increased responsiveness of target cells to neurotransmitters following denervation.

sympathetic nervous system A division of the peripheral autonomic nervous system in vertebrates comprising, for the most part, adrenergic ganglion cells located relatively far from the related end organs (derived from thoracolumbar neural crest).

synapse A specialized apposition between a neuron and its target cell for transmission of information by release and reception of a chemical transmitter agent.

syncytium A group of cells in protoplasmic continuity.

tadpole A larval frog.

taxonomy The discipline of classifying plants and animals (see Figure 1).

telencephalon The part of the brain that includes the cerebral hemispheres (derived from the anterior part of the embryonic forebrain vesicle).

teleost A bony fish (as opposed to a cartilagenous fish like a shark) (technically, a member of the class Osteichthyes).

totipotent The ability of a cell or group of cells to give rise to a whole organism.

transmitter (neurotransmitter) A chemical agent that is released by a presynaptic cell and influences the conductance of a postsynaptic cell.

trophic The ability of one tissue or cell to support another; usually applied to long-term interactions between presynaptic and postsynaptic cells.

tropic An influence of one cell or tissue on the direction of movement (or outgrowth) of another.

tropism Orientation of growth in response to an external stimulus.

tunicate Any marine animal with a saclike body and a leathery tunic (technically, a member of the subphylum Urochordata).

urodele A tailed amphibian. Examples are salamanders and newts (technically, a member of the order Urodela).

vegetal pole The pole of the egg opposite the animal pole; adjacent structures give rise to "vegetal" organs such as the gut (cf. **animal pole**).

ventral Referring to the belly.

ventricles The cavities in the vertebrate brain that contain cerebrospinal fluid.

vertebrate An animal with a backbone (technically, a member of the subphylum Vertebrata).

vesicle Literally a small sac. Used to refer to any of the three dilations of the anterior end of the neural tube that give rise to the three major subdivisions of the brain. Also used to refer to the organelles that store and release transmitter at nerve endings.

vitalism The mystical view that nonmaterial forces must be invoked to explain biological phenomena.

yolk The parts of an egg (or its progeny) that contain stored nutrition.

zygote The fertilized egg.

Bibliography

THE NUMBERS THAT FOLLOW EACH ENTRY
IDENTIFY THE CHAPTER(S) IN WHICH THE REFERENCE IS CITED.

Abercrombie, M. (1946). Estimation of nuclear population from microtome sections. *Anat. Rec. 94*: 239–247. [6]

Abercrombie, M. (1961). The bases of the locomotory behavior of fibroblasts. *Exp. Cell Res. 8(Suppl)*: 188–198. [4]

Abercrombie, M. (1980). The crawling movement of metazoan cells. *Proc. R. Soc. Lond. [Biol.] 207*: 129–147. [4]

Abercrombie, M. (1982). The crawling movement of metazoan cells. In: *Cell Behavior*, R. Bellairs, A. Curtis and G. Dunn, eds. Cambridge: Cambridge University Press, pp. 19–48. [4]

Abercrombie, M. and J. E. M. Heaysman. (1954). Observations on the social behaviour of cells in tissue culture. II. "Monolayering" of fibroblasts. *Exp. Cell Res. 6*: 293–306. [4]

Abercrombie, M., J. E. M. Heaysman and S. M. Pegrum. (1970). The locomotion of fibroblasts in culture. II. "Ruffling." *Exp. Cell Res. 60*: 437–444 [4]

Abercrombie, M. and C. A. Middleton. (1968). Epithelial–mesenchymal interactions affecting locomotion of cells in culture. In: *Epithelial–Mesenchymal Interactions*, R. Fleischmajer and R. E. Billingham, eds. Baltimore: Williams and Wilkins, pp. 56–63 [4]

Acheson, G. H., E. S. Lee and R. S. Morison. (1942). A deficiency in the phrenic respiratory discharges parallel to retrograde degeneration. *J. Neurophysiol. 5*: 269–273. [13]

Adams, I. and D. G. Jones. (1982). Quantitative ultrastructural changes in rat cortical synapses during early-, mid- and late-adulthood. *Brain Res. 239*: 349–363. [9]

Adler, J. (1976). The sensing of chemicals by bacteria. *Sci. Am. 234(4)*: 40–47. [4]

Adler, R., K. B. Landa, M. Manthorpe and S. Varon. (1979). Cholinergic neurontrophic factors: Intraocular distribution of trophic activity for ciliary neurons. *Science 204*: 1434–1436. [7]

Aghajanian, G. K. and F. E. Bloom. (1967). The formation of synaptic junctions in developing rat brain: A quantitative electron microscopic study. *Brain Res. 6*: 716–727. [9]

Aguayo, A. J., G. M. Bray, C. S. Perkins and I. D. Duncan. (1979). Axon–sheath cell interactions in peripheral and central nervous system transplants. *Soc. Neurosci. Symp. 4*: 361–383. [5]

Aguayo, A., S. David, P. Richardson and G. Bray. (1982a). Axonal elongation in peripheral and central nervous system transplants. *Adv. Cell Neurobiol. 3*: 215–234. [5]

Aguayo, A. J., P. M. Richardson and M. Benrey. (1982b). Transplantation of neurons and sheath cells—A tool for the study of regeneration. In: *Repair and Regeneration of the Nervous System, Life Sciences Research Report 24*, J. G. Nicholls, ed., Berlin: Springer-Verlag, pp. 91–106. [5]

Aguayo, A. J., L. C. Terry and G. M. Bray. (1973). Spontaneous loss of axons in sympathetic unmylinated nerve fibers of the rat during development. *Brain Res. 54*: 360 -364. [6]

Aguilar, C. E., M. A. Bisby, E. Cooper and J. Diamond. (1973). Evidence that axoplasmic transport of trophic factors is involved in the regulation of peripheral nerve fields in salamanders. *J. Physiol. (Lond.) 234*: 449–464. [13]

Alberts, B., D. Bray, J. Lewis, M. Raff, K. Roberts and J. D. Watson. (1983). *Molecular Biology of the Cell.* New York: Garland. [3, 4]

Albertson, D. G. and J. N. Thomson. (1976). The pharynx of *Caenorhabditis elegans*. *Philos. Trans. R. Soc. Lond [Biol.] 275*: 299–325. [2]

Albrecht-Buehler, G. (1977). Daughter 3T3 cells. Are they mirror images of each other? *J. Cell Biol. 72*: 595–603. [4]

Albrecht-Buehler, G. (1978). The tracks of moving cells. *Sci. Am. 245(4)*: 68–76. [4]

Albuquerque, E. X. and R. J. McIsaac. (1970). Fast and slow mammalian muscles after denervation. *Exp. Neurol. 26*: 183–202 [8]

Albuquerque, E. X., F. T. Schuh and F. C. Kauffman. (1971). Early membrane depolarization of the fast mammalian muscle after denervation. *Pflügers Arch. 328*: 36–50. [8]

Albuquerque, E. X., J. E. Warnick, J. R. Tasse and F. M. Sansone. (1972). Effects of vinblastine and colchicine on neural regulation of the fast and slow skeletal muscles of the rat. *Exp. Neurol. 37*: 607–634. [8]

Alderman, A. L. (1935). The determination of the eye in the anuran, *Hyla regilla*. *J. Exp. Zool.* 70: 205–232. [3]

Allen, B. M. (1918). The results of thyroid removal in the larvae of *Rana pipiens*. *J. Exp. Zool.* 24: 499–519. [1]

Allen, B. M. (1938). The endocrine control of amphibian metamorphosis. *Biol. Rev.* 13: 1–19. [1]

Allen, R. D., N. S. Allen and J. L. Travis. (1981). Video-enhanced contrast, differential interference contrast (AVEC-DIC) microscopy: A new method capable of analyzing microtuble-related motility in the reticulopodial network of *Allogromia laticollaris*. *Cell Motil.* 1: 291–302. [8]

Allen, R. D., G. B. David and G. Nomarski. (1969). The Zeiss-Nomarski differential interference equipment for transmitted-light microscopy. *A. Wiss. Mikrosk.* 69: 193 - 221. [8]

Allen, R. D. and D. L. Taylor. (1975). The molecular basis of amoeboid movement. In: *Molecules and Cell Movement*, S. Inoue and R. E. Stephens, eds. New York: Raven Press, pp. 239–257. [4]

Alley, K. E. (1974). Morphogenesis of the trigeminal mesencephalic nucleus in the hamster: Cytogenesis and neurone death. *J. Embryol. Exp. Morphol.* 31: 99 - 121. [6]

Aloe, L., C. Cozzari, P. Calilssano and R. Levi-Montalcini. (1981). Somatic and behavioural postnatal effects of fetal injections of nerve growth factor antibodies in the rat. *Nature* 291: 413–415. [7]

Aloe, L. and R. Levi-Montalcini. (1977). Mast cells increase in tissues of neonatal rats injected with the nerve growth factor. *Brain Res.* 133: 358–366. [7]

Aloe, L. and R. Levi-Montalcini. (1979). Nerve growth factor-induced transformation of immature chromaffin cells *in vivo* into sympathetic neurons: Effect of antiserum to nerve growth factor. *Proc. Natl. Acad. Sci. USA* 76: 1246–1250. [7]

Aloe, L., E. Mugnaini and R. Levi-Montalcini. (1975). Light and electron microscopic studies on the excessive growth of sympathetic ganglia in rats injected daily from birth with 6-OHDA and NGF. *Arch. Ital. Biol.* 113: 326–353. [7]

Altman, J. (1972). Postnatal development of the cerebellar cortex in the rat. III. Maturation of the components of the granular layer. *J. Comp. Neurol.* 145: 465–514. [9]

Anderson, C. B. and S. Meier. (1981). The influence of the metameric pattern in the mesoderm on migration of cranial neural crest cells in the chick embryo. *Dev. Biol.* 85: 385–402. [4]

Anderson, H., J. S. Edwards and J. Palka. (1980). Developmental neurobiology of invertebrates. *Annu. Rev. Neurosci.* 3: 97–139. [10]

Anderson, M. J. and M. W. Cohen. (1974). Fluorescent staining of acetylcholine receptors in vertebrate skeletal muscle. *J. Physiol. (Lond.)* 237: 385–400. [9]

Anderson, M. J. and M. W. Cohen. (1977). Nerve-induced and spontaneous redistribution of acetylcholine receptors on cultured muscle cells. *J. Physiol. (Lond.)* 268: 757–773. [9]

Anderson, M. J., M. W. Cohen and E. Zorychta. (1977). Effects of innervation on the distribution of acetylcholine receptors on cultured muscle cells. *J. Physiol. (Lond.)* 268: 731–756. [9]

Andres, R. Y., I. Jeng and R. A. Bradshaw. (1977). Nerve growth factor receptors: Identification of distinct classes in plasma membranes and nuclei of embryonic dorsal root neurons. *Proc. Natl. Acad. Sci. USA* 74: 2785–2789. [7]

Angeletti, P. U., R. Levi-Montalcini and F. Caramia. (1971). Ultrastructural changes in sympathetic neurons of newborn and adult mice treated with nerve growth factor. *J. Ultrastruct. Res.* 36: 24–36. [7]

Angeletti, R. H., P. U. Angeletti and R. Levi-Montalcini. (1972). Selective accumulation of [125I]-labelled nerve growth factor in a sympathetic ganglion. *Brain Res.* 46: 421–425. [7]

Angeletti, R. H. and R. A. Bradshaw. (1971). Nerve growth factor from mouse submaxillary gland: Amino acid sequence. *Proc. Natl. Acad. Sci. USA* 68: 2417–2420. [7]

Angeletti, R. H., M. A. Hermodson and R. A. Bradshaw. (1973). Amino acid sequences of mouse 2.5S nerve growth factor. II. Isolation and characterization of the thermolytic and peptic peptides and the complete covalent structure. *Biochemistry* 12: 100–115. [7]

Anzil, A. P., A. Beiser and A. Wernig. (1984). Light and electron microscopic identification of nerve terminal sprouting and retraction in normal adult frog muscle. *J. Physiol. (Lond.)* 350: 393–399. [13]

Archer, S. M., M. W. Dubin and L. A. Stark. (1982). Abnormal development of kitten retino-geniculate connectivity in the absence of action potentials. *Science* 217: 743–745. [12]

Ariëns Kappers, C. U., G. C. Huber and E. C. Crosby. (1936). *The Comparative Anatomy of the Nervous System of Vertebrates, Including Man* (2 volumes). New York: Macmillan. [5]

Armstrong, R. C. and P. G. H. Clarke. (1979). Neuronal death and the development of the pontine nuclei and inferior olive in the chick. *Neuroscience* 4: 1635–1647. [6]

Armstrong-James, M. and R. Johnson. (1970). Quantitative studies of postnatal changes in synapses in rat superficial motor cerebral cortex. An electron microscopical study. *A. Zellforsch. Microsk. Anat.* 110: 559–568. [9]

Arnold, A. P. (1980). Effects of androgens on volumes of sexually dimorphic brain regions in the zebra finch. *Brain Res.* 185: 441–444. [14]

Atsumi, S. (1971). The histogenesis of motor neurons with special reference to the correlation of their endplate formation. I. The development of endplates in the intercostal muscle in the chick embryo. *Acta Anat. (Basel)* 80: 161–182. [9]

Atsumi, S. (1977). Development of neuromuscular junctions of fast and slow muscles in the chick embryo: A light and electron microscopic study. *J. Neurocytol.* 6: 691–709. [9]

Attardi, D. G. and R. W. Sperry. (1963). Preferential selection of central pathways by regenerating optic fibers. *Exp. Neurol.* 7: 46–64. [11]

Axelsson, J. and S. Thesleff. (1959). A study of super-sensitivity in denervated mammalian skeletal muscle. *J. Physiol. (Lond.) 147*: 178–193. [8]

Bader, C. R., D. Bertrand, E. Dupin and A. C. Kato. (1983). Development of electrical membrane properties in cultured avian neural crest. *Nature 305*: 808–810. [2]

Bagust, J., D. M. Lewis and R. A. Westerman. (1973). Polyneuronal innervation of kitten skeletal muscle. *J. Physiol. (Lond.) 229*: 241–255. [12]

Bailey, C. H. and M. Chen. (1983). Morphological basis of long-term habituation and sensitization in *Aplysia*. *Science 220*: 91–93. [13]

Balinsky, B. I. (1975). *An Introduction to Embryology*, 4th Ed. Philadelphia: Saunders. [1]

Balsamo, J. and J. Lilien. (1975). The binding of tissue-specific adhesive molecules to the cell surface. A molecular basis for specificity. *Biochemistry 14*: 167–171. [11]

Balsamo, J., J. McDonough and J. Lilien. (1976). Retinal–tectal connections in the embryonic chick: Evidence for regionally specific cell surface components which mimic the pattern of innervation. *Dev. Biol. 49*: 338–346. [11]

Baltzer, F. (1967). *Theodor Boveri: Life and Work of a Great Biologist, 1862–1915*. Translated by D. Rudnick. Berkeley: University of California Press. [3]

Banker, B. Q. (1982). Physiologic death of neurons in the developing anterior horn of the mouse. In: *Human Motor Neuron Diseases*, L. P. Rowland, ed. New York: Raven Press, pp. 473–485. [6]

Banker, B. Q., S. S. Kelly and N. Robbins. (1983). Neuromuscular transmission and correlative morphology in young and old mice. *J. Physiol. (Lond.) 339*: 353–375. [13]

Banker, G. A. and W. M. Cowan. (1979). Further observations on hippocampal neurons in dispersed cell culture. *J. Comp. Neurol. 187*: 469–494. [2]

Barbera, A. J. (1975). Adhesive recognition between developing retinal cells and the optic tecta of the chick embryo. *Dev. Biol. 46*: 167–191. [11]

Barbera, A. J., R. B. Marchase and S. Roth. (1973). Adhesive recognition and retinotectal specificity. *Proc. Natl. Acad. Sci. USA 70*: 2482–2486. [11]

Barde, Y.-A., D. Edgar and H. Thoenen. (1980). Sensory neurons in culture: Changing requirements for survival factors during embryonic development. *Proc. Natl. Acad. Sci. USA 77*: 1199–1203. [7]

Barde, Y.-A., D. Edgar and H. Thoenen. (1982). Purification of a new neurotrophic factor from mammalian brain. *EMBO J. 1*: 549–553. [7]

Barde, Y.-A., D. Edgar and H. Thoenen (1983). New neurotrophic factors. *Annu. Rev. Physiol. 45*: 601–612. [7]

Barker, D. and M. C. Ip. (1966). Sprouting and degeneration of mammalian motor axons in normal and de-afferentated skeletal muscle. *Proc. R. Soc. Lond. [Biol.] 163*: 538–554. [13]

Barlow, H. B. (1975). Visual experience and cortical development. *Nature 258*: 199–204. [14]

Barnstable, C. J. (1980). Monoclonal antibodies which recognize different cell types in the rat retina. *Nature 286*: 231–235. [11]

Barth, L. (1964). *Development: Selected Topics*. Reading, MA: Addison-Wesley. [2]

Bate, C. M. (1976). Pioneer neurones in an insect embryo. *Nature 260*: 54–56. [5]

Bate, C. M., C. S. Goodman and N. C. Spitzer. (1981). Embryonic development of identified neurons: Segment-specific differences in the H cell homologues. *J. Neurosci. 1*: 103–106. [6]

Bate, C. M. and E. B. Grunewald. (1981). Embryogenesis of an insect nervous system. II. A second class of neuron precursor cells and the origin of the intersegmental connectives. *J. Embryol. Exp. Morphol. 61*: 317–330. [6]

Bauer, H. C., M. P. Daniels, P. A. Pudimat, L. Jacques, H. Sugiyama and C. N. Christian. (1981). Characterization and partial purification of a neuronal factor which increases acetylcholine receptor aggregation on cultured muscle cells. *Brain Res. 209*: 395–404. [9]

Bayer, S. A., J. W. Yackel and P. S. Puri. (1982). Neurons in the rat dentate gyrus granular layer substantially increase during juvenile and adult life. *Science 216*: 890–892. [6]

Baylor, D. A. and J. G. Nicholls. (1971). Patterns of regeneration between individual nerve cells in the central nervous system of the leech. *Nature 232*: 268–270. [10]

Bayne, E. K., J. Gardner and D. M. Fambrough. (1981). Monoclonal antibodies to extracellular matrix antigens in chicken skeletal muscle. In: *Monoclonal Antibodies to Neural Antigens*, R. McKay, M. Raff and L. Reichardt, eds. Cold Spring Harbor, NY: Cold Spring Harbor Laboratories, pp. 259–270. [9]

Beams, H. W. and R. G. Kessel. (1976). Cytokinesis: A comparative study of cytoplasmic division in animal cells. *Am. Sci. 64*: 279–290. [1]

Beaudoin, A. R. (1956). The development of lateral motor column cells in the lumbo-sacral cord in *Rana pipiens*. II. Development under the influence of thyroxin. *Anat. Rec. 125*: 247–259. [6]

Beermann, S. (1977). The diminution of heterochromatic chromosomal segments in *cyclops* (crustacea, copepoda). *Chromasoma 60*: 297–344. [2]

Beerman, W. and U. Clever. (1964). Chromosome puffs. *Sci. Am. 210(4)*: 50–58. [1]

Beidler, L. M. (1963). Dynamics of taste cells. In: *Olfaction and Taste*, Y. Zotterman, ed. Oxford: Pergamon Press, pp. 133–148. [8]

Beidler, L. M. and R. L. Smallman. (1965). Renewal of cells within taste buds. *J. Cell Biol. 27*: 263–272. [8]

Bekoff, A. (1976). Ontogeny of leg motor output in the chick embryo: A neural analysis. *Brain Res. 106*: 271–291. [14]

Bekoff, A. (1978). A neuroethological approach to the study of the ontogeny of coordinated behavior. In: *The Development of Behavior: Comparative and Evolutionary Aspects*, G. M. Burghardt and M. Bekoff, eds. New York: Garland Press, pp. 19–41. [14]

Bekoff, A., P. S. G. Stein and V. Hamburger. (1975). Coordinated motor output in the hindlimb of the 7-day chick embryo. *Proc. Natl. Acad. Sci. USA 72*: 1245–1248. [14]

Bender, W., M. Akam, F. Karch, P. A. Beachy, M. Peifer, P. Spierer, E. B. Lewis and D. S. Hogness. (1983). Molecular genetics of the bithorax complex in *Drosophilia melanogaster*. *Science 221*: 23–29. [3]

Benfey, M. and A. J. Aguayo. (1982). Extensive elongation of axons from rat brain into peripheral grafts. *Nature 296*: 150–152. [5]

Benjamin, T. L., E. J. Furshpan, D. H. Hubel, E. P. Kennedy, E. A. Kravitz, H. C. Meadow, D. D. Potter and T. N. Weisel. (1983). Stephen Kuffler. *Harvard Gazette*, March 18, p. 6. [8]

Bennet-Clark, H. C. and A. W. Ewing. (1970). The love song of the fruit fly. *Sci. Am. 223(1)*: 85–92. [14]

Bennett, M. R. (1981). The development of neuromuscular synapses. *Proc. Aust. Physiol. Pharmacol. Soc. 12 (2)*: 41–58. [5]

Bennett, M. R., D. F. Davey and K. E. Uebel. (1980). The growth of segmental nerves from the brachial myotomes into the proximal muscles of the chick forelimb during development. *J. Comp Neurol. 189*: 335–357. [5]

Bennett, M. R. and K. Lai. (1981a). The development of topographical distributions of cutaneous sensory neurons in amphibian ganglia. *Dev. Biol. 86*: 212–223. [6]

Bennett, M. R. and K. Lai. (1981b). Cell death during development of the topographical distributions of cutaneous sensory neurons in amphibian ganglia. *Dev. Biol. 86*: 224–226. [6]

Bennet, M. R., K. Lai and V. Nurcombe. (1980). Identification of embryonic motoneurons *in vitro*: Their survival is dependent on skeletal muscle. *Brain Res. 190*: 537–542. [7]

Bennett, M. R. and N. A. Lavidis. (1981). Development of the topographical projection of motor neurons to amphibian muscle accompanies motor neuron death. *Dev. Brain Res. 2*: 448–452. [6]

Bennett, M. R. and N. A. Lavidis. (1984). Development of the topographical projection of motor neurons to a rat muscle accompanies loss of polyneuronal innervation. *J. Neurosci.* (in press). [12]

Bennett, M. R., P. A. McGrath and D. F. Davey. (1979). The regression of synapses formed by a foreign nerve in a mature axolotl striated muscle. *Brain Res. 173*: 451–469. [10]

Bennett, M. R., P. A. McGrath, D. F. Davey and I. Hutchinson. (1983). Death of motor neurons during the postnatal loss of polyneuronal innervation of rat muscles. *J. Comp. Neurol. 218*: 351–363. [12]

Bennett, M. R., E. M. McLachlan and R. S. Taylor. (1937b). The formation of synapses in mammalian striated muscle reinnervated with autonomic preganglionic nerves. *J. Physiol. (Lond.) 233*: 501–517. [9]

Bennett, M. R. and A. G. Pettigrew. (1974). The formation of synapses in striated muscle during development. *J. Physiol. (Lond.) 241*: 515–545. [9,12]

Bennett, M. R. and A. G. Pettigrew. (1975). The formation of synapses in amphibian striated muscle during development. *J. Physiol. (Lond.) 252*: 203–239. [9]

Bennett, M. R. and A. G. Pettigrew. (1976). The formation of neuromuscular synapses. *Cold Spring Harbor Symp. Quant. Biol. 40*: 409–424. [9,12]

Bennett, M. R. and J. Raftos. (1977). The formation and regression of synapses during the re-innervation of axolotl striated muscle. *J. Physiol. (Lond.) 265*: 261–295. [10]

Benoit, P. and J.-P. Changeux. (1975). Consequences of tenotomy on the evolution of multi-innervation in developing rat soleus muscle. *Brain Res. 99*: 354–358. [12]

Benoit, P. and J.-P. Changeux. (1978). Consequences of blocking the nerve with a local anaesthetic on the evolution of multi-innervation at the regenerating neuromuscular junction of the rat. *Brain Res. 149*: 89–96. [12]

Benowitz, L. I. and L. A. Greene. (1979). Nerve growth factor in the goldfish brain: Biological assay studies using pheochromocytoma cells. *Brain Res. 162*: 164–168. [7]

Bentley, D. and M. Caudy. (1983). Pioneer axons lose directed growth after selective killing of guidepost cells. *Nature 304*: 62–65. [5]

Bentley, D. and R. R. Hoy. (1974). The neurobiology of cricket song. *Sci. Am. 231(2)*: 34–44. [14]

Bentley, D. and H. Keshishian. (1982). Pioneer neurons and pathways in insect appendages. *Trends Neurosci. 5*: 354–358. [5]

Benzer, S. (1971). From the gene to behavior. *J. Am. Med. Assoc. 218*: 1015–1022. [2]

Berg. D. K. (1982). Cell death in neuronal development. Regulation by trophic factors. In: *Neuronal Development*, N. C. Spitzer, ed. New York: Plenum Press, pp. 297–331. [7]

Berg. D. K. (1984). New neuronal growth factors. *Annu. Rev. Neurosci. 7*: 149–170. [7]

Berg. D. K. and Z. W. Hall. (1975). Increased extrajunctional acetylcholine sensitivity produced by chronic postsynaptic neuromuscular blockade. *J. Physiol. (Lond.) 244*: 659–676. [8]

Berger, E. A. and E. M. Shooter. (1978). Biosynthesis of β nerve growth factor in mouse submaxillary glands. *J. Biol. Chem. 253*: 804–810. [7]

Berlot, J. and C. S. Goodman. (1984). Guidance of peripheral pioneer neurons in the grasshopper: Adhesive hierarchy of epithelial and neuronal surfaces. *Science 223*: 493–496. [5]

Berman, N. and N. W. Daw. (1977). Comparison of the critical periods for monocular and directional deprivation in cats. *J. Physiol. (Lond.) 265*: 249–259. [14]

Bernstein, J. J. and L. Guth (1961). Nonselectivity in establishment of neuromuscular connections following nerve regeneration in the rat. *Exp. Neurol. 4*: 262–275. [5,10]

Bessou, P., Y. Laporte and B. Pagès. (1966). Observations sur la ré-innervation de fuseaux neuro–musculaires de chat. *C. R. Soc. Biol. (Paris) 160*: 408–411. [5]

Betz, W. J. and J. H. Caldwell. (1984). Mapping electric currents around skeletal muscle with a vibrating probe. *J. Gen. Physiol. 83*: 143–156. [5]

Betz, W. J., J. H. Caldwell and S. C. Kinnamon. (1984). Physiological basis of a steady endogenous current in rat lumbrical muscle. *J. Gen. Physiol. 83*: 175–192. [5]

Betz, W. J., J. H. Caldwell and R. R. Ribchester. (1979). The size of motor units during post-natal development of rat lumbrical muscle. *J. Physiol. (Lond.)* 297: 463–478. [12]

Betz, W. J., J. H. Caldwell and R. R. Ribchester. (1980). The effects of partial denervation at birth on the development of muscle fibres and motor units in rat lumbrical muscle. *J. Physiol. (Lond.)* 303: 265–279. [12]

Betz, W. J., J. H. Caldwell and R. R. Ribchester, K. R. Robinson and R. F. Stump. (1980). Endogenous electric field around muscle fibres depends on the Na^+-K^+ pump. *Nature* 287: 235–237. [5]

Bevan, S and J. H. Steinbach. (1977). The distribution of α-bungarotoxin binding sites on mammalian skeletal muscle developing *in vivo*. *J. Physiol. (Lond.)* 267: 195–213. [9]

Bieser, A., A. Wernig and H. Zucker. (1984). Different quantal responses within single frog neuromuscular junctions. *J. Physiol. (Lond.)* 350: 401–412. [13]

Birse, S. C., R. B. Leonard and R. E. Coggeshall. (1980). Neuronal increase in various areas of the nervous system of the guppy, *Lebistes*. *J. Comp. Neurol.* 194: 291–301. [6]

Bishop, G. H. and P. Heinbecker. (1932). A functional analysis of the cervical sympathetic nerve supply to the eye. *Am. J. Physiol.* 100: 519–532. [10]

Bishop, J. M. (1982). Retroviruses and cancer genes. *Adv. Cancer Res.* 37: 1–32. [7]

Bixby, J. L. (1981). Ultrastructural observations on synapse elimination in neonatal rabbit skeletal muscle. *J. Neurocytol.* 10: 81–100. [12]

Bixby, J. L. and D. C. Van Essen. (1979a). Competition between foreign and original nerves in adult mammalian skeletal muscle. *Nature* 282: 726–728. [10]

Bixby, J. L. and D. C. Van Essen. (1979b). Regional differences in the timing of synapse elimination in skeletal muscles of the neonatal rabbit. *Brain Res.* 169: 275–286. [12]

Björklund, A. and U. Stenevi. (1972). Nerve growth factor: Stimulation of regenerative growth of central noradrenergic neurons. *Science* 175: 1251–1253. [7]

Black, I. B. and S. C. Geen. (1973). Trans-synaptic regulation of adrenergic neuron development: Inhibition by ganglionic blockade. *Brain Res.* 63: 291–302. [8]

Black, I. B. (1978). Regulation of autonomic development. *Annu. Rev. Neurosci.* 1: 183–214. [8]

Black, I. B. (1979). Idiopathic autonomic insufficiency (idiopathic orthostatic hypotension, Shy-Drager syndrome). In: *Textbook of Medicine*, 15th Ed., Vol. 1, P. B. Beeson, W. McDermott, and J. B. Wyngaarden, eds. Philadelphia, Saunders, pp. 762–763. [8]

Black, I. B., E. M. Bloom and R. W. Hamill. (1976). Central regulation of sympathetic neuron development. *Proc. Natl. Acad. Sci. USA* 78: 3575–3578. [8]

Black, I. B., I. A. Hendry and L. L. Iverson. (1972a). Effects of surgical decentralization and nerve growth factor on the maturation of adrenergic neurons in a mouse sympathetic ganglion. *J. Neurochem.* 19: 1367–1377. [8]

Black, I. B., I. A. Hendry and L. L. Iversen. (1972b). The role of post-synaptic neurones in the biochemical maturation of presynaptic cholinergic nerve terminals in a mouse sympathetic ganglion. *J. Physiol. (Lond.)* 221: 149–159. [9]

Blackshaw, S. E., J. G. Nicholls and I. Parnas. (1982). Expanded receptive fields of cutaneous mechanoreceptor cells after single neurone deletion in leech central nervous system. *J. Physiol. (Lond.)* 326: 261–268. [13]

Blackshaw, S. E. and A. E. Warner. (1976). Low resistance junctions between mesoderm cells during development of trunk muscles. *J. Physiol. (Lond.)* 255: 209–230. [9]

Blair, S. S. (1983). Blastomere ablation and the developmental origin of identified monoamine-containing neurons in the leech. *Dev. Biol.* 95: 65–72. [2]

Blakemore, C. (1974). Developmental factors in the formation of feature extracting neurons. In: *The Neurosciences: Third Study Program*, F. O. Schmitt and F. G. Worden, eds. Cambridge, MA: MIT Press, pp. 105–113. [14]

Blakemore, C. and G. F. Cooper. (1970). Development of the brain depends on the visual environment. *Nature* 228: 477–478. [14]

Blakemore, C. and D. E. Mitchell. (1973). Environmental modification of the visual cortex and the neural basis of learning and memory. *Nature* 241: 467–468. [14]

Blinzinger, K. and G. Kreutzberg. (1968). Displacement of synaptic terminals from regenerating motoneurons by microglial cells. *Z. Zellforsch. Mikrosk. Anat.* 85: 145–157. [13]

Bliss, T. V. P. and A. R. Gardner-Medwin. (1973). Long-lasting potentiation of synaptic transmission in the dentate area of the unanaesthetized rabbit following stimulation of the perforant path. *J. Physiol. (Lond.)* 232: 357–374. [13]

Bliss, T. V. P. and T. Lømo. (1973). Long-lasting potentiation of synaptic transmission in the dentate area of the anaesthetized rabbit following stimulation of the perforant path. *J. Physiol. (Lond.)* 232: 357–374. [13]

Blue, M. E. and J. G. Parnavelas. (1983). The formation and maturation of synapses in the visual cortex of the rat. II. Quantitative analysis. *J. Neurocytol.* 12: 697–712. [9]

Bocchini, V. and P. U. Angeletti. (1969). The nerve growth factor: Purification as a 30,000-molecular-weight-protein. *Proc. Natl. Acad. Sci. USA* 64: 787–794. [7]

Bodenmüller, H., H. C. Schaller and G. Darai. (1980). Human hypothalamus and intestine contain a hydra-neuropeptide. *Neurosci. Lett.* 16: 71–74. [3]

Bodmer, R., D. Dagan, and I. B. Levitan. (1984). Chemical and electrotonic connections between *Aplysia* neurons in primary culture. *J. Neurosci.* 4: 228–233. [10]

Boeckh, J., V. Boeckh and A. Kühn. (1977). Further data on the topography and physiology of central olfactory neurons in insects., *Olfaction and Taste (Paris)* 6: 315–321. [14]

Boeke, J. (1932). Nerve endings, motor and sensory. In: *Cytology and Cellular Pathology of the Nervous System*, Vol. 1, W. Penfield, ed. Facsimile of the 1932 Edition. New York: Hafner Press, 1965, pp. 243–315. [12]

Bohn, H. (1976). Tissue interactions in the regenerating cockroach leg. In: *Insect Development, Royal Entomological Society Symposium, No. 8.*, P. A. Lawrence, ed. Oxford, England: B. Blackwell Scientific, for the Royal Entomological Society, pp. 170–185. [3]

Bonhoeffer, F. and J. Huf. (1980). Recognition of cell types by axonal growth cones *in vitro*. *Nature 288*: 162–164. [11]

Bonhoeffer, F. and J. Huf. (1982). *In vitro* experiments on axon guidance demonstrating an anterior–posterior gradient on the tectum. *EMBO J. 1*: 427–431. [11]

Bonyhady, R. E., I. A. Hendry, C. E. Hill and I. S. McLennan. (1980). Characterization of a cardiac muscle factor required for the survival of cultured parasympathetic neurones. *Neurosci. Lett. 18*: 197–201. [7]

Borgens, R. B. (1982). Mice regrow the tips of their foretoes. *Science 217*: 747–750. [3]

Borgens, R. B., E. Roederer and M. J. Cohen. (1981). Enhanced spinal cord regeneration in lamprey by applied electric fields. *Science 213*: 611–617. [5]

Boucaut, J. C., T. Darribère, H. Boulekbache and J.-P. Thiery. (1984). Prevention of gastrulation but not neurulation by antibodies to fibronectin in amphibian embryos. *Nature 307*: 364–367. [4]

Boveri, T. (1901). Über die Polarität des Seeigeleies. *Eisverh. Phys. Med. Ges. (Würzburg) 34*: 145–175. [3]

Boyd, A. and M. Simon. (1982). Bacterial chemotaxis. *Annu. Rev. Physiol. 44*: 501–517. [4]

Bradshaw, R. A. (1978). Nerve growth factor. *Annu. Rev. Biochem. 47*: 191–216. [7]

Bradshaw, R. A. and M. Young (1976). Nerve growth factor—Recent developments and perspectives. *Biochem. Pharmacol. 25*: 1445–1449. [7]

Bray, D. (1970). Surface movements during the growth of single explanted neurons. *Proc. Natl. Acad. Sci. USA 65*: 905–910. [4]

Bray, D. (1973a). Branching patterns of individual sympathetic neurons in culture. *J. Cell Biol. 56*: 702–712. [4]

Bray, D. (1973b). Model for membrane movements in the neural growth cone. *Nature 244*: 93–96. [4]

Bray, D. (1979). Mechanical tension produced by nerve cells in tissue culture. *J. Cell Sci. 37*: 391–410. [4,5]

Bray, D. (1982a). The mechanism of growth cone movements. *Neurosci. Res. Program Bull. 20*: 821–829. [4]

Bray, D. (1982b). Filopodial contraction and growth cone guidance. In: *Cell Behavior: A Tribute to Michael Abercrombie*, R. Bellairs, A. Curtis and G. Dunn, eds. Cambridge: Cambridge University Press, pp. 299–317. [4,5]

Bray, D. (1984). Axonal growth in response to experimentally applied mechanical tension. *Dev. Biol. 102*: 379–389. [4,5]

Bray, D. and M. B. Bunge. (1973). The growth cone in neurite extension. *Ciba Found. Symp. 14*. Amsterdam: Elsevier, pp. 195–209. [4]

Bray, D. and D. Gilbert. (1981). Cytoskeletal elements in neurons. *Annu. Rev. Neurosci. 4*: 505–523. [4]

Bray, D., C. Thomas and G. Shaw. (1978). Growth cone formation in cultures of sensory neurons. *Proc. Natl. Acad. Sci. USA 75*: 5226–5229. [4]

Bray, G. M., M. Rasminsky and A. J. Aguayo. (1981). Interactions between axons and their sheath cells. *Annu. Rev. Neurosci. 4*: 127–162. [5]

Breitschmid, P. and H. R. Brenner. (1981). Channel gating at frog neuromuscular junctions formed by different cholinergic neurones. *J. Physiol. (Lond.) 312*: 237–252. [9]

Brenner, H. R. and E. W. Johnson. (1976). Physiological and morphological effects of postganglionic axotomy on presynaptic nerve terminals. *J. Physiol. (Lond.) 26*: 143–158. [13]

Brenner, S. (1973). The genetics of behavior. *Br. Med. Bull. 29*: 269–271. [2]

Briggs, R. and T. J. King. (1952). Transplantation of living nuclei from blastula cells into enucleated frogs' eggs. *Proc. Natl. Acad. Sci. USA 38*: 455–463. [2]

Brockes, J. P. and Z. W. Hall. (1979a). Acetylcholine receptors in normal and denervated rat diaphragm muscle. II. Comparison of junctional and extrajunctional receptors. *Biochemistry 20*: 2100–2106. [9]

Brockes, J. P. and Z. W. Hall. (1979b). Synthesis of acetylcholine receptor by denervated rat diaphragm muscle. *Proc. Natl. Acad. Sci. USA 72*: 1368–1372. [8]

Brockes, J. P., G. E. Lemke and D. R. Balzer. (1980). Purification and preliminary characterization of a glial growth factor from the bovine pituitary. *J. Biol. Chem. 255*: 8374–8377. [8]

Brody, H. (1955). Organization of the cerebral cortex. III. A study of aging in the human cerebral cortex. *J. Comp. Neurol. 102*: 511–556. [13]

Brown, A. G. and R. E. W. Fyffe. (1981). Direct observations on the contacts made between Ia afferent fibres and α-motoneurones in the cat's lumbosacral spinal cord. *J. Physiol. (Lond.) 313*: 121–140. [10]

Brown, D. D. (1981). Gene expression in eukaryotes. *Science 211*: 667–674. [2]

Brown, G. L. (1937). The actions of acetylcholine on denervated mammalian and frog's muscle. *J. Physiol. (Lond.) 89*: 438–461. [8]

Brown, M. C. and C. M. Booth. (1983a). Segregation of motor nerves on a segmental basis during synapse elimination in neonatal muscles. *Brain Res. 273*: 188–190. [12]

Brown, M. C. and C. M. Booth. (1983b). Postnatal development of the adult pattern of motor axon distribution in rat muscle. *Nature 304*: 741–742. [12]

Brown, M. C. and R. G. Butler. (1976). Regeneration of afferent and efferent fibres to muscle spindles after nerve injury in adult cats. *J. Physiol. (Lond.) 260*: 253–266. [5]

Brown, M. C., R. L. Holland and W. G. Hopkins. (1981a). Excess neuronal inputs during development. In: *Development in the Nervous System*, D. R. Garrod and J. D. Feldman, eds. Cambridge: Cambridge University Press, pp. 245–262. [12]

Brown, M. C., R. L. Holland and W. G. Hopkins. (1981b). Motor nerve sprouting. *Annu. Rev. Neurosci. 4*: 17–42. [13]

Brown, M. C., R. L. Holland and R. Ironton. (1978). Degenerating nerve products affect innervated muscle fibres. *Nature* 275: 652–654. [8,13]

Brown, M. C., W. G. Hopkins and R. J. Keynes. (1982). Short- and long-term effects of paralysis on the motor innervation of two different neonatal mouse muscles. *J. Physiol. (Lond.)* 329: 439–450. [12]

Brown, M. C. and R. Ironton. (1977). Motor neurone sprouting induced by prolonged tetrodotoxin block of nerve action potentials. *Nature* 265: 459–461. [13]

Brown, M. C. and R. Ironton. (1978). Sprouting and regression of neuromuscular synapses in partially denervated mammalian muscles. *J. Physiol. (Lond.)* 278: 325–348. [13]

Brown, M. C., J. K. S. Jansen and D. Van Essen. (1976). Polyneuronal innervation of skeletal muscle in new-born rats and its elimination during maturation. *J. Physiol. (Lond.)* 261: 387–422. [12]

Brown, M. E. (1946). The histology of the tadpole tail during metamorphosis with special reference to the nervous sytem. *Am. J. Anat.* 78: 79–113. [6]

Brown, T. H. and D. A. McAfee. (1982). Long-term synaptic potentiation in the superior cervical ganglion. *Science* 215: 1411–1413. [13]

Brunelli, M., V. Castellucci and E. R. Kandel. (1976). Synaptic facilitation and behavioral sensitization in *Aplysia*: Possible role of serotonin and cyclic AMP. *Science* 194: 1178–1181. [13]

Brunso-Bechtold, J. K. and V. Hamburger. (1979). Retrograde transport of nerve growth factor in chicken embryo. *Proc. Natl. Acad. Sci. USA* 76: 1494–1496. [7]

Brunt, P. W. and V. A. McKusick. (1970). Familial dysautonomia. A report of genetic and clinical studies, with a review of the literature. *Medicine (Balt.)* 49: 343–374. [7]

Brushart, T. M., E. G. Henry and M.-M. Mesulam. (1981). Reorganization of muscle afferent projections accompanies peripheral nerve regeneration. *Neuroscience* 6: 2053–2061. [10]

Brushart, T. M. and M.-M. Mesulam. (1980). Alteration in connections between muscle and anterior horn motoneurons after peripheral nerve repair. *Science* 208: 603–605. [5,10]

Brushart, T. M., E. C. Tarlov and M.-M. Mesulam. (1983). Specificity of muscle reinnervation after epineurial and individual fascicular suture of the rat sciatic nerve. *J. Hand Surg.* 8: 248–253. [10]

Bryant, P. M., S. V. Bryant and V. French. (1977). Biological regeneration and pattern formation. *Sci. Am.* 237(1): 66–81. [3]

Bryant, S. V., V. French and P. J. Bryant. (1981). Distal regeneration and symmetry. *Science* 212: 993–1002. [3]

Buc-Caron, M. H., P. Nystrom and G. D. Fischbach. (1983). Induction of acetylcholine receptor synthesis and aggregation: Partial purification of low molecular weight activity. *Dev. Biol.* 95: 378–386. [9]

Bueker, E. D. (1945). Hyperplastic changes in the nervous system of a frog (*Rana*) as associated with multiple functional limbs. *Anat. Rec.* 93: 323–331. [6]

Bueker, E. D. (1948). Implantation of tumors in the hind limb field of the embryonic chick and the developmental response of the lumbosacral nervous system. *Anat. Rec.* 102: 369–390. [7]

Buell, S. J. and P. D. Coleman. (1979). Dendritic growth in the aged human brain and failure of growth in senile dementia. *Science* 206: 854–856. [13]

Buell, S. J. and P. D. Coleman. (1981). Quantitative evidence for selective dendritic growth in normal human aging but not in senile dementia. *Brain Res.* 214: 23–41. [13]

Buller, A. J., J. C. Eccles and R. M. Eccles. (1960a). Differentiation of fast and slow muscles in the cat hind limb. *J. Physiol. (Lond.)* 150: 399–416. [8]

Buller, A. J., J. C. Eccles and R. M. Eccles. (1960b). Interactions between motoneurones and muscles in respect of the characteristic speeds of their responses. *J. Physiol. (Lond.)* 150: 417–439. [8]

Buller, A. J. and R. Pope. (1977). Plasticity in mammalian skeletal muscle. *Philos. Trans. R. Soc. Lond. [Biol.]* 278: 295–305. [8]

Bunge, M. B. (1977). Initial endocytosis of peroxidase or ferritin by growth cones of cultured nerve cells. *J. Neurocytol.* 6: 407–439. [4]

Bunge, M. B., M. I. Johnson and V. J. Argiro. (1983). Studies of regenerating nerve fibers and growth cones. In: *Spinal Cord Reconstruction*, C. C. Kao, R. P. Bunge and P. J. Reier, eds. New York: Raven Press, pp. 99–120. [4]

Bunge, R., M. Johnson and C. D. Ross. (1978). Nature and nurture in development of the autonomic neuron. *Science* 199: 1409–1416. [2]

Burden, S. (1977a). Development of the neuromuscular junction in the chick embryo: The number, distribution, and stability of acetylcholine receptors. *Dev. Biol.* 57: 317–329. [9]

Burden, S. (1977b). Acetylcholine receptors at the neuromuscular junction: Developmental change in receptor turnover. *Dev. Biol.* 61: 79–85. [9]

Burden, S. J., P. B. Sargent and U. J. McMahan. (1979). Acetylcholine receptors in regenerating muscle accumulate at original synaptic sites in the absence of the nerve. *J. Cell Biol.* 82: 412–425. [9]

Burgess, P. R., K. B. English, K. W. Horch and L. J. Stensaas. (1974). Patterning in the regeneration of type I cutaneous receptors. *J. Physiol. (Lond.)* 236: 57–82. [5]

Burgess, P. R. and K. W. Horch. (1973). Specific regeneration of cutaneous fibers in the cat. *J. Neurophysiol.* 36: 101–114. [5]

Burke, R. E., B. Walmsley and J. A. Hodgson. (1979). HRP anatomy of group Ia afferent contacts on alpha motoneurones. *Brain Res.* 160: 347–352. [10]

Burnside, M. B. and A. G. Jacobson. (1968). Analysis of morphogenetic movements in the neural plate of the newt *Taricha torosa*. *Dev. Biol.* 18: 537–552. [1]

Buskirk, D. R., J.-P. Thiery, U. Rutishauser and G. M. Edelman. (1980). Antibodies to a neural cell adhesion molecule disrupt histogenesis in cultured chick retinae. *Nature* 285: 488–489. [11]

Butler, J., E. Cosmos and J. Brierley. (1982). Differentiation of muscle fiber types in aneurogenic brachial muscles of the chick embryo. *J. Exp. Zool.* 224: 65–80. [8]

Cairns, J. M. and J. W. Saunders (1954). The influence of embryonic mesoderm on the regional specification of epidermal derivatives in the chick. *J. Exp. Zool.* 127: 221–248. [2]

Caldwell, J. H. and W. J. Betz. (1984). Properties of an endogenous steady current in rat muscle. *J. Gen Physiol* 83: 157–174. [5]

Caldwell, J. H. and R. M. A. P. Ridge. (1983). The effects of deafferentation and spinal cord transection on synapse elimination in developing rat muscles. *J. Physiol. (Lond.)* 339: 145–159. [12]

Camardo, J., E. Proshansky and S. Schacher. (1983). Identified *Aplysia* neurons form specific chemical synapses in culture. *J. Neurosci.* 3: 2614–2620. [10]

Campenot, R. B. (1977). Local control of neurite development by nerve growth factor. *Proc. Natl. Acad. Sci. USA* 74: 4516–4519. [5,7]

Campenot, R. B. (1981). Regeneration of neurites long-term cultures of sympathetic neurons deprived of nerve growth factor. *Science* 214: 579–581. [7]

Campenot, R. B. (1982a). Development of sympathetic neurons in compartmentalized cultures. I. Local control of neurite growth by nerve growth factor. *Dev. Biol.* 93: 1–12. [7]

Campenot, R. B. (1982b). Development of sympathetic neurons in compartmentalized cultures. II. Local control of neurite survival by nerve growth factor. *Dev. Biol.* 93: 13–21. [7]

Cangiano, A. and L. Lutzemberger. (1977). Partial denervation affects both denervated and inervated fibers in mammalian skeletal muscle. *Science* 196: 542–545. [8]

Cangiano, A. and L. Lutzemberger. (1980). Partial denervation in inactive muscle affects innervated and denervated fibres equally. *Nature* 285: 233–235. [8]

Cannon, W. B. (1949). *Denervation Supersensitivity.* London: Macmillan. [8]

Caramia, F., P. V. Angeletti and R. Levi-Montalcini. (1962). Experimental analysis of the mouse submaxillary salivary gland in relationship to its nerve growth factor content. *Endocrinology* 70: 915–922. [7]

Cardasis, C. A. and H. A. Padykula. (1981). Ultrastructural evidence indicating reorganization at the neuromuscular junction in the normal rat soleus muscle. *Anat. Rec.* 200: 41–59. [13]

Carr, V. M. and S. B. Simpson. (1978a). Proliferative and degenerative events in the early development of chick dorsal root ganglia. I. Normal development. *J. Comp. Neurol.* 182: 727–739. [6]

Carr, V. M. and S. B. Simpson. (1978b). Proliferative and degenerative events in the early development of chick dorsal root ganglia. II. Responses to altered peripheral fields. *J. Comp. Neurol.* 182: 741–755. [6]

Carr, V. M. and S. B. Simpson. (1982). Rapid appearance of labeled degenerating cells in the dorsal root ganglia after exposure of chick embryos to tritiated thymidine. *Dev. Brain Res.* 2: 157–162. [6]

Cass, D. T. and R. F. Mark. (1975). Re-innervation of axolotl limbs. I. Motor nerves. *Proc. R. Soc. Lond. [Biol.]* 190: 45–58. [10]

Cass, D. T., T. J. Sutton and R. F. Mark. (1973). Competition between nerves for functional connexions with Axolotl muscles. *Nature* 243: 201–203. [5,10]

Castellucci, V. F., T. J. Carew and E. R. Kandel. (1978). Cellular analysis of long- term habituation of the gill-withdrawal reflex of *Aplysia californica. Science* 202: 1306–1308. [13]

Castellucci, V. F. and E. R. Kandel. (1974). A quantal analysis of the synaptic depression underlying habituation of the gill-withdrawal reflex in *Aplysia. Proc. Natl. Acad. Sci. USA* 71: 5004–5008. [13]

Castellucci, V. F. and E. R. Kandel. (1976). Presynaptic facilitation as a mechanism for behavioral sensitization in *Aplysia. Science* 194: 1176–1178. [13]

Castellucci, V. F., E. R. Kandel, J. H. Schwartz, F. D. Wilson, A. C. Nairn and P. Greengard. (1980). Intracellular injection of the catalytic subunit of cyclic AMP-dependent protein kinase stimulates facilitation of transmitter release underlying behavioral sensitization in *Aplysia. Proc. Natl. Acad. Sci. USA* 77: 7492–7496. [13]

Castellucci, V. F., A. Nairn, P. Greengard, J. H. Schwartz and E. R. Kandel. (1982). Inhibitor of adenosine 3′:5′-monophosphate-dependent protein kinase blocks presynaptic facilitation in *Aplysia. J. Neurosci.* 2: 1673–1681. [13]

Castellucci, V. F., H. Pinsker, I. Kupfermann and E. R. Kandel. (1970). Neuronal mechanisms of habituation and dishabituation of the gill-withdrawal reflex in *Aplysia. Science* 167: 1745–1748. [13]

Caviness, V. S. (1976). Patterns of cell and fiber distribution in the neocortex of the reeler mutant mouse. *J. Comp. Neurol.* 170: 435–448. [5]

Caviness, V. S., M. C. Pinto-Lord and P. Evrard. (1981). The development of laminated pattern in the mammalian neocortex. In: *Morphogenesis and Pattern Formation*, T. G. Connelly, L. L. Brinkley and B. M. Carlson, eds. New York: Raven Press, pp. 103–126. [4]

Caviness, V. S. and P. Rakic. (1978). Mechanisms of cortical development: A view from mutations in mice. *Annu. Rev. Neurosci.* 1: 297–326. [5]

Ceccarelli, B., W. P. Hurlbut and A. Mauro. (1973). Turnover of transmitter and synaptic vesicles at the frog neuromuscular junction. *J. Cell Biol.* 57: 499–524. [5]

Chalfie, M., H. R. Horvitz and J. E. Sulston. (1981). Mutations that lead to reiterations in the cell lineages of *C. elegans. Cell* 24: 59–69. [2]

Changeux, J.-P. (1972). Le cerveau et l'événement. *Extrait de Comm.* 18: 37–47. [12]

Changeux, J.-P., P. Courrege and A. Danchin. (1973). A theory of the epigenesis of neuronal networks by selective stabilization of synapses. *Proc. Natl. Acad. Sci. USA* 70: 2974–2978. [12]

Changeux, J.-P. and A. Danchin. (1976). Selective stabilization of developing synapses as a mechanism for the specification of neuronal networks. *Nature* 264: 705–712. [12]

Changeux, J.-P. and K. Mikoshiba. (1978). Genetic and "epigenetic" factors regulating synapse formation in vertebrate cerebellum and neuromuscular junction. *Prog. Brain Res.* 48: 43–64. [12]

Child, C. M. (1941). *Patterns and Problems of Development*. Chicago: University of Chicago Press. [3]

Chitwood, B. G. and M. B. Chitwood. (1974). *Introduction to Nematology*. Baltimore: University Park Press. [2]

Chiu, A. Y. and J. R. Sanes. (1984). Development of basal lamina in synaptic and extrasynaptic portions of embryonic rat muscle. *Dev. Biol* 103: 456–467. [9]

Chow, I. and M. W. Cohen. (1983). Developmental changes in the distribution of acetylocholine receptors in the myotomes of *Xenopus laevis*. *J. Physiol. (Lond.)* 339: 553–571. [9]

Christ, B., H. J. Jacob and M. Jacob. (1977). Experimental analysis of the origin of the wing musculature in avian embryos. *Anat. Embryol. (Berl.)* 150: 171–186. [5]

Christian, C. N., M. P. Daniels, H. Sugiyama, Z. Vogel, L. Jacques and P. G. Nelson. (1978). A factor from neurons increases the number of acetylcholine receptor aggregates on cultured muscle cells. *Proc. Natl. Acad. Sci. USA* 75: 4011–4015. [9]

Chuang, H. H. (1939). Induktion Sleistungen von frischen und gekochten Organteilen (Niere, Leber) nach ihrer verpflanzung in Explante und versheidene Wirtsregionen von Tritonkeimen. *Wilhelm Roux Arch. Entwicklungsmech. Org.* 139: 556–638. [4]

Chun, L. L. Y. and P. H. Patterson. (1977a). Role of nerve growth factor in the development of rat sympathetic neurons *in vitro*. I. Survival, growth and differentiation of catecholamine production. *J. Cell Biol.* 75: 694–704. [7]

Chun, L. L. Y. and P. H. Patterson. (1977b). Role of nerve growth factor in the development of rat sympathetic neurons *in vitro*. II. Developmental studies. *J. Cell Biol.* 75: 705–711. [7]

Chun, L. L. Y. and P. H. Patterson. (1977c). Role of nerve growth factor in the development of rat sympathetic neurons *in vitro*. III. Effect on acetylcholine production. *J. Cell Biol.* 75: 712–718. [7]

Chung, S. H., M. J. Keating and T. V. P. Bliss. (1974). Functional synaptic relations during the development of the retino-tectal projections in amphibians. *Proc. R. Soc. Lond [Biol.]* 187: 449–459. [11]

Chu-Wang, I.-W. and R. W. Oppenheim. (1978). Cell death of motoneurons in the chick embryo spinal cord. II. A quantitative and qualitative analysis of degeneration in the ventral root, including evidence for axon outgrowth and limb innervation prior to cell death. *J. Comp. Neurol.* 177: 59–85. [6]

Close, R. (1965). Effects of cross-union of motor nerves to fast and slow skeletal muscles. *Nature* 206: 831–832. [8]

Close, R. (1969). Dynamic properties of fast and slow skeletal muscles of the rat after nerve cross-union. *J. Physiol. (Lond)*. 204: 331–346. [8]

Close, R. (1972). Dynamic properties of mammalian skeletal muscle. *Physiol. Rev.* 52: 129–197. [8]

Coghill, G. E. (1929). *Anatomy and the Problem of Behavior*. New York: Hafner Press (republished in 1965). [14]

Cohen, M. W. (1972). The development of neuromuscular connexions in the presence of *d*-tubocurarine. *Brain Res.* 41: 457–465. [9]

Cohen, M. W., M. J. Anderson, E. Zorychta and P. R. Weldon. (1979). Accumulation of acetylcholine receptors at nerve–muscle contacts in culture. *Prog. Brain. Res.* 49: 335–349. [9]

Cohen, M. W., M. Greschner and M. Tucci. (1984). In vivo development of cholinesterase at a neuromuscular junction in the absence of motor activity in *Xenopus laevis*. *J. Physiol. (Lond.)* 348: 57–66 [9]

Cohen, S. (1959). Purification and metabolic effects of a nerve growth-promoting protein from snake venom. *J. Biol. Chem.* 234: 1129–1137. [7]

Cohen, S. (1960). Purification and metabolic effects of a nerve growth-promoting protein from the mouse salivary gland and its neuro-cytotoxic antiserum. *Proc. Natl. Acad. Sci. USA* 46: 302–311. [7]

Cohen, S. and R. Levi-Montalcini. (1956). A nerve growth stimulating factor isolated from snake venom. *Proc. Natl. Acad. Sci. USA* 42: 571–574. [7]

Cohen, S. and R. Levi-Montalcini and V. Hamburger. (1954). A nerve growth-stimulating factor isolated from sarcomas 37 and 180. *Proc. Natl. Acad. Sci. USA* 40: 1014–1018. [7]

Cole, W. V. (1955). Motor endings in the striated muscle of vertebrates. *J. Comp. Neurol.* 102: 671–716. [10]

Collin, R. (1906). Recherches cytologiques sur le developpment de la cellule nerveuse. *Le Nevraxe* 8: 181–307. [6]

Collins, F. and J. E. Garrett. (1980). Elongating nerve fibres are guided by a pathway of material released from embryonic non-neuronal cells. *Proc. Natl. Acad. Sci. USA.* 77: 6226–6228. [5]

Conklin, E. G. (1905). The organization and cell-lineage of the ascidian egg. *J. Acad. Nat. Sci. (Phila.)* 13: 1–119. [1]

Conklin, E. G. (1931). The development of centrifuged eggs of ascidians. *J. Exp. Zool.* 60: 1–119. [1]

Conklin, E. G. (1932). The embryology of *Amphioxus*. *J. Morphol.* 54: 69–133. [1]

Connor, J. R., M. C. Diamond and R. E. Johnson. (1980). Occipital cortical morphology of the rat: Alterations with age and environment. *Exp. Neurol.* 68: 158–170. [13]

Constantine-Paton, M. and M. I. Law. (1978). Eye-specific termination bands in tecta of three-eyed frogs. *Science* 202: 639–641. [12]

Cook, W. H., J. H. Walker and M. L. Barr. (1951). A cytological study of transneuronal atrophy in the cat and rabbit. *J. Comp. Neurol.* 94: 267–291. [8]

Cooke, J. (1980). Clones and compartments in the vertebrate central nervous system—a valid approach to the development of the neural plate? *Trends Neurosci.* 3: 100. [3]

Cooke, J. (1982). Vitamin A, limb patterns and the search for the positional code. *Nature* 296: 603–605. [3]

Cooper, E. (1984). Synapse formation among developing sensory neurones from rat nodose ganglia grown in tissue culture. *J. Physiol. (Lond)* 351: 263–274. [9]

Cotman, C. W. and J. V. Nadler. (1978). Reactive synaptogenesis in the hippocampus. In: *Neuronal Plasticity*, C. W. Cotman, ed. New York: Raven Press, pp. 227–271. [13]

Cotman, C. W., M. Nieto-Sampedro and E. W. Harris. (1981). Synapse replacement in the nervous system of adult vertebrates. *Physiol. Rev.* 61: 684–784. [13]

Coughlin, M. D., E. M. Bloom and I. B. Black. (1981). Characterization of neuronal growth factor from mouse heart-cell-conditioned medium. *Dev. Biol.* 82: 56-68. [7]

Courtney, J. and J. H. Steinbach: (1981). Age changes in neuromuscular junction morphology and acetylcholine receptor distribution on rat skeletal muscle fibres. *J. Physiol. (Lond.)* 320: 435–447. [3]

Courtney, K. and S. Roper. (1976). Sprouting and synapses after partial denervation of frog cardiac ganglion. *Nature* 259: 317–319. [13]

Cowan, W. M. (1970). Anterograde and retrograde transneuronal degeneration in the central and peripheral nervous system. In: *Contemporary Research Methods in Neuroanatomy*, S. Ebbesson and W. J. H. Nauta, eds. New York: Springer-Verlag, pp. 217–251. [8]

Cowan, W. M. (1978). Aspects of neural development. In: *Neurophysiology III. International Review of Physiology*, Vol. 17, R. Porter, ed. Baltimore: University Park Press, pp. 149–191. [1, 2]

Cowan, W. M. (1979). The development of the brain. *Sci. Am.* 241(3): 106–117. [1, 4]

Cowan, W. M. and P. G. H. Clarke. (1976). The development of the isthmo-optic nucleus. *Brain Behav. Evol.* 13: 345–375. [6]

Cowan, W. M. and E. Wenger. (1967). Cell loss in the trochlear nucleus of the chick during normal development and after radical extirpation of the optic vesicle. *J. Exp. Zool.* 164: 267–280. [6]

Cowan, W. M. and E. Wenger. (1968). Degeneration in the nucleus of origin of the preganglionic fibers to the chick ciliary ganglion following early removal of the optic vesicle. *J. Exp. Zool.* 168: 105–124. [6]

Cragg, B. G. (1975). The development of synapses in the visual system of the cat. *J. Comp. Neurol.* 160: 147–166. [9]

Creazzo, T. L. and G. S. Sohal. (1979). Effects of chronic injections of α-bungarotoxin on embryonic cell death. *Exp. Neurol.* 66: 135–145. [6]

Crepel, F., N. Delhaye-Bouchaud, J. M. Guastavino and I. Sampaio. (1980). Multiple innervation of cerebellar Purkinje cells by climbing fibers in *staggerer* mutant mouse. *Nature* 283: 483–484. [12]

Crepel, F., J. Mariani and N. Delhaye-Bouchaud. (1976). Evidence for a multiple innervation of Purkinje cells by climbing fibers in the immature rat cerebellum. *J. Neurobiol.* 7: 567–578. [12]

Crick, F. H. C. (1970). Diffusion in embryogenesis. *Nature* 225: 420–422. [3]

Crick, F. H. C. and P. A. Lawrence. (1975). Compartments and polyclones in insect development. *Science* 189: 340–347. [3]

Cull-Candy, S. G. (1978). Glutamate sensitivity and distribution of receptors along normal and denervated locust muscle fibres. *J. Physiol. (Lond.)* 276: 165–181. [8]

Cunningham, T. J. (1982). Naturally occurring neuron death and its regulation by developing neural pathways. *Int. Rev. Cytol.* 74: 163–186. [6]

Cunningham, T. J., C. Huddelston and M. Murray. (1979). Modification of neuron numbers in the visual system of the rat. *J. Comp. Neurol.* 184: 423–434. [6]

Currie, J. and W. M. Cowan. (1974). Some observations on the early development of the optic tectum in the frog (*Rana pipiens*) with special reference to the effects of early eye removal on mitotic activity in the larval tectum. *J. Comp. Neurol.* 156: 123–142. [6]

Curtis, A. S. G. (1964). The mechanism of adhesion of cells to glass. A study by interference reflection microscopy. *J. Cell Biol.* 20: 199–215. [4]

Cynader, M., N. Berman and A. Hein. (1973). Cats reared in stroboscopic illumination: Effects on receptive fields. *Proc. Natl. Acad. Sci. USA* 70: 1353–1354. [14]

Dagan, D. and I. B. Levitan. (1981). Isolated identified *Aplysia* neurons in cell culture. *J. Neurosci.* 1: 736–740. [10]

Danielli, J. F. and M. A. Di Berardino (eds.) (1979). *Nuclear Transplantation. Int. Rev. Cytol*, Suppl. 9. New York: Academic Press, pp. 1–9. [2]

Darwin, C. (1859). *The Origin of Species*. London: John Murray. [14]

Davey, B., L. H. Younkin and S. G. Younkin. (1979). Neural control of skeletal muscle cholinesterase: A study using organ-cultured rat muscle. *J. Physiol. (Lond.)* 289: 501–515. [9]

Davey, D. F. and M. R. Bennett. (1982). Variation in the size of synaptic contacts along developing and mature motor terminal branches. *Dev. Brain Res.* 5: 11–22. [12]

Davies, D. C. (1978). Neuronal numbers in the superior cervical ganglion of the neonatal rat. *J. Anat.* 127: 43–51. [6]

Daw, N. W. and H. G. Wyatt. (1976). Kittens reared in a unidirectional environment: Evidence for a critical period. *J. Physiol. (Lond.)* 257: 155–170. [14]

Decker, R. S. (1976). Influence of thyroid hormones on neuronal death and differentiation in larval *Rana pipiens*. *Dev. Biol.* 49: 101–118. [6]

DeGroot, D. and G. Vrensen. (1978). Postnatal development of synaptic contact zones in the visual cortex of rabbits. *Brain Res.* 147: 362–369. [9]

Del Castillo, J. and B. Katz. (1954). Statistical factors involved in neuromuscular facilitation and depression. *J. Physiol. (Lond.)* 124: 574–585. [13]

DeLong, G. R. and R. L. Sidman. (1962). Effects of eye removal at birth on histogenesis of the mouse superior colliculus: An autoradiographic analysis with tritiated thymidine. *J. Comp. Neurol.* 118: 205–219. [6]

Denburg, J. L., R. L. Seecof and G. A. Horridge. (1977). The path and rate of growth of regenerating motor neurons in the cockroach. *Brain Res.* 125: 213–226. [10]

Dennis, M. J. and R. Miledi. (1974). Non-transmitting neuromuscular junctions during an early stage of end-plate reinnervation. *J. Physiol. (Lond.) 239*: 553–570. [9]

Dennis, M. J. and C. A. Ort. (1977). The distribution of acetylcholine receptors on muscle fibres of regenerating salamander limbs. *J. Physiol. (Lond.) 266*: 765–776. [9]

Dennis, M. J. and P. B. Sargent. (1979). Loss of extra-synaptic acetylcholine sensitivity upon reinnervation of parasympathetic ganglion cells. *J. Physiol. (Lond.) 289*: 263–275. [8]

Dennis, M. J. and J. W. Yip. (1978). Formation and elimination of foreign synapses on adult salamander muscle. *J. Physiol. (Lond.) 274*: 299–310. [10]

Dennis, M. J., L. Ziskind-Conhaim and A. J. Harris. (1981). Development of neuromuscular junctions in rat embryos. *Dev. Biol. 81*: 266–279. [9, 12]

Denny-Brown, D. E. (1929). The histological features of striped muscle in relation to its functional activity. *Proc. R. Soc. Lond. [Biol.] 104*: 371–411. [8]

Deppe, U., E. Schierenberg, T. Cole, C. Krieg, D. Schmitt, B. Yoder and G. Von Ehrenstein. (1978). Cell lineages of the embryo of the nematode *Caenorhabditis elegans. Proc. Natl. Acad. Sci. USA 75*: 376–380. [2]

Derby, M. A. (1978). Analysis of glycosaminoglycans within the extracellular environments encountered by migrating neural crest cells. *Dev. Biol. 66*: 321-336. [4]

DeRobertis, E. M., J. B. Gurdon, G. A. Partington, J. E. Mirtz and R. A. Laskey. (1977). Injected amphibian oocytes: A living test tube for the study of eukaryotic gene transcription. *Biochem. Soc. Symp. 42*: 181–191. [2]

Desaki, J. and Y. Uehara. (1981). The overall morphology of neuromuscular junctions as revealed by scanning electron microscopy. *J. Neurocytol. 10*: 101–110. [9]

DeSilva, H. R. and W. D. Ellis. (1934). Changing conceptions in physiological psychology. *J. Gen. Psychol. 11*: 145–159. [11]

Detwiler, S. R. (1920). On the hyperplasia of nerve centers resulting from excessive peripheral loading. *Proc. Natl. Acad. Sci. USA 6*: 96–101. [6]

Detwiler, S. R. (1936). *Neuroembryology: An Experimental Study.* New York: Macmillan. [1, 5, 6]

DeVoogd, T. J. and F. Nottebohm. (1981a). Sex differences in dendritic morphology of a song control nucleus in the canary: A quantitative Golgi study. *J. Comp. Neurol. 196*: 309–316. [14]

DeVoogd, T. J. and F. Nottebohm. (1981b). Gonadal hormones induce dendritic growth in the adult avian brain. *Science 214*: 202–204. [14]

Dennis, M. J. (1975). Physiological properties of junctions between nerve and muscle developing during salamander limb regeneration. *J. Physiol. (Lond.) 244*: 683–702. [9]

Dennis, M. J. (1981). Development of the neuromuscular junction. *Annu. Rev. Neurosci. 4*: 43–68. [9]

Dennis, M. J., A. J. Harris and S. W. Kuffler. (1971). Synaptic transmission and its duplication by focally applied acetylcholine in parasympathetic neurons in the heart of the frog. *Proc. R. Soc. Lond. [Biol.] 177*: 509–539. [8]

Devor, M. and P. D. Wall. (1978). Reorganisation of spinal cord sensory map after peripheral nerve injury. *Nature 276*: 75–76. [10]

Devreotes, P. N. and D. M. Fambrough. (1976). Synthesis of acetylcholine receptors by cultured chick myotubes and denervated mouse extensor digitorum longus muscles. *Proc. Natl. Acad. Sci. USA 73*: 161–164. [8]

Diamond, J. (1982). The patterning of neuronal connections. *Am Zool. 22*: 153–172. [13]

Diamond, J., E. Cooper, C. Turner and L. MacIntyre. (1976). Trophic regulation of nerve sprouting. *Science 193*: 371–377. [13]

Diamond, J. and P. C. Jackson. (1980). Regeneration and collateral sprouting of peripheral nerves. In: *Nerve Repair and Regeneration, Its Clinical and Experimental Basis*, D. L. Jewett and H. R. McCarroll, eds. St. Louis: Mosby, pp. 115–127. [13]

Diamond, J. and R. Miledi. (1962). A study of fetal and new-born rat muscle fibres. *J. Physiol. (Lond.) 162*: 393–408. [9]

Dichter, M. A. (1978). Rat cortical neurons in cell culture: Culture methods, cell morphology, electrophysiology, and synapse formation. *Brain Res. 149*: 279–293. [2]

Dijkstra, C. (1933). Die De- und Regeneration der sensiblen Endkörperchen des Entenschnabels (Grandry- und Herbstörperchen) nach Durchschneidung des Nerven, nach Fortnahme der ganzen Haut und nach Transplantation des Hautstückens. *Z. Mikrosk. Anat. Forsch. 34*: 75–158. [8]

Ding, R., J. K. S. Jansen, N. G. Laing and H. Tønnesen. (1983). The innervation of skeletal muscles in chickens curarized during early development. *J. Neurophysiol. 12*: 887–919. [5]

Dodd, J. and J. P. Horn. (1983). A reclassification of B and C neurones in the ninth and tenth paravertebral sympathetic ganglia of the bullfrog. *J. Physiol. (Lond.) 334*: 255–269. [10]

Donaldson, P. L. and R. K. Josephson. (1981). Collateral sprouting of insect motoneurons. *J. Comp. Neurol, 196*: 317–327. [10]

Doolittle, R. F., M. W. Hunkapiller, L. B. Hood, S. G. Devare, K. C. Robbins, S. A. Aaronson and H. N. Antoniades. (1982). Simian sarcoma virus *onc* gene, *v-sis*, is derived from the gene (or genes) encoding a platelet-derived growth factor. *Science 221*: 275–277. [7]

Douglas, and Goddard. (1975). Long-term potentiation of the perforant path-granule cell synapse in the rat hippocampus. *Brain Res. 86*: 205–215. [13]

Doupe, A. J., S. C. Landis and P. H. Patterson. (1984a). The long-term culture of rat adrenal chromaffin cells and their interconversions with other neural crest phenotypes: The role of glucocorticoids and growth factors. *J. Neurosci.* (in press). [2]

Doupe, A. J., P. H. Patterson and S. C. Landis. (1984b). Differentiation of small intensely fluorescent (SIF) cells in vitro and their interconversion with other neural crest phenotypes. *J. Neurosci.* (in press). [2]

Downman, C. B. B., J. C. Eccles and A. K. McIntyre. (1953). Functional changes in chromatolysed motoneurones. *J. Comp. Neurol. 98*: 9–36. [13]

Downward, J., Y. Yarden, E. Mayes, G. Scrace, N. Totty, P. Stockwell, A. Ullrich, J. Schlessinger and M. D. Waterfield. (1984). Close similarity of epidermal growth factor receptor and *v-erb-B* oncogene protein sequences. *Nature* 307: 521–527. [7]

Drachman, D. B. and F. C. A. Romanul. (1970). Effect of neuromuscular blockade on enzymatic activities of muscles. *Arch. Neurol.* 23: 85–89. [8]

Dribin, L. B. and J. N. Barrett. (1980). Conditioned medium enhances neuritic outgrowth from rat spinal cord explants. *Dev. Biol.* 74: 184–195. [7]

Dribin, L. B. and J. N. Barrett. (1982). Two components of conditioned medium increase neuritic outgrowth from rat spinal cord explants. *J. Neurosci. Res.* 8: 271–280. [7]

Driesch, H. (1892). Entwicklungsmechanische Studien. I. Der Werth der beiden ersten Furchungszellen in der Echinodermenentwicklung. Experimentelle Erzeugen von Theil- und Doppelbildung. *Zeitschrift für wissenschaftliche Zoologie* 53: 160–178; 183–184. Tafel VII. Abridged and translated by L. Mezger, M. Hamburger, V. Hamburger, and T. S. Hall. In: *Foundations of Experimental Embryology*, 2nd Ed., 1974, B. H. Willier and J. M. Oppenheimer, eds. New York: Hafner Press, pp. 38–50. [1]

Duchen, L. W. and S. J. Strich. (1968). The effects of botulinum toxin on the pattern of innervation of skeletal muscle in the mouse. *Q. J. Exp. Physiol.* 53: 84–89. [13]

Dudel, J. and S. W. Kuffler. (1961). Mechanism of facilitation at the crayfish neuromuscular junction. *J. Physiol. (Lond.)* 155: 530–542. [13]

Dumas, M., M. E. Schwab and H. Thoenen. (1979). Retrograde axonal transport of specific macromolecules as a tool for characterizing nerve terminal membranes. *J. Neurobiol.* 10: 179–197. [7]

Dunn, G. A. (1982). Contact guidance of cultured tissue cells: A survey of potentially relevant properties of the substratum. In: *Cell Behaviour*. R. Bellairs, A. Curtis and G. Dunn, eds. Cambridge: Cambridge University Press. pp. 247–280. [4]

Dunnebacke, T. H. (1953). The effects of the extirpation of the superior oblique muscle on the trochlear nucleus in the chick embryo. *J. Comp. Neurol.* 98: 155–177. [6]

Easter, S. S. (1983). Postnatal neurogenesis and changing connections. *Trends Neurosci.* 6: 53–56. [11]

Easter, S. S. and C. A. O. Stuermer. (1984). An evaluation of the hypothesis of shifting terminals in goldfish optic tectum. *J. Neurosci.* 4: 1052–1063. [11]

Easter, S. S., A. C. Rusoff and P. E. Kish. (1981). The growth and organizaiton of the optic nerve and tract in juvenile and adult goldfish. *J. Neurosci.* 1: 793–811. [11]

Ebbott, S. and I. Hendry. (1978). Retrograde transport of nerve growth factor in the rat central nervous system. *Brain Res.* 139: 160–163. [7]

Ebendal, T. (1977). Extracellular matrix fibrils and cell contacts in the chick embryo. *Cell Tiss. Res.* 175: 439–459. [4]

Ebendal, T., M. Belew, C.-O. Jacobson and J. Porath. (1979). Neurite outgrowth elicited by embryonic chick heart: Partial purification of the active factor. *Neurosci. Lett.* 14: 91–95. [7]

Ebendal, T. and C.-O. Jacobson. (1977). Tissue explants affecting extension and orientation of axons in cultured chick embryo ganglia. *Exp. Cell Res.* 105: 379–387. [5]

Ebendal, T., G. Norrgren and K.-O. Hedlund. (1983). Nerve growth promoting activity in the chick embryo: Quantitative aspects. *Med. Biol.* 61: 65–72. [7]

Ebendal, T., L. Olson, Å. Seiger and K.-O. Hedlund. (1980). Nerve growth factors in the rat iris. *Nature* 286: 25–28. [6, 7]

Eccles, J. C. (1935). The action potential of the superior cervical ganglion. *J. Physiol. (Lond.)* 85: 179–206. [10]

Eccles, J. C., R. M. Eccles and A. Lundberg. (1957). The convergence of monosynaptic excitatory afferents onto many different species of alpha motoneurones. *J. Physiol. (Lond.)* 137: 22–50. [10]

Eccles, J. C., B. Libet and R. R. Young. (1958). The behaviour of chromatolysed motoneurones studied by intracellular recording. *J. Physiol. (Lond.)* 143: 11–40. [13]

Eccles, J. C., R. Llinás and K. Sasaki. (1966). The excitatory synaptic action of climbing fibres on the Purkinje cells of the cerebellum. *J. Physiol. (Lond.)* 182: 268–296. [12]

Edds, M. V. (1953). Collateral nerve regeneration. *Q. Rev. Biol.* 28: 260–276. [13]

Ede, D. A., J. R. Hinchliffe and M. Bell. (eds.). (1977). *Vertebrate Limb and Somite Morphogenesis*. Cambridge: Cambridge University Press. [3]

Edelman, G. M. (1983). Cell adhesion molecules. *Science* 219: 450–457. [4, 11]

Edelman, G. M. (1984). Cell-adhesion molecules: A molecular basis for animal form. *Sci. Am.* 250(4): 118–129. [1, 4]

Edelman, G. M. and C.-M. Chuong. (1982). Embryonic to adult conversion of neural cell adhesion molecules in normal and staggerer mice. *Proc. Natl. Acad. Sci. USA* 72: 7036–7040. [11]

Edelman, G. M., W. J. Gallin, A. Delouvée, B. A. Cunningham and J.-P. Thiery. (1983). Early epochal maps of two different cell adhesion molecules. *Proc. Natl. Acad. Sci. USA* 80: 4384–4388. [4]

Edgar, D., Y. A. Barde and H. Thoenen. (1981). Subpopulations of cultured chick sympathetic neurones differ in their requirements for survival factors. *Nature* 289: 294–295. [7]

Edwards, J. S. (1977). Pathfinding by arthropod sensory nerves. In: *Identified Neurons and Behavior of Arthropods*, G. Hoyle, ed. New York: Plenum Press, pp. 284–493. [5]

Edwards, J. S., S.-W. Chen and M. W. Berns. (1981). Cercal sensory development following laser microlesions of embryonic apical cells in *Acheta domesticus. J. Neurosci.* 1: 250–258. [5]

Elliott, E. J. and K. J. Muller. (1983). Accurate regeneration of an electrical synapse between two leech neurons after destruction of the ensheathing glial cell. *J. Physiol. (Lond.)* 344: 243–255. [10]

Ellis, R. S. (1920). Norms for some structural changes in the human cerebellum from birth to old age. *J. Comp. Neurol.* 32: 1–34. [13]

Elul, R., R. Miledi and E. Stefani. (1970). Neural control of contracture in slow muscle fibres of the frog. *Acta Physiol. Lat. Am. 20*: 194–226. [10]

Emerson, A. E. (1958). The evolution of behavior among social insects. In: *Behavior and Evolution*, A. Roe and G. G. Simpson, eds. New Haven: Yale University Press, pp. 311–335. [14]

Emmelin, N. and L. Malm. (1965). Development of supersensitivity as dependent on the length of degenerating nerve fibres. *Q. J. Exp. Physiol. 50*: 142–145. [8]

Ennis, M., F. L. Pearce and C. A. Vernon. (1979). Some studies on the mechanism of action of antibodies to nerve growth factor. *Neuroscience 4*: 1391–1398. [7]

Eränkö, O., L. Eränkö, C. E. Hill and G. Burnstock. (1972). Hydrocotisone–induced increase in the number of small intensely fluorescent cells and their histochemically demonstrable catecholamine content in cultures of sympathetic ganglia of the newborn rat. *Histochem. J. 4*: 49–58. [2]

Etkin, W. (1964). Metamorphosis. In: *Physiology of the Amphibia*, J. A. Moore, ed. New York: Academic Press, pp. 427–468. [1]

Fahim, M. A., J. A. Holley and N. Robbins. (1983). Scanning and light microscopic study of age changes at a neuromuscular junction in the mouse. *J. Neurocytol. 12*: 13–25. [13]

Fahim, M. A., and N. N. Robbins. (1982). Ultrastructural studies of young and old mouse neuromuscular junctions. *J. Neurocytol. 11*: 641–656. [13]

Fallon, J. F. and A. I. Caplan (eds.). (1983). *Limb Development and Regeneration*. Part A. New York: Alan R. Liss. [3]

Fambrough, D. M. (1970). Acetylcholine sensitivity of muscle fiber membranes: Mechanism of regulation by motoneurons. *Science 168*: 372–373. [8]

Fambrough, D. M. (1981). Denervation: Cholinergic receptors of skeletal muscle. In: *Receptors and Recognition Series*, Vol. 13, R. J. Lefkowitz, ed. London: Chapman and Hall, pp. 125–142. [8]

Fangboner, R. F. and J. W. Vanable. (1975). Formation and regression of inappropriate nerve sprouts during trochlear nerve regeneration in *Xenopus laevis. J. Comp. Neurol. 157*: 391–406. [5]

Fankhauser, G. (1955). The role of nucleus and cytoplasm in development. In: *Analysis of Development*, B. H. Willier, R. Weiss and V. Hamburger, eds. Philadelphia: Saunders, pp. 126–150. [2]

Farbman, A. I. (1971). Development of the taste bud. In: *Handbook of Sensory Physiology*, Vol. 4, Part 2, L. M. Beidler, ed. Berlin: Springer-Verlag. pp. 51–62. [8]

Fawcett, J. W. and D. J. Willshaw. (1982). Compound eyes project stripes on the optic tectum in *Xenopus. Nature 296*: 350–352. [12]

Fernández, J. and G. S. Stent. (1980). Embryonic development of the glossiphoniid leech *Theromyzon rude*: Structure and development of the germinal bands. *Dev. Biol. 78*: 407–434. [1]

Filogamo, G. (1950). Consequenze della demolizione dell'abbozzo dell'occhio sullo sviluppo del lobo ottico nell'embrione di pollo. *Riv Biol. Colonaile (Rome) 42*: 73–80. [6]

Finlay, B. L. and M. Slattery. (1983). Local differences in the amount of early cell death in neocortex predict local specialization. *Science 219*: 1349–1351. [6]

Fischbach, G. D. (1970). Synaptic potentials recorded in cell cultures of nerve and muscle. *Science 169*: 1331–1333. [2]

Fischbach, G. D. and S. A. Cohen. (1973). The distribution of acetylcholine sensitivity over uninnervated and innervated muscle fibers grown in cell culture. *Dev. Biol. 31*: 147–162. [9]

Fischbach, G. D., E. Frank, T. M. Jessell, L. L. Rubin and S. M. Schuetze. (1979). Accumulation of acetylcholine receptors and acetylcholinesterase at newly formed nerve-muscle synapses. *Pharmacol. Rev. 30*: 411–428. [9]

Fischbach, G. D. and S. M. Schuetze. (1980). A postnatal decrease in acetylcholine channel open time at rat endplates. *J. Physiol. (Lond.) 303*: 125–137. [9]

Fletcher, W. M. (1925). Obituary of J. N. Langley. *Proc. R. Soc. Lond. CI*: xxiii–xli. [10]

Fletcher, W. M. (1926). John Newport Langley. In Memorium. *J. Physiol. (Lond.) 61*: 1–27. [10]

Forehand, C. J. and D. Purves. (1984). Regional innervation of rabbit ciliary ganglion cells by the terminals of preganglionic axons. *J. Neurosci. 4*: 1–12. [12]

Foster, M. and C. S. Sherrington. (1897). *A Textbook of Physiology*, Part III. *The Central Nervous System*, 7th Ed. London: Macmillan. [9]

Fouvet, B. (1973). Innervation et morphogenése de la patte chez l'embryon de Poulet. I. Mise en place de l'innervation normale. *Arch. Anat. microsc. Morphol. expér. 62*: 269–280. [5]

Fox, H. and J. M. Moulton. (1968). Mauthner cells and the thyroid hormonal level in larvae of *Rana temporaria. Arch. Anat. microsc. Morphol. expér. 57*: 107–120. [6]

Frank, E. (1974). The sensitivity to glutamate of denervated muscles of the crayfish. *J. Physiol. (Lond.) 242*: 371–382. [8]

Frank, E. and G. D. Fischbach. (1979). Early events in neuromuscular junction formation *in vitro*: Induction of acetylcholine receptor clusters in the postsynaptic membrane and morphology of newly formed synapses. *J. Cell Biol. 83*: 143–158. [9]

Frank, E. and J. K. S. Jansen. (1976). Interaction between foreign and original nerves innervating gill muscles in fish. *J. Neurophysiol. 39*: 84–90. [10]

Frank, E. and M. Westerfield. (1982). Synaptic organization of sensory and motor neurones innervating triceps brachii muscles in the bullfrog. *J. Physiol. (Lond.) 324*: 479–494. [10, 11]

Frank, E. and M. Westerfield. (1983). Development of sensory–motor synapses in the spinal cord of the frog. *J. Physiol. (Lond.) 343*: 593–610. [12]

Frazier, W. A., R. H. Angeletti and R. A. Bradshaw. (1972). Nerve growth factor and insulin. Structural similarities indicate an evolutionary relationship reflected by physiological action. *Science 176*: 482–488. [7]

Frazier, W. A. and L. Glaser. (1979). Surface components and cell recognition. *Annu. Rev. Biochem.* 48: 491–523. [11]

French, V. (1981). Pattern regulation and regeneration. *Philos. Trans. R. Soc. Lond. [Biol.]* 295: 601–617. [3]

French, V., P. J. Bryant and S. V. Bryant. (1976). Pattern regulation in epimorphic fields. *Science* 183: 969–981. [3]

Fuchs, P. A., L. P. Henderson and J. G. Nicholls. (1982). Chemical transmission between individual Retzius and sensory neurones of the leech in culture. *J. Physiol. (Lond.)* 323: 145–210. [10]

Fuchs, P. A., J. G. Nicholls and D. F. Ready. (1981). Membrane properties and selective connexions of identified leech neurones in culture. *J. Physiol. (Lond.)* 316: 203–223. [10]

Fujisawa, H. (1981a). Persistence of disorganized pathways and tortuous trajectories of regenerating retinal fibers in the adult newt *Cynops pyrrhogaster*. *Dev. Growth Differ.* 23: 215–219. [11]

Fujisawa, H. (1981b). Retinotopic analysis of fiber pathways in the regenerating retinotectal system of the adult newt *Cynops pyrrhogaster*. *Brain Res.* 206: 27–37. [11]

Fujisawa, H., N. Tani, K. Watanabe and Y. Ibata. (1982). Branching of regenerating retinal axons and preferential selection of appropriate branches for specific neuronal connection in the newt. *Dev. Biol.* 90: 43–57. [11]

Fujisawa, H., S. Thanos and U. Schwarz. (1984). Mechanisms in the development of retinotectal projections in the chick embryo studied by surgical deflection of the retinal pathway. *Dev. Biol.* 102: 356–367. [11]

Fujisawa, H., K. Watanabe, N. Tani and Y. Ibata. (1981). Retinotopic analysis of fiber pathways in amphibians. II. The frog *Rana nigromaculata*. *Brain Res.* 206: 21–26. [11]

Fujita, S. (1963). The matrix cell cytogenesis in the developing central nervous system. *J. Comp. Neurol.* 120: 37–42. [11]

Fukada, K. (1980). Hormonal control of neurotransmitter choice in sympathetic neurone cultures. *Nature* 287: 553–555. [2]

Fukada, K. (1983). Studies on the cholinergic differentiation factor for sympathetic neurons. *Soc. Neurosci. Abs.* 9: 614. [2]

Fulton, J. F. (1949). *Physiology of the Nervous System*, 3rd Ed. New York: Oxford University Press. [9]

Furshpan, E. J., P. R. MacLeish, P. H. O'Lague and D. D. Potter. (1976). Chemical transmission between rat sympathetic neurons and cardiac myocytes developing in microcultures: Evidence for cholinergic, adrenergic, and dual-function neurons. *Proc. Natl. Acad. Sci. USA* 73: 4225–4229. [9]

Gallin, J. I. and P. G. Quie (eds.). (1978). *Leucocyte Chemotaxis*. New York: Raven Press. [4]

Garber, B. B. and A. A. Moscona. (1972a). Reconstruction of brain tissue from cell suspensions. I. Aggregation patterns of cells dissociated from different regions of the developing brain. *Dev Biol.* 27: 217–234. [11]

Garber, B. B. and A. A. Moscona. (1972b). Reconstruction of brain tissue from cell suspensions. II. Specific enhancement of aggregation of embryonic cerebral cells by supernatant from homologous cell cultures. *Dev Biol.* 27: 235–243. [11]

Garcia-Bellido, A. (1975). Genetic control of wing disc development in *Drosophila*. *CIBA Found. Symp.* 29: 161–182. [3]

Garcia-Bellido, A., P. A. Lawrence and G. Morata. (1979). Compartments in animal development. *Sci. Am.* 241(1): 102–110. [3]

Gauthier, G. F., S. Lowey, P. A. Benfield and A. W. Hobbs. (1982). Distribution and properties of myosin isozymes in developing avian and mammalian skeletal muscle fibres. *J. Cell Biol.* 92: 471–484. [8]

Gaze, R. M., M. Jacobson and G. Székely. (1963). The retino-tectal projection in *Xenopus* with compound eyes. *J. Physiol. (Lond.)* 165: 484–499. [11]

Gaze, R. M., M. Jacobson and G. Székely. (1965). On the formation of connexions by compound eyes in *Xenopus*. *J. Physiol. (Lond.)* 176: 409–417. [11]

Gaze, R. M., M. J. Keating and S.-H. Chung. (1974). The evolution of the retinotectal map during development in *Xenopus*. *Proc. R. Soc. Lond. [Biol.]* 185: 301–330. [11]

Gaze, R. M., M. J. Keating, A. Ostberg and S.-H. Chung. (1979). The relationship between retinal and tectal growth in larval *Xenopus*: Implications for the development of retino-tectal projection. *J. Embryol. Exp. Morphol.* 53: 103–143. [11]

Gaze, R. M. and S. C. Sharma. (1970). Axial differences in the reinnervation of the goldfish optic tectum by regenerating optic nerve fibres. *Exp. Brain Res.* 10: 171–181. [11]

Gaze, R. M. and C. Straznicky. (1980). Regeneration of optic nerve fibres from a compound eye to both tecta in *Xenopus*: Evidence relating to the state of specification of the eye and the tectum. *J. Embryol. Exp. Morphol.* 60: 125–140. [11]

Geinisman, Y. (1979). Loss of axosomatic synapses in the dentate gyrus of aged rats. *Brain Res.* 168: 485–492. [13]

Geinisman, Y. (1981). Loss of axon terminals contacting neuronal somata in the dentate gyrus of aged rats. *Brain Res.* 212: 136–139. [13]

Genat, B. R. and R. F. Mark. (1977). Electrophysiological experiments on the mechanism and accuracy of neuromuscular specificity in the axolotl. *Philos. Trans. R. Soc. Lond. [Biol.].* 278: 335–347. [10]

Gerding, R., N. Robbins and J. Antosiak. (1977). Efficiency of reinnervation of neonatal rat muscle by original and foreign nerves. *Dev. Biol.* 61: 177–183. [10]

Ghysen, A. (1978). Sensory neurones recognise defined pathways in *Drosophila* central nervous system. *Nature* 274: 869–872. [5]

Gierer, A. (1974). Hydra as a model for the development of biological form. *Sci. Am.* 231(6): 44–54. [3]

Gierer, A. (1977). Biological features and physical concepts of pattern formation exemplified by hydra. *Curr. Top. Dev. Biol.* 1: 17–59. [3]

Gimlich, R. L. and J. Cooke. (1983). Cell lineage and the induction of second nervous systems in amphibian development. *Nature* 306: 471–473. [3]

Ginetsinskii, A. G. and N. M. Shamarina. (1942). The tonomotor phenomenon in denervated muscle. (Department of Scientific and Industrial Research, Translation RTS 1710.) *Osp. Sourem. Biol.* 15: 283–294. [8]

Ginsborg, B. L. and B. MacKay. (1960). A histochemical demonstration of two types of motor innervation in avian skeletal muscle. *Histochemistry of Cholinesterase Symp. Basel. Bibl. Anat.* 2: 174–181. [12]

Glicksman, M. A. and J. R. Sanes. (1983). Differentiation of motor nerve terminals formed in the absence of muscle fibres. *J. Neurocytol.* 12: 661–671. [9]

Glücksmann, A. (1951). Cell deaths in normal vertebrate ontogeny. *Biol. Rev.* 26: 59–86. [6]

Goedert, M., U. Otten, T. Schäfer, M. Schwab and H. Thoenen. (1980). Immunosympathectomy: Lack of evidence for a complement-mediated cytotoxic mechanism. *Brain Res.* 201: 399–409. [7]

Goldman, S. A. and F. Nottebohm. (1983). Neuronal production, migration, and differentiation in a vocal control nucleus of the adult female canary brain. *Proc. Natl. Acad. Sci. USA* 80: 2390–2394. [14]

Goldowitz, D. and R. J. Mullen. (1982). Granule cell as a site of gene action in *Weaver* mouse cerebellum: Evidence for heterozygous mutant chimeras. *J. Neurosci.* 2: 1474–1485. [4]

Goodman, C. S. (1982). Embryonic development of identified neurons in the grasshopper. In: *Neuronal Development*, N. C. Spitzer, ed. New York: Plenum Press, pp. 171–212. [2]

Goodman, C. S and M. Bate. (1981). Neuronal development in the grasshopper. *Trends Neurosci.* 4: 163–169. [6]

Goodman, C. S., R. K. Ho and E. E. Ball. (1982a). Pathfinding by growth cones in grasshopper embryos: Guidance cues in the ectoderm and mesoderm. *Neurosci. Res. Program Bull.* 20: 847–859. [5]

Goodman, C. S., J. Raper, R. Ho and S. Chang. (1982b). Pathfinding by neuronal growth cones in grasshopper embryos. In: *Cytochemical Methods in Neuroanatomy*, V. Chan-Palay and S. L. Palay, eds. New York: Alan R. Liss, pp. 461–494. [5]

Goodman, C. S. and N. C. Spitzer. (1979). Embryonic development of identified neurones: Differentiation from neuroblast to neurone. *Nature* 280: 208–214. [2]

Goodman, C. S. and N. C. Spitzer. (1980). Embryonic development of neurotransmitter receptors in grasshoppers. In: *Receptors for Neurotransmitters, Hormones and Pheromones in Insects*, D. B. Satelle, L. M. Hall and J. G. Hildebrand, eds. Amsterdam: Elsevier/North Holland Biomedical Press, pp. 195–207. [2]

Goodman, C. S. and N. C. Spitzer. (1981a). Embryonic development of identified neurons: Segment specific differences in the H-cell homologues. *J. Neurosci.* 1: 103–106. [12]

Goodman, C. S. and N. C. Spitzer. (1981b). The mature electrical properties of identified neurones in grasshopper embryos. *J. Physiol. (Lond.)* 313: 369–384. [2]

Goodman, C. S. and N. C. Spitzer. (1981c). The development of electrical properties of identified neurones in grasshopper embryos. *J. Physiol. (Lond.)* 313: 385–403. [2]

Gordon, H. and D. C. Van Essen. (1983). The relation of neuromuscular synapse elimination to spinal position of rabbit and rat soleus motoneurones. *J. Physiol. (Lond.)* 339: 591–597. [12]

Gordon, T., N. Niven-Jenkins and G. Vrbová. (1980). Observations on neuromuscular connection between the vagus nerve and skeletal muscle. *J. Neurosci.* 5: 597–610. [9]

Gordon, T., R. Perry, A. R. Tuffery and G. Vrbová. (1974). Possible mechanisms determining synapse formation in developing skeletal muscles of the chick. *Cell Tissue Res.* 155: 13–25. [9,12]

Gorin, P. D. and E. M. Johnson. (1979). Experimental autoimmune model of nerve growth factor deprivation: Effects on developing peripheral sympathetic and sensory neurons. *Proc. Natl. Acad. Sci. USA* 76: 5382–5386. [7]

Gorio, A., G. Carmignoto, M. Finesso, P. Polato and M. G. Nunzi. (1983). Muscle reinnervation. II. Sprouting, synapse formation and repression. *Neuroscience* 8: 403–416. [13]

Goss, R. J. (1969). *Principles of Regeneration.* New York: Academic Press. [8]

Gottlieb, D. I. and C. Arington. (1979). Patterns of adhesive specificity in the developing central nervous system of the chick. *Dev. Biol* 71: 260–273. [11]

Gottlieb, D. I. and L. Glaser. (1980). Cellular recognition during neural development. *Annu. Rev. Neurosci.* 3: 303–318. [11]

Gottlieb, D. I., R. Merrell and L. Glaser. (1974). Temporal changes in embryonal cell surface recognition. *Proc. Natl. Acad. Sci. USA* 71: 1800–1802. [11]

Gottlieb, D. I., K. Rock and L. Glaser. (1976). A gradient of adhesive specificity in developing avian retina. *Proc. Natl. Acad. Sci. USA* 73: 410–414. [11]

Gould, S. J. (1977). *Ontogeny and Phylogeny.* Cambridge, MA: Harvard University Press. [1]

Gouze, J.-L., J. M. Lasry and J.-P. Changeux. (1983). Selective stabilization of muscle innervation during development: A mathematical model. *Biol. Cybern.* 46: 207–215. [12]

Govind, C. K. and K. S. Kent. (1982). Transformation of fast fibres to slow prevented by lack of activity in developing lobster muscle. *Nature* 298: 755–757. [8]

Grampp, W., J. B. Harris and S. Thesleff. (1972). Inhibition of denervation changes in skeletal muscle by blockers of protein synthesis. *J. Physiol. (Lond.)* 221: 743–754. [8]

Grantyn, R., A. I. Shapovalov and B. I. Shiriaev. (1982). Combined morphological and electrophysiological description of connections between single primary afferent fibers and individual motoneurons in the frog spinal cord. *Exp. Brain Res.* 48: 459–462. [12]

Grantyn, R., A. I. Shapovalov and B. I. Shiriaev. (1984). Tracing of frog sensory–motor synapses by intracellular injection of horseradish peroxidase. *J. Physiol. (Lond.)* 349: 441–458. [10]

Graziadei, P. P. C. and G. A. Monti Graziadei. (1978). Continuous nerve cell renewal in the olfactory system. In: *Handbook of Sensory Physiology*, Vol. 9, M. Jacobson, ed. Berlin: Springer-Verlag, pp. 55–83. [6]

Graziadei, P. P. C. and G. A. Monti Graziadei. (1979a). Neurogenesis and neuron regeneration in the olfactory system of mammals. I. Morphological aspects of differentiation and structural organization of the olfactory sensory neurons. *J. Neurocytol. 8*: 1–18. [6]

Graziadei, P. P. C. and G. A. Monti Graziadei. (1979b). Neurogenesis and neuron regeneration in the olfactory system of mammals. II. Degeneration and reconstitution of the olfactory sensory neurons after axotomy. *J. Neurocytol. 8*: 197–213. [6]

Greene, L. A. (1977a). Quantitative *in vitro* studies on the nerve growth factor (NGF) requirement of neurons. I. Sympathetic neurons. *Dev. Biol 58*: 96–105. [7]

Greene, L. A. (1977b). Quantitative *in vitro* studies on the nerve growth factor (NGF) requirement of neurons. II. Sensory neurons. *Dev. Biol 58*: 106–113. [7]

Greene, L. A., D. E. Burstein, J. C. McGuire and M. M. Black. (1979). Cell culture studies on the mechanism of action of nerve growth factor. *Soc. Neurosci. Symp. 4*: 153–171. [7]

Greene, L. A. and E. M. Shooter. (1980). The nerve growth factor: Biochemistry, synthesis and mechanism of action. *Annu. Rev. Neurosci. 3*: 353–402. [7]

Greene, L. A., S. Varon, A. J. Piltch and E. M. Shooter. (1971). Substructure of the β-subunit of mouse 7S nerve growth factor. *Neurobiology 1*: 37–48. [7]

Greengard, P. (1976). Possible role for cyclic nucleotides and phosphorylated membrane proteins in postsynaptic actions of neurotransmitters. *Nature 260*: 101–108. [13]

Greengard, P. (1981). Intracellular signals in the brain. *Harvey Lect. 75*: 277–331. [13]

Greenwald, I. S., P. W. Sternberg and H. R. Horvitz. (1983). The *lin-12* locus specifies cell fate in *Caenorhabditis elegans*. *Cell 34*: 435–444. [2]

Grimm, L. M. (1971). An evaluation of myotypic respecification in axolotls. *J. Exp. Zool. 178*: 479–496. [5]

Grinnell, A. D. and A. A. Herrera. (1981). Specificity and plasticity of neuromuscular connections: Long-term regulation of motoneuron function. *Prog. Neurobiol. 17*: 203–282. [8]

Grinnell, A. D., M. S. Letinsky and M. B. Rheuben. (1979). Competitive interaction between foreign nerves innervating frog skeletal muscle. *J. Physiol. (Lond.) 289*: 241–262. [10, 13]

Grinnell, A. D. and M. B. Rheuben. (1979). The physiology, pharmacology and tropic effectiveness of synapses formed by autonomic preganglionic nerves on frog skeletal muscles. *J. Physiol. (Lond.) 289*: 219–240. [9]

Guillery, R. W. (1972). Binocular competition in the control of geniculate cell growth. *J. Comp. Neurol. 144*: 117–130. [8]

Guillery, R. W. (1973a). The effect of lid suture upon the growth of cells in the dorsal lateral geniculate nucleus of kittens. *J. Comp. Neurol. 148*: 412–422. [8]

Guillery, R. W. (1973b). Quantitative studies of transneuronal atrophy in the dorsal lateral geniculate nucleus of cats and kittens. *J. Comp. Neurol. 149*: 423–438. [8]

Guillery, R. W. (1974). Visual pathways in albinos. *Sci. Am. 230(5)*: 44–54. [2]

Guillery, R. W., V. A Casagrande and M. D. Oberdorfer. (1974). Congenitally abnormal vision in Siamese cats. *Nature 252*: 195–199. [2]

Gundersen, R. W. and J. N. Barrett. (1979). Neuronal chemotaxis: Chick dorsal-root axons turn toward high concentrations of nerve growth factor. *Science 206*: 1079–1080. [5, 7]

Gundersen, R. W. and J. N. Barrett. (1980). Characterization of the turning response of dorsal root neurites toward nerve growth factor. *J. Cell. Biol. 87*: 546–554. [5, 7]

Gurdon, J. B. (1968). Transplanted nuclei and cell differentiation. *Sci. Am. 219(6)*: 24–35. [2]

Gurdon, J. B. (1974). *The Control of Gene Expression in Animal Development*. Cambridge, MA: Harvard University Press. [2]

Gurdon, J. B., R. A. Laskey and O. R. Reeves. (1975). The developmental capacity of nuclei transplanted from keratinized skin cells of adult frogs. *J. Embryol. Exp. Morphol. 34*: 92–112. [2]

Gurdon, J. B. and H. R. Woodland. (1968). The cytoplasmic control of nuclear activity in animal development. *Biol. Rev. 43*: 233–267. [2]

Gurney, M. E. (1981). Hormonal control of cell form and number in the zebra finch song system. *J. Neurosci. 1*: 658–673. [14]

Gurney, M. E. (1984). Suppression of terminal sprouting at the neuromuscular junction by immune sera. *Nature 307*: 546–548. [7, 13]

Gurney, M. E. and M. Konishi. (1980). Hormone-induced sexual differentiation of brain and behavior in zebra finches. *Science 208*: 1380–1383. [14]

Guth, L. (1957). The effects of glossopharyngeal nerve transection on the circumvallate papilla of the rat. *Anat. Rec. 128*: 715–731. [8]

Guth, L. (1958). Taste buds on the cat's circumvallate papilla after reinnervation by glossopharyngeal, vagus and hypoglossal nerves. *Anat. Rec. 130*: 25–37. [8]

Guth, L. (1971). Degeneration and regeneration of taste buds. In: *Handbook of Sensory Physiology*, Vol. 4, Part 2, L. Beidler, ed. Berlin: Springer-Verlag, pp. 63–74. [8]

Guth, L. and J. J. Bernstein. (1961). Selectivity in the reestablishment of synapses in the superior cervical sympathetic ganglion of the cat. *Exp. Neurol. 4*: 59–69. [10, 13]

Guth, L. and K. Frank. (1959). Restoration of diaphragmatic function following vago–phrenic anastomosis in the rat. *Exp. Neurol. 1*: 1–12. [9]

Guth, L. and P. K. Watson. (1967). The influence of innervation on the soluble proteins of slow and fast muscles of the rat. *Exp. Neurol. 17*: 107–117. [8]

Gutmann, E. and V. Hanzliková. (1965). Age changes of motor endplates in muscle fibers of the rat. *Gerontologia 11*: 12–24. [9]

Gutmann, E. and J. Z. Young. (1944). Reinnervation of muscle after various periods of atrophy. *J. Anat. 78*: 15–43. [5, 9]

Hadorn, E. (1968). Transdetermination in cells. *Sci. Am. 219(5)*: 110–120. [3]

Haimann, C., A. Mallart, J. Tomás i Ferré and N. F. Zilber-Gachelin. (1981). Patterns of motor innervation in the pectoral muscle of adult *Xenopus laevis*: Evidence for possible synaptic remodelling. *J. Physiol. (Lond.) 310*: 241–256. [13]

Halfter, W., M. Claviez and U. Schwarz. (1981). Preferential adhesion of tectal membranes to anterior embryonic chick retina neurites. *Nature 292*: 67–70. [11]

Hall, J. C. (1977). Portions of the central nervous system controlling reproductive behavior in *Drosophila melanogaster*. *Behav. Genet. 7*: 291–312. [14]

Hall, J. C. (1979). Control of male reproductive behavior by the central nervous sytem of *Drosophila*: Dissection of a courtship pathway by genetic mosaics. *Genetics 92*: 437–457. [14]

Hall, Z. W., M.-P. Rosin, Y. Gu and P. D. Gorin. (1983). A developmental change in the immunological properties of acetylcholine receptors at the rat neuromuscular junction. *Cold Spring Harbor Symp. Quant. Biol. 48*: 101–108. [9]

Hamburger, V. (1934). The effects of wing bud extirpation on the development of the central nervous system in chick embryos. *J. Exp. Zool. 68*: 449–494. [6, 7]

Hamburger, V. (1939a). The development and innervation of transplanted limb primordia of chick embryos. *J. Exp. Zool. 80*: 347–389. [5, 8]

Hamburger, V. (1939b). Motor and sensory hyperplasia following limb-bud transplantations in chick embryos. *Physiol. Zool. 12*: 268–284. [6]

Hamburger, V. (1947). *A Manual of Experimental Embryology*. Chicago: University of Chicago Press. [1]

Hamburger, V. (1948). The mitotic patterns in the spinal cord of the chick embryo and their relation to histogenetic processes. *J. Comp. Neurol. 88*: 221–284. [1]

Hamburger, V. (1958). Regression versus peripheral control of differentiation in motor hypoplasia. *Am. J. Anat. 102*: 365–409. [6]

Hamburger, V. (1963a). Embryology, Experimental. *Encyclopedia Britannica*, 1963 Ed. [1, 2, 3]

Hamburger, V. (1963b). Some aspects of the embryology of behavior. *Q. Rev. Biol. 38*: 342–265. [14]

Hamburger, V. (1968). Emergence of nervous coordination. Origins of integrated behavior. *Dev. Biol 2(Suppl.)*: 251–271. [14]

Hamburger, V. (1969). Hans Spemann and the organizer concept. *Experientia 25*: 1121–1125. [3]

Hamburger, V. (1975). Cell death in the development of the lateral motor column of the chick embryo. *J. Comp. Neurol. 160*: 535–546. [6]

Hamburger, V. (1977). The developmental history of the motor neuron. The F. O. Schmitt lecture in neuroscience, 1976. *Neurosci. Res. Program Bull. 15(Suppl. III)*: 1–37. [6]

Hamburger, V. (1979). Roger Sperry. *Neurosci. Neslett. 10*: 5–6. [11]

Hamburger, V. (1980a). S. Ramón y Cajal, R. G. Harrison and the beginnings of neuroembryology. *Perspect. Biol. Med. 23*: 600–616. [4]

Hamburger, V. (1980b). Trophic interactions in neurogenesis: A personal historical account. *Annu. Rev. Neurosci. 3*: 269–278. [7]

Hamburger, V. (1981). Historical landmarks in neurogenesis. *Trends Neurosci. 4*: 151–155. [1, 3]

Hamburger, V. (1983). Oral history interview. Washington University Library Archives. [7]

Hamburger, V. and M. Balaban. (1963). Observations and experiments on spontaneous rhythmical behavior in the chick embryo. *Dev. Biol 7*: 533–545. [14]

Hamburger, V., M. Balaban, R. Oppenheim and E. Wenger. (1965). Periodic motility of normal and spinal chick embryos between 8 and 17 days of incubation. *J. Exp. Zool. 159*: 1–13. [14]

Hamburger, V., J. K. Brunso-Bechtold and J. W. Yip. (1981). Neuronal death in the spinal ganglia of the chick embryo and its reduction by nerve growth factor. *J. Neurosci.1*: 60–71. [6, 7]

Hamburger, V. and H. L. Hamilton. (1951). A series of normal stages in the development of the chick embryo. *J. Morphol. 88*: 49–92. [1, 6]

Hamburger, V. and R. Levi-Montalcini. (1949). Proliferation, differentiation and degeneration in the spinal ganglia of the chick embryo under normal and experimental conditions. *J. Exp. Zool. 111*: 457–501. [6]

Hamburger, V. and R. Levi-Montalcini. (1950). Some aspects of neuroembryology. In: *Genetic Neurology*, P. Weiss, ed. Chicago: University of Chicago Press, pp. 128–165. [4]

Hamburger, V. and R. W. Oppenheim. (1982). Naturally occurring neuronal death in vertebrates. *Neurosci. Comment. 1*: 39–55. [6]

Hamburger, V., E. Wenger and R. Oppenheim. (1966). Motility in the chick embryo in the absence of sensory input. *J. Exp. Zool. 162*: 133–160. [6, 14]

Hamburger, V. and J. W. Yip. (1984). Reduction of experimentally induced neuronal death in spinal ganglia of the chick embryo by nerve growth factor. *J. Neurosci. 4*: 767–774. [7]

Hamill, R. W., E. M. Bloom and I. B. Black. (1977). The effect of spinal cord transection on the development of cholinergic and adrenergic sympathetic neurons. *Brain Res. 134*: 269–278. [8]

Harlow, H. F. (1958). The nature of love. *Am. Psych. 13*: 673–685. [14]

Harlow, H. F. (1959). Love in infant monkeys. *Sci. Am. 200(6)*: 68–74. [14]

Harlow, H. F. and M. K. Harlow (1973). Social deprivation in monkeys. In: *Readings from the Scientific American. The Nature and Nurture of Behavior*. San Francisco: W. H. Freeman Co., pp. 108–116. [14]

Harlow, H. F. and R. R. Zimmermann. (1959). Affectional responses in the infant monkey. *Science 130*: 421–432. [14]

Harper, G. P., Y.-A. Barde, G. Burnstock, J. R. Carstairs, M. E. Dennison, K. Suda and C. A. Vernon. (1979). Guinea-pig prostate is a rich source of nerve growth factor. *Nature* 279: 160–162. [7]

Harper, G. P., Y.-A. Barde, D. Edgar, D. Ganten, F. Hefti, R. Heumann, K. W. Naujoks, H. Rohrer, J. E. Turner and H. Thoenen. (1983). Biological and immunological properties of the nerve growth factor from bovine seminal plasma: Comparison with the properties of mouse nerve growth factor. *Neuroscience* 8: 375–387. [7]

Harper, G. P., R. W. Glanville and H. Thoenen. (1982). The purification of nerve growth factor from bovine seminal plasma. Biochemical characterization and partial amino acid sequence. *J. Biol. Chem* 257: 8541–8548. [7]

Harper, G. P. and H. Thoenen. (1980). Nerve growth factor: Biological significance, measurement, and distribution. *J. Neurochem.* 34: 5–16. [7]

Harris, A. J. (1974). Inductive functions of the nervous system. *Annu. Rev. Physiol.* 36: 251–305. [8]

Harris, A. J. (1981). Embryonic growth and innervation of rat skeletal muscles. I. Neural regulation of muscle fibre numbers. II. Neural regulation of muscle cholinesterase. III. Neural regulation of junctional and extra-junctional acetylcholine receptor clusters. *Philos. Trans. R. Soc. Lond.* [*Biol*] 293: 257–314. [8, 9, 12]

Harris, A. J., S. W. Kuffler and M. J. Dennis. (1971). Differential chemosensitivity of synaptic and extrasynaptic areas on the neuronal surface membrane in parasympathetic neurons of the frog, tested by microapplication of acetylcholine. *Proc. R. Soc. Lond.* [*Biol.*] 177: 541–553. [8]

Harris, A. K. (1982). Traction, and its relation to contraction in tissue cell locomotion. In: *Cell Behaviour: A Tribute to Michael Abercrombie*, R. Bellairs, A. Curtis and G. Dunn, eds. Cambridge: Cambridge University Press, pp. 109–134. [4]

Harris, J. B. and S. Thesleff. (1971). Studies on tetrodotoxin resistant action potentials in denervated skeletal muscle. *Acta Physiol. Scand.* 83: 382–388. [8]

Harris, W. A. (1980). The effects of eliminating impulse activity on the development of the retinotectal projection in salamanders. *J. Comp. Neurol.* 194: 303–317. [11]

Harris, W. A. (1984). Axonal pathfinding in the absence of normal pathways and impulse activity. *J. Neurosci.* 4: 1153–1162. [11]

Harrison, R. G. (1903). Experimentelle Untersuchungen über die Entwicklung der Sinnesorgane der Seitenlinie bei den Amphibien. *Arch. Mikrosk. Anat. Entwicklungsmech.* 63: 35–149. [4]

Harrison, R. G. (1907a). Experiments in transplanting limbs and their bearing upon the problems of the development of nerves. *J. Exp. Zool.* 4: 239–281. [5]

Harrison, R. G. (1907b). Observations on the living developing nerve fiber. *Anat. Rec.* 1: 116–118. [4]

Harrison, R. G. (1910). The outgrowth of the nerve fiber as a mode of protoplasmic movement. *J. Exp. Zool.* 9: 787–846. [4]

Harrison, R. G. (1914). The reaction of embryonic cells to solid structures. *J. Exp. Zool.* 17: 521–544. [4]

Harrison, R. G. (1918). Experiments on the development of the fore limb of *Amblystoma*, a self-differentiating equipotential system. *J. Exp. Zool.* 25: 413–461. [4]

Harrison, R. G. (1921). On relations of symmetry in transplanted limbs. *J. Exp. Zool.* 32: 1–136. [4]

Harrison, R. G. (1924). Neuroblast versus sheath cell in the development of peripheral nerves. *J. Comp. Neurol.* 37: 123–206. [4]

Harrison, R. G. (1935). On the origin and development of the nervous system studied by the methods of experimental embryology. The Croonian Lecture. *Proc. R. Soc. Lond.* [*Biol.*] 118: 155–196. [4]

Harrison, R. G. (1937). Embryology and its relations. *Science* 85: 369–374. [2]

Harrison, R. G. (1947). Wound healing and reconstitution of the central nervous system of the amphibian embryo after removal of parts of the neural plate. *J. Exp. Zool.* 106: 27–83. [3]

Hartzell, H. C. and D. M. Fambrough. (1972). Acetylcholine receptors. Distribution and extrajunctional density in rat diaphragm after denervation correlated with acetylcholine sensitivity. *J. Gen. Physiol.* 60: 248–262. [8]

Hausen, K. and N. J. Strausfeld. (1980). Sexually dimorphic interneuron arrangements in the fly visual system. *Proc. R. Soc. Lond.* [*Biol.*] 208: 57–71. [14]

Hawrot, E. (1980). Cultured sympathetic neurons: Effects of cell-derived and synthetic substrate on survival and development. *Dev. Biol* 74: 136–151. [2]

Heaton, M. B., S. A. Moody and M. E. Kosier. (1978). Peripheral innervation by migrating neuroblasts in the chick embryo. *Neurosci. Lett.* 10: 55–59. [5]

Hebb, D. O. (1937). The innate organization of visual activity. *J. Genet. Psychol.* 51: 101–126. [14]

Hebb, D. O. (1949). *The Organization of Behavior*. New York: J. Wiley & Sons. [12]

Hedgecock, E. M., J. E. Sulston and J. N. Thomson. (1983). Mutations affecting programmed cell deaths in the nematode *Caenorhabditis elegans*. *Science* 220: 1277–1279. [6]

Heimer, L. and M. J. Robards. (1981). *Neuroanatomical Tract Tracing Methods*. New York: Plenum Press. [5]

Heinroth, O. (1911). Beiträge zur Biologie, namenlich Ethologie und Psychologie der Anatiden. *Verh. Inter. Ornith. Kongr.* 5: 589–702. [14]

Henderson, C. E., M. Huchet and J.-P. Changeux. (1981). Neurite outgrowth from embryonic chicken spinal neurons is promoted by media conditioned by muscle cells. *Proc. Natl. Acad. Sci. USA* 78: 2625–2629. [7]

Henderson, L. P., D. P. Kuffler, J. Nicholls and R.-J. Zhang. (1983). Structural and functional analysis of synaptic transmission between identified leech neurones in culture. *J. Physiol. (Lond.)* 340: 347–358. [10]

Hendry, I. A. (1975). The response of adrenergic neurons to axotomy and nerve growth factor. *Brain Res.* 94: 87–97. [7]

Hendry, I. A. and J. Campbell. (1976). Morphometric analysis of the rat superior cervical ganglion after axotomy and nerve growth factor treatment. *J. Neurocytol.* 5: 351–360. [6, 7]

Hendry, I. A. and L. L. Iversen. (1973). Reduction in the concentration of nerve growth factor in mice after sialectomy and castration. *Nature* 243: 500–504. [7]

Hendry, I. A., R. Stach and K. Herrup. (1974a). Characteristics of the retrograde axonal transport system for nerve growth factor in the sympathetic nervous system. *Brain. Res.* 82: 117–128. [7]

Hendry, I. A., K. Stöckel, H. Thoenen and L. L. Iversen. (1974b). The retrograde axonal transport of nerve growth factor. *Brain Res.* 68: 103–121. [7]

Herrup, K. and E. M. Shooter. (1975). Properties of the β-nerve growth factor receptor in development. *J. Cell. Biol.* 67: 118–125. [7]

Hess, A. (1961). Structural differences of fast and slow extrafusal muscle fibres and their nerve endings in chickens. *J. Physiol. (Lond.)* 157: 221–231. [9]

Heumann, D. and T. Rabinowicz. (1980). Postnatal development of the dorsal lateral geniculate nucleus in the normal and enucleated albino mouse. *Exp. Brain Res. 38*: 75–85. [6]

Heumann, R., M. Schwab and H. Thoenen. (1981). A second messenger required for nerve growth factor biological activity? *Nature* 292: 838–840. [7]

Heuser, J. E. and T. S. Reese. (1973). Evidence for recycling of synaptic vesicle membrane during transmitter release at the frog neuromuscular junction. *J. Cell Biol.* 57: 315–344. [5]

Hibbard, E. (1965). Orientation and directed growth of Mauthner's cell axons from duplicated vestibular nerve roots. *Exp. Neurol. 13*: 289–301. [5]

Hildebrand, J. G., S. G. Matsumoto, S. M. Camazine, L. P. Tolbert, S. Blank, H. Ferguson and V. Ecker. (1980). Organization and physiology of antennal centres in the brain of the moth *Manduca sexta*. In: *Insect Neurobiology and Pesticide Action*, F. E. Rickett, ed. London: Society for Chemical Industry, pp. 375–382. [14]

Hill, C. E., I. A. Hendry and R. E. Bonyhady. (1981). Avian parasympathetic neurotropic factors: Age-related increases and lack of regional specificity. *Dev. Biol. 85*: 258–261. [7]

Hinchliffe, J. R. and D. R. Johnson. (1980). *The Development of the Vertebrate Limb*. Oxford: Clarendon Press. [3]

Hinde, R. A. and Y. Spencer-Booth. (1971). Effects of brief separation from mother on rhesus monkeys. *Science* 173: 111–118. [14]

Hinds, J. W. and N. A. McNelly. (1977). Aging of the rat olfactory bulb: Growth and atrophy of constituent layers and changes in size and number of mitral cells. *J. Comp. Neurol, 171*: 345–368. [13]

Hinkle, L., C. D. McCaig and K. R. Robinson. (1981). The direction of growth of differentiating neurones and myoblasts from frog embryos in an applied electric field. *J. Physiol. (Lond.) 314*: 121–135. [5]

Hirano, A. and H. M. Dembitzer. (1973). Cerebellar alterations in the weaver mouse. *J. Cell Biol. 56*: 478–486. [9]

Hirokawa, N. and J. E. Heuser. (1982). Internal and external differentiations of the postsynaptic membrane at the neuromuscular junction. *J. Neurocytol.* 11: 487–510. [9]

Hirose, G. and M. Jacobson. (1979). Clonal organization of the central nervous system of the frog. I. Clones stemming from individual blastomeres of the 16-cell and earlier stages. *Dev. Biol. 71*: 191–202. [3]

Hirsch, H. V. B. and D. N. Spinelli. (1971). Modification of the distribution of receptive field orientation in cats by selective visual exposure during development. *Exp. Brain Res. 13*: 509–527. [14]

His, W. (1874). *Unsers Körperform und das physiologische Problem ihrer Entstehung*. Leipzig: F. C. W. Vogel. [1]

His, W. (1887). Die Entwicklung der ersten Nervenbahnnon beim menschlichen Embryo: Ueber sichtliche Darstellung. *Arch. Anat. Physiol. Anat. Abt. 92*: 368–378. [2]

Ho, R. K. and C. S. Goodman. (1982). Peripheral pathways are pioneered by an array of central and peripheral neurones in grasshopper embryos. *Nature 279*: 404–406. [5]

Hoffman, H. (1951). A study of the factors influencing innervation of muscles by implanted nerves. *Austral. J. Exp. Bio. Med. Sci. 29*: 289–308. [13]

Hofmann, W. W. and S. Thesleff. (1972). Studies on the trophic influence of nerve on skeletal muscle. *Eur. J. Pharmacol. 20*: 256–260. [8]

Hogan, E. L., D. M. Dawson and F. C. A. Romanul. (1965). Enzymatic changes in denervated muscle. II. Biochemical studies. *Arch. Neurol. 13*: 274–282. [8]

Holland, R. L. and M. C. Brown. (1980). Postsynaptic transmission block can cause terminal sprouting of a motor nerve. *Science 207*: 649–651. [13]

Hollyday, M. (1980a). Motoneuron histogenesis and the development of limb innervation. *Curr. Top. Dev. Neurobiol. 15*: 181–215. [5]

Hollyday, M. (1980b). Organization of motor pools in the chick lumbar lateral motor column. *J. Comp. Neurol. 194*: 143–170. [5]

Hollyday, M. (1983). Development of motor innervation of chick limbs. In: *Limb Development and Regeneration, Part A*, New York: Alan R. Liss, pp. 183–193. [5]

Hollyday, M. and V. Hamburger. (1976). Reduction of the naturally occurring motor neuron loss by enlargement of the periphery. *J. Comp. Neurol. 170*: 311–320. [6]

Hollyday, M. and V. Hamburger. (1977). An autoradiographic study of the formation of the lateral motor column in the chick embryo. *Brain Res. 132*: 197–208. [5]

Hollyday, M., V. Hamburger and J. M. G. Farris. (1977). Localization of motor neuron pools supplying identified muscles in normal and supernumerary legs of chick embryo. *Proc. Natl. Acad. Sci. USA 74*: 3582–3586. [5, 6]

Holtfreter, J. (1933). Nachweis der Induktionsfähigkeit abgetöteter Keimteile. Isolations und Transplantationsversuche. *Wilhelm Roux Arch. Entwicklungsmech. Org. 128*: 584–633. [3]

Holtfreter, J. (1938). Differenzierungspotenzen isoerter Tiele der Urodelen gastrula. *Wilhelm Roux Arch. Entwicklungsmech. Org. 138*: 522–656. [4]

Holtfreter, J. (1939). Gewebeaffinität, ein Mittel der embryonalen Formbildung. *Arch. exp. Zellforsch.* 23: 169–209. [4]

Holtfreter, J. (1944). Neural differentiation of ectoderm through exposure to saline solution. *J. Exp. Zool.* 95: 307–343. [4]

Holtfreter, J. (1968). Address in honor of Viktor Hamburger. In: *27th Symposium of the Society for Developmental Biology, The Emergence of Order in Developing Systems.* M. Locke, ed. New York: Academic Press, pp. IX–XX. [6]

Holtzman, E., A. R. Freeman and L. A. Kashner. (1971). Stimulation dependent alterations in peroxidase uptake at lobster neuromuscular junctions. *Science* 173: 733–736. [5]

Honig, M. G. (1982). The development of sensory projection patterns in embryonic chick hind limb. *J. Physiol. (Lond.)* 330: 175–202. [5]

Hope, R. A., B. J. Hammond and R. M. Gaze. (1976). The arrow model: Retinotectal specificity and map formation in the goldfish visual system. *Proc. R. Soc. Lond. [Biol.]* 194: 447–466. [11]

Horder, T. J. (1971). Retention by fish optic nerve fibres regenerating to new terminal sites in the tectum of "chemospecific" affinity for their original sites. *J. Physiol. (Lond.)* 216: 53–55P. [11]

Horder, T. J. (1978). Functional adaptability and morphogenetic opportunism, the only rules for limb development? In: *Formshaping Movements in Neurogenesis,* C. Jacobson and T. Ebendal, eds. Stockholm: Amlgvist and Wiksell, pp. 181–192. [5]

Horder, T. J. and K. A. C. Martin. (1979). Morphogenetics as an alternative to chemospecificity in the formation of nerve connections. *Symp. Soc. Exp. Biol.* 32: 275–359. [5, 11]

Horn, G. (1981). Neural mechanisms of learning: An analysis of imprinting in the domestic chick. *Proc. R. Soc. Lond. [Biol.]* 213: 101–137. [14]

Horton, J. C., M. M. Greenwood and D. H. Hubel. (1979). Non-retinotopic arrangement of fibres in cat optic nerve. *Nature* 282: 720 -722. [11]

Horvitz, H. R. (1981). Neuronal cell lineages in the nematode *Caenorhabditis elegans.* In: *Development of the Nervous System,* D. Garrod and J. Feldman, eds. Cambridge: Cambridge University Press, pp. 331–345. [2, 6]

Horvitz, H. R., H. M. Ellis and P. W. Sternberg. (1982). Programmed cell death in nematode development. *Neurosci. Comment.* 1: 56–65. [6]

Hotta, Y. and S. Benzer. (1976). Courtship in *Drosophila* mosaics: Sex specific loci for sequential action patterns. *Proc. Natl. Acad. Sci. USA* 73: 4154–4158. [14]

Hoy, R. R. and R. C. Paul (1973). Genetic control of song specificity in crickets. *Science* 180: 82–83. [14]

Hoyle, G. (1983). *Muscles and Their Neural Control.* Somerset, NJ: John Wiley & Sons. [10]

Hubel, D. H. (1963). The visual cortex of the brain. *Sci. Am.* 209(5): 54–62. [14]

Hubel, D. H. (1979). The brain. *Sci. Am.* 241(3): 39–47. [13]

Hubel, D. H. (1982a). Cortical neurobiology: A slanted historical perspective. *Annu. Rev. Neurosci.* 5: 363–370. [12]

Hubel, D. H. (1982b). Exploration of the primary visual cortex, 1955–1978. *Nature* 299: 515–524. [14]

Hubel, D. H. and T. N. Wiesel. (1959). Receptive fields of single neurones in the cat's striate cortex. *J. Physiol. (Lond.)* 148: 574–591. [14]

Hubel, D. H. and T. N. Wiesel. (1962). Receptive fields, binocular interaction and functional architecture in the cat's visual cortex. *J. Physiol. (Lond.)* 160: 106–154. [14]

Hubel, D. H. and T. N. Wiesel. (1963). Receptive fields of cells in striate cortex of very young, visually inexperienced kittens. *J. Neurophysiol.* 26: 994–1002. [14]

Hubel, D. H. and T. N. Wiesel. (1965). Binocular interaction in striate cortex of kittens reared with artificial squint. *J. Neurophysiol.* 28: 1041–1059. [12]

Hubel, D. H. and T. N. Wiesel. (1970). The period of susceptibility to the physiological effects of unilateral eye closure in kittens. *J. Physiol. (Lond.)* 206: 419–436. [14]

Hubel, D. H., T. N. Wiesel and S. LeVay. (1977). Plasticity of ocular dominance columns in the monkey striate cortex. *Philos. Trans. R. Soc. Lond. [Biol.].* 278: 377–409. [8, 12, 14]

Hughes, A. F. (1953). The growth of embryonic neurites. A study on cultures of chick neural tissue. *J. Anat.* 87: 150–162. [4]

Hughes, A. (1968). *Aspects of Neural Ontogeny.* New York: Academic Press. [6]

Hughes, A. and D. New (1959). Tail regeneration in the Geckonid lizard *Sphaerodactylus. J. Embryol. Exp. Morphol.* 7: 281–302. [8]

Hughes, W. F. and S. C. McLoon. (1979). Ganglion-cell death during normal retinal development in the chick: Comparisons with cell death induced by early target field destruction. *Exp. Neurol.* 66: 587–601. [6]

Hume, R. I. and D. Purves. (1981). Geometry of neonatal neurones and the regulation of synapse elimination. *Nature* 293: 469–471. [12]

Hume, R. I. and D. Purves. (1983). Apportionment of the terminals from single preganglionic axons to target neurones in the rabbit ciliary ganglion. *J. Physiol. (Lond.)* 338: 259–275. [12]

Humphreys, T. (1963). Chemical dissolution and *in vitro* reconstruction of sponge cell adhesions. I. Isolation and functional demonstration of the components involved. *Dev. Biol.* 8: 27–47. [4]

Huttenlocher, P. R., C. de Courten, L. J. Garey and H. Van der Loos. (1982). Synaptogenesis in the human visual cortex—evidence for synapse elimination during normal development. *Neurosci. Lett.* 33: 247–252. [9]

Hutter, O. F. (1952). Post-tetanic restoration of neuromuscular transmission blocked by d-tubocurarine. *J. Physiol. (Lond.)* 118: 216–227. [13]

Ide, C. F., S. E. Fraser and R. L. Meyer. (1983). Eye dominance columns from an isogenic double-nasal frog eye. *Science* 221: 293–296. [12]

Iles, J. F. (1976). Central termination of muscle afferents

on motoneurones in the cat spinal cord. *J. Physiol. (Lond.)* 262: 91–117. [10]

Illingworth, C. M. (1974). Trapped fingers and amputated finger tips in children. *J. Pediatr. Surg.* 9: 853–858. [3]

Illmensee, K. (1973). The potentialities of transplanted early gastrula nuclei of *Drosophila melanogaster*. *Wilhelm Roux Arch. Entwicklungsmech. Org.* 171: 331–343. [2]

Immelmann, K. (1969). Song development in the zebra finch and other estrildid finches. In: *Bird Vocalisations*, R. A. Hinde, ed. New York: Cambridge University Press, p. 61. [14]

Innocenti, G. M. (1981). Growth and reshaping of axons in the establishment of visual callosal connections. *Science* 212: 824–827. [12]

Innocenti, G. M. (1982). Development of interhemispheric cortical connections. *Neurosci. Res. Program Bull.* 20: 532–540. [12]

Innocenti, G. M., L. Fiore and R. Caminiti. (1977). Exuberant projection into the corpus callosum from the visual cortex of newborn cats. *Neurosci. Lett.* 4: 237–242. [12]

Isenberg, G., P. C. Rathke, N. Hülsmann, W. W. Franke and K. E. Wohlfarth-Bottermann. (1976). Cytoplasmic actomyosin fibrils in tissue culture cells: Direct proof of contractility by visualization of ATP-induced contraction in fibrils isolated by laser micro-beam dissection. *Cell Tissue Res.* 166: 427–443. [4]

Iversen, L. L., K. Stöckel and H. Thoenen. (1975). Autoradiographic studies of the retrograde axonal transport of nerve growth factor in mouse sympathetic neurones. *Brain Res.* 88: 37–43. [7]

Ivy, G. O., R. M. Akers and H. P. Killackey. (1979). Differential distribution of callosal projection neurons in the neonatal and adult rat. *Brain Res.* 173: 532–537. [12]

Ivy, G. O. and H. P. Killackey. (1981). The ontogeny of the distribution of callosal projection neurons in the rat parietal cortex. *J. Comp. Neurol.* 195: 367–389. [12]

Ivy, G. O. and H. P. Killackey. (1982). Ontogenetic changes in the projections of neocortical neurons. *J. Neurosci.* 2: 735–743. [12]

Izzard, C. S. and L. R. Lochner. (1976). Cell-to-substrate contacts in living fibroblasts: An interference reflexion study with an evaluation of the technique. *J. Cell Sci.* 21: 129–159. [4]

Jackson, H. and T. N. Parks. (1982). Functional synapse elimination in the developing avian cochlear nucleus with simultaneous reduction in cochlear–nerve axon branching. *J. Neurosci.* 2: 1736–1743. [12]

Jackson, P. C. (1983). Reduced activity during development delays the normal rearrangement of synapses in the rabbit ciliary ganglion. *J. Physiol. (Lond.)* 345: 319–327. [12]

Jackson, P. C. and J. Diamond. (1980). Regenerating axons reclaim sensory targets from collateral nerve sprouts. *Science* 214: 926–928. [13]

Jacob, F. (1982). *The Logic of Life*. New York: Pantheon. [1]

Jacobson, A. G. (1966). Inductive processes in embryonic development. *Science* 152: 25–35. [2]

Jacobson, A. G. (1978). Some forces that shape the nervous system. *Zoon* 6: 13–22. [1]

Jacobson, A. G. (1981). Morphogenesis of the neural plate and tube. In: *Morphogenesis and Pattern Formation*, T. G. Connelly, L. L. Brinkley and B. M. Carlson, eds. New York: Raven Press, pp. 179–203. [1]

Jacobson, C.-O. (1959). The localization of the presumptive cerebral regions in the neural plate of axolotl larva. *J. Embryol. Exp. Morphol.* 7: 1–21. [3]

Jacobson, M. (1978). Clonal origins of the central nervous system: Towards a developmental neuroanatomy. *Zoon* 6: 149–156. [2]

Jacobson, M. (1980). Clones and compartments in the vertebrate central nervous system. *Trends Neurosci.* 3: 3–5. [2, 3]

Jacobson, M. (1982). Origins of the nervous system in amphibians. In: *Neuronal Development*, N. C. Spitzer, ed. New York: Plenum Press, pp. 45–99. [2, 3]

Jacobson, M. (1983). Clonal organization of the central nervous system of the frog. III. Clones stemming from individual blastomeres of the 128-, 256-, and 512-cell stages. *J. Neurosci.* 3: 1019–1038. [2, 3]

Jacobson, M. (1984). Cell lineage analysis of neural induction: Origins of cells forming the induced nervous system. *Dev. Biol.* 102: 122–129. [3]

Jacobson, M. and G. Hirose. (1981). Clonal organization of the central nervous system of the frog. II. Clones stemming from individual blastomeres of the 32- and 64-cell stages. *J. Neurosci.* 1: 271–284. [3]

Jaffe, L. F. (1979). Control of development by ionic currents. In: *Membrane Transduction Mechanisms*, R. A. Cone and J. E. Dowling, eds. New York: Raven Press, pp. 199–231. [5]

Jaffe, L. F. (1981). The role of ionic currents in establishing developmental pattern. *Philos. Trans. R. Soc. Lond.* [Biol.]. 295: 553–566. [5]

Jaffe, L. F. and R. Nuccitelli. (1974). An ultrasensitive vibrating probe for measuring steady extracellular currents. *J. Cell Biol.* 63: 614–628. [5]

Jaffe, L. F. and M.-M Poo. (1979). Neurites grow faster towards the cathode than the anode in a steady field. *J. Exp. Zool.* 209: 115–128. [5]

Jakoi, E. R. and R. B. Marchase. (1979). Ligatin from embryonic chick neural retina. *J. Cell Biol.* 80: 642–650. [11]

Jansen, J. K. S. and J. G. Nicholls. (1972). Regeneration and changes in synaptic connections between individual nerve cells in the central nervous system of the leech. *Proc. Natl. Acad. Sci. USA* 69: 636–639. [10]

Jansen, J. K. S., W. Thompson and D. P. Kuffler. (1978). The formation and maintenance of synaptic connections as illustrated by studies of the neuromuscular junction. *Prog. Brain res.* 48: 3–19. [12]

Jeanmonod, D., F. L. Rice and H. Van der Loos. (1981). Mouse samatosensory cortex: Alterations in the barrelfield following receptor injury at different early postnatal ages. *Neuroscience* 6: 1503–1535. [8]

Jessell, T. M., R. E. Siegel and G. D. Fischbach. (1979). Induction of acetylcholine receptors on cultured skeletal muscle by a factor extracted from brain and spinal cord. *Proc. Natl. Acad. Sci. USA* 76: 5397–5401. [9]

Johns, P. R. (1977). Growth of the adult goldfish eye. III. Source of the new retinal cells. *J. Comp. Neurol*, 176: 343–358. [11]

Johns, P. R. (1981). Growth of fish retinas. *Am. Zool.* 21: 441–458. [6]

Johnson, D. A. and D. Purves. (1981). Postnatal reduction of neural unit size in the rabbit ciliary ganglion. *J. Physiol. (Lond.)* 318: 143–159. [12]

Johnson, D. A. and D. Purves. (1983). Tonic and reflex synaptic activity recorded in ciliary ganglion cells of anaesthetized rabbits. *J. Physiol. (Lond.)* 339: 599–563. [12]

Johnson, E. M., R. Y. Andres and R. A. Bradshaw. (1978). Characterization of the retrograde transport of nerve growth factor (NGF) using high specific activity [125I] NGF. *Brain Res.* 150: 319–331. [7]

Johnson, E. M., P. D. Gorin, L. D. Brandeis and J. Pearson. (1980). Dorsal root ganglion neurons are destroyed by exposure *in utero* to maternal antibody to nerve growth factor. *Science* 210: 916–918. [7]

Johnson, K. E. (1969). Altered contact behavior of presumptive mesodermal cells from hybrid amphibian embryos arrested at gastrulation. *J. Exp. Zool.* 170: 325–332. [4]

Johnson, K. E. (1970). The role of changes in cell contact behavior in amphibian gastrulation. *J. Exp. Zool.* 175: 391–428. [4]

Johnson, M., D. Ross, M. Meyers, R. Rees, R. Bunge, E. Wakshull and H. Burton. (1976). Synaptic vesicle cytochemistry changes when cultured sympathetic neurons develop cholinergic interactions. *Nature* 262: 308–310. [2]

Johnston, B. T., J. E. Schrameck and R. F. Mark. (1975). Re-innervation of axolotl limbs. II. Sensory nerves. *Proc. R. Soc. Lond. [Biol.]* 190: 59–75. [10]

Johnston, R. N. and N. K. Wessells. (1980). Regulation of the elongating nerve fiber. *Curr. Top. Dev. Biol.* 16: 165–206. [4]

Jolesz, F. and F. A. Sréter. (1981). Development, innervation and activity-pattern induced changes in skeletal muscle. *Annu. Rev. Physiol.* 43: 531–552. [8]

Jonakait, G. M., M. C. Bohn and I. B. Black. (1980). Maternal glucocorticoid hormones influence neurotransmitter phenotypic expresion in embryos. *Science* 210: 551–553. [2]

Jonakait, G. M., J. Wolf, P. Cochard, M. Goldstein and I. B. Black. (1979). Selective loss of noradrenergic phenotypic characters in neuroblasts of the rat embryo. *Proc. Natl. Acad. Sci. USA* 76: 4683–4686. [2]

Jones, D. G. and A. M. Cullen. (1979). A quantitative investigation of some presynaptic terminal parameters during synaptogenesis. *Exp. Neurol.* 64: 245–259. [9]

Jones, D. G. and R. M. Devon. (1980). An analysis of the association between various synaptic parameters during cortical development. *Cell. Tissue Res.* 208: 237–246. [9]

Jones, R. and G. Vrbová. (1970). Effect of muscle activity on denervation hypersensitivity. *J. Physiol. (Lond.)* 210: 144–145. [8]

Jones, R. and G. Vrbová. (1974). Two factors responsible for the development of denervation hypersensitivity. *J. Physiol. (Lond.)* 236: 517–538. [8,13]

Jørgensen, J. M. and Å. Flock. (1976). Non-innervated sense organs of the lateral line: Development in the regenerating tail of the salamander *Ambystoma mexicanum*. *J. Neurocytol.* 5: 33–41. [8]

Kaczmarek, L. K., M. Finbow, J. P. Revel and F. Strumwasser. (1979). The morphology and coupling of *Aplysia* bag cells within the abdominal ganglion and in cell culture. *J. Neurobiol.* 10: 535–550. [10]

Kandel, E. R. (1976). *Cellular Basis of Behavior: An Introduction to Behavioral Neurobiology*. New York: W. H. Freeman and Co. [13]

Kandel, E. R. (1979a). Psychotherapy and the single synapse. *N. Engl. J. Med.* 301: 1028–1037. [13]

Kandel, E. R. (1979b). Small systems of neurons. *Sci. Am.* 241(3): 60–70. [13]

Kandel, E. R. (1979c). Cellular insights into behavior and learning. *Harvey Lect.* 73: 19–92. [13]

Kandel, E. R., T. Abrams, L. Bernier, T. J. Carew, R. D. Hawkins and J. H. Schwartz. (1983). Classical conditioning and sensitization share aspects of the same molecular cascade in *Aplysia*. *Cold Spring Harbor Symp. Quant. Biol.* 48: 821–830. [13]

Kandel, E. R. and J. H. Schwartz. (1982). Molecular biology of learning: Modulation of transmitter release. *Science* 218: 433–443. [13]

Kandel, E. R. and L. Tauc. (1965). Heterosynaptic facilitation in neurones of the abdominal ganglion of *Aplysia depilans*. *J. Physiol. (Lond.)* 181: 1–27. [13]

Kano, M. (1975). Development of excitability in embryonic chick skeletal muscle cells. *J. Cell. Physiol.* 86: 503–510. [2]

Kaplan, M. S. and J. W. Hinds. (1977). Neurogenesis in the adult rat: Electronmicroscopic analysis of light radioautographs. *Science* 197: 1092–1094. [6]

Karkinen-Jääskeläinen, M. (1978). Permissive and directive interactions in lens induction. *J. Embryol. Exp. Morphol.* 44: 167–179. [2]

Karp, G. and N. J. Berrill. (1981). *Development*, 2nd Ed. New York: McGraw-Hill. [2, 3]

Karpati, G. and W. K. Engel. (1967). Transformation of the histochemical profile of skeletal muscle by "foreign" innervation. *Nature* 215: 1509–1510. [8]

Katz, B. (1960). Book Reviews. *Perspect. Biol. Med.* 3: 563–565. [13]

Katz, B. (1969). *The Release of Neural Transmitter Substances*. Liverpool: Liverpool University Press. [13]

Katz, B. (1982). Stephen William Kuffler 1913–1980. *Biogr. Mem. Fellows R. Soc.* 28: 225–259. [8]

Katz, B. and R. Miledi. (1967a). The timing of calcium action during neuromuscular transmission. *J. Physiol. (Lond.)* 189: 535–544. [13]

Katz, B. and R. Miledi. (1976b). A study of synaptic transmission in the absence of nerve impulses. *J. Physiol. (Lond.)* 192: 407–436. [13]

Katz, B. and R. Miledi. (1968). The role of calcium in neuromuscular facilitation. *J. Physiol. (Lond.)* 195: 481–492. [13]

Katz, B. and R. Miledi. (1969). Tetrodotoxin resistant electric activity in presynaptic terminals. *J. Physiol. (Lond.)* 203: 459–487. [13]

Kaufman, L. M. and J. N. Barrett. (1983). Serum factor supporting long-term survival of rat central neurons in culture. *Science* 220: 1394–1396. [7]

Kay, R. R. and K. A. Jermyn. (1983). A possible morphogen controlling differentiation in *Dictyostelium*. *Nature* 303: 242–244. [2]

Kelley, R. O. and J. F. Fallon. (1981). The developing limb: An analysis of interacting cells and tissues in a model morphogenetic system. In: *Morphogenesis and Pattern Formation*. T. C. T. Connelly, L. L. Brinkley and B. M. Carlson, eds. New York: Raven Press, pp. 49–86. [3]

Kelley, R. O., D. F. Goetinck and J. A. MacCabe. (1983). *Limb Development and Regeneration*. New York: Alan R. Liss. [3]

Kelly, A. M. and S. I. Zacks. (1969). The fine structure of motor endplate morphogenesis. *J. Cell Biol.* 42: 154–169. [9]

Kelly, J. P. and W. M. Cowan. (1972). Studies on the development of the chick optic tectum. III. Effects of early eye removal. *Brain Res.* 42: 263–283. [8]

Kelly, S. J. (1977). Studies of the developmental potential of 4- and 8-cell stage mouse blastomeres. *J. Exp. Zool.* 200: 365–376. [2]

Kelly, S. S. (1978). The effect of age on neuromuscular transmission. *J. Physiol. (Lond.)* 274: 51–62. [9]

Kelly, S. S. and N. Robbins. (1983). Progression of age changes in synaptic transmission at mouse neuromuscular junctions. *J. Physiol. (Lond.)* 343: 375–383. [13]

Kerns-Viets, B. and F. Bonhoeffer. (1984). Recognition of cell position and cell type specific membrane components by growing axons. (in preparation). [11]

Kimble, J. E. (1981). Strategies for control of pattern formation in *Caenorhabditis elegans*. *Philos. Trans. R. Soc. Lond. [Biol.]* 295: 539–551. [2]

Kimble, J. E. and D. Hirsh. (1979). The postembryonic cell lineages of the hermaphrodite and male gonads in *Caenorhabditis elegans*. *Dev. Biol.* 70: 396–417. [2]

Kimble, J. E., J. Sulston and J. White. (1979). Regulative development in the post-embryonic lineages of *Caenorhabditis elegans*. In: *Cell Lineage, Stem Cells and Cell Determination, INSERM Symp. No. 10*, N. LeDouarin, ed. Amsterdam: Elsevier, pp. 59–68. [2]

Klein, M. and E. R. Kandel. (1978). Presynaptic modulation of voltage-dependent Ca^{2+} current: Mechanism for behavioral sensitization in *Aplysia californica*. *Proc. Natl. Acad. Sci. USA* 75: 3512–3516. [13]

Klein, M. and E. R. Kandel. (1980). Mechanism of calcium current modulation underlying presynaptic facilitation and behavioral sensitization in *Aplysia*. *Proc. Natl. Acad. Sci. USA* 77: 6912–6916. [13]

Klein, M., E. Shapiro and E. R. Kandel. (1980). Synaptic plasticity and the modulation of the Ca^{2+} current. *J. Exp. Biol.* 89: 117–157. [13]

Knudsen, E. I., S. D. Esterly and P. F. Knudsen. (1984a). Monaural occlusion alters sound localization during a sensitive period in the barn owl. *J. Neurosci.* 4: 1001–1011. [14]

Knudsen, E. I., P. F. Knudsen and S. D. Esterly. (1984b). A critical period for the recovery of sound localization accuracy following monaural occlusion in the barn owl. *J. Neurosci.* 4: 1012–1020. [14]

Köhler, G. and C. Milstein. (1976). Derivation of specific antibody-producing tissue culture and tumor lines by cell fusion. *Eur. J. Immunol.* 6: 511–519. [11]

Kohler, I. (1962). Experiments with goggles. *Sci. Am.* 206(5): 62–72. [13]

Kollar, E. J. and C. Fisher. (1980). Tooth induction in chick epithelium: Expression of quiescent genes for enamel synthesis. *Science* 207: 993–995. [2]

Kollros, J. J. (1968). Endocrine influences in neural development. In: *Growth of the Nervous System, Ciba Found. Symp.*, G. W. Wolstenholme and M. O'Conner, eds. Boston: Little, Brown & Company, pp. 179–199. [6]

Kollros, J. J. (1981). Transitions in the nervous system during amphibian metamorphosis. In: *Metamorphosis: A Problem in Developmental Biology*, 2nd Ed., L. I. Gilbert and E. Frieden, eds. New York: Plenum Press, pp. 445–459. [6]

Kollros, J. J. and V. M. McMurray. (1956). The mesencephalic V nucleus in anurans. II. The influence of thyroid hormone on cell size and cell number. *J. Exp. Zool.* 131: 1–26. [6]

Konishi, M. (1965). The role of auditory feedback in the control of vocalization in the white-crowned sparrow. *Z. Tierpsychol.* 22: 770–783. [14]

Konishi, M. and M. E. Gurney. (1982). Sexual differentiation of brain and behaviour. *Trends Neurosci.* 5: 20–23. [14]

Kornberg, T. (1981). *Engrailed*: A gene controlling compartment and segment formation in *Drosophila*. *Proc. Natl. Acad. Sci. USA* 78: 1095–1099. [3]

Korneliussen, H. and J. K. S. Jansen. (1976). Morphological aspects of the elimination of polyneuronal innervation of skeletal muscle fibres in newborn rats. *J. Neurocytol.* 5: 591–604. [12]

Korneliussen, H. and H. Sommerschild. (1976). Ultrastructure of the new neuromuscular junctions formed during reinnervation of rat soleus muscle by a "foreign" nerve. *Cell Tissue Res.* 167: 439–452. [9]

Korsching, S. and H. Thoenen. (1983). Nerve growth factor in sympathetic ganglia and corresponding target organs of the rat: Correlation with density of sympathetic innervation. *Proc. Natl. Acad. Sci. USA* 80: 3513–3516. [7]

Koshland, D. E. (1981). Biochemistry of sensing and adaptation in a simple bacterial system. *Annu. Rev. Biochem.* 50: 765–782. [4]

Kramer, A. P. and J. Y. Kuwada. (1983). Formation of

the receptive fields of leech mechanosensory neurons during embryonic development. *J. Neurosci.* 3: 2474–2486. [13]

Krasne, F. B. (1976). Invertebrate systems as a means of gaining insight into the nature of learning and memory. In: *Neural Mechanisms of Learning and Memory*, M. R. Rosensweig and E. L. Bennett, eds. Cambridge, MA: MIT Press, pp. 401–429. [13]

Krayanek, S. and S. Goldberg. (1981). Oriented extracellular channels and axonal guidance in the embryonic chick retina. *Dev. Biol. 84*: 41–50. [5]

Kriegstein, A. R. and M. A. Dichter. (1983). Morphological classification of rat cortical neurons in cell culture. *J. Neurosci. 3*: 1634–1647. [2]

Kristensson, K. and Y. Olsson. (1971). Retrograde axonal transport of protein. *Brain Res. 29*: 363–365. [5]

Kuczmarski, E. R. and J. L. Rosenbaum. (1979). Studies on the organization and localization of actin and myosin in neurons. *J. Cell Biol. 80*: 356–371. [4]

Kuffler, D., W. Thompson and J. K. S. Jansen. (1977). The elimination of synapses in multiply-innervated skeletal muscle fibres of the rat: Dependence on distance between end-plates. *Brain Res. 38*: 353–358. [12]

Kuffler, D., W. Thompson and J. K. S. Jansen. (1980). The fate of foreign endplates in cross-innervated rat soleus muscle. *Proc. R. Soc. Lond. [Biol.] 208*: 189–222. [12]

Kuffler, S. W. (1943). Specific excitability of the endplate region in normal and denervated muscle. *J. Neurophysiol. 6*: 99–110. [8]

Kuffler, S. W., M. J. Dennis and A. J. Harris. (1971). The development of chemosensitivity in extrasynaptic areas of the neuronal surface after denervation of parasympathetic ganglion cells in the heart of the frog. *Proc. R. Soc. Lond. [Biol.] 177*: 555–563. [8]

Kuffler, S. W. and J. G. Nicholls. (1976). *From Neuron to Brain.* Sunderland, MA: Sinauer Associates. [9]

Kuffler, S. W. and E. M. Vaughn-Williams. (1953a). Properties of the "slow" skeletal muscle fibres of the frog. *J. Physiol. (Lond.) 121*: 318–340. [10]

Kuffler, S. W. and E. M. Vaughan-Williams. (1953b). Small nerve junctional potentials. The distribution of small motor nerves to frog skeletal muscle, and the membrane characteristics of the fibres they innervate. *J. Physiol. (Lond.) 121*: 289–317. [10]

Kuffler, S. W. and D. Yoshikami. (1975). The distribution of acetylcholine sensitivity at the post-synaptic membrane of vertebrate skeletal twitch muscles: Iontophoretic mapping in the micron range. *J. Physiol. (Lond.) 244*: 703–730. [12]

Kugelberg, E., L. Edström and M. Abbruzzese. (1970). Mapping of motor units in experimentally reinnervated rat muscle. Interpretation of histochemical and atrophic fibre patterns in neurogenic lesions. *J. Neurol. Neurosurg. Psychiatry 33*: 319–329. [10]

Kullberg, R. W., T. L. Lentz and M. W. Cohen. (1977). Development of the myotomal neuromuscular junction in *Xenopus laevis*: An electrophysiological and fine-structural study. *Dev. Biol. 60*: 101–129. [9]

Kuno, M. and R. Llinás. (1970). Alterations of synaptic action in chromatolysed motoneurones of the cat. *J. Physiol. (Lond.) 210*: 823–838. [13]

Kuno, M., S. A. Turkanis and J. N. Weakly. (1971). Correlation between nerve terminal size and transmitter release at the neuromuscular junction of the frog. *J. Physiol. (Lond.) 213*: 545–556. [9]

Kupfer, C. and P. Palmer. (1964). Lateral geniculate nucleus: Histological and cytochemical changes following afferent denervation and visual deprivation. *Exp. Neurol. 9*: 400–409. [8]

Kupfermann, I., V. Castellucci, H. Pinsker and E. R. Kandel. (1970). Neuronal correlates of habituation and dishabituation of the gill-withdrawal reflex in *Aplysia*. *Science 167*: 1743–1745. [13]

Laing, N. G. (1982). Timing of motoneuron death in the brachial and lumbar regions of the chick embryo. *Dev. Brain Res. 5*: 181–186. [6]

Laing, N. G. and M. C. Prestige. (1978). Prevention of spontaneous motoneurone death in chick embryos. *J. Physiol. (Lond.) 282*: 33–34P. [6]

Lamb, A. H. (1976). The projection patterns of the ventral horn to the hind limb during development. *Dev. Biol. 54*: 82–99. [5, 6]

Lamb, A. H. (1977). Neuronal death in the development of the somatotopic projections of the ventral horn in *Xenopus*. *Brain Res. 134*: 145–150. [6]

Lamb, A. H. (1979). Evidence that some developing limb motoneurons die for reasons other than peripheral competition. *Dev. Biol. 71*: 8–21. [6]

Lamb, A. H. (1980). Motoneurone counts in *Xenopus* frogs reared with one bilaterally-innervated hindlimb. *Nature 284*: 347–350. [6]

Lamb, A. H. (1981a). Selective bilateral motor innervation in *Xenopus* tadpoles with one hind limb. *J. Embryol. Exp. Morphol. 65*: 149–163. [6]

Lamb, A. H. (1981b). Target dependency of developing motoneurons in *Xenopus laevis*. *J. Comp. Neurol. 203*: 157–171. [6]

Lamb, A. H. (1984). Motoneuron death in the embryo. *Critical Reviews in Clinical Neurobiology* (in press). [6]

Lamborghini, J. E. (1980). Rohon-Beard cells and other large neurons in *Xenopus* embryos originate during gastrulation. *J. Comp. Neurol. 189*: 323–333. [2]

Lance-Jones, C. and L. Landmesser. (1980a). Motoneurone projection patterns in embryonic chick limbs following partial deletions of the spinal cord. *J. Physiol. (Lond.) 302*: 559–580. [5]

Lance-Jones, C. and L. Landmesser. (1980b). Motoneurone projection patterns in chick hind limb following partial reversals of the spinal cord. *J. Physiol. (Lond.) 302*: 581–602. [5]

Lance-Jones, C. and L. Landmesser. (1981a). Pathway selection by chick lumbosacral motoneurons during normal development. *Proc. R. Soc. Lond. [Biol.] 214*: 1–18. [5]

Lance-Jones, C. and L. Landmesser. (1981b). Pathway selection by embryonic chick motoneurons in an experimentally altered environment. *Proc. R. Soc. Lond. [Biol.] 214*: 19–52. [5]

Land, P. W. and R. D. Lund. (1979). Development of the rat's uncrossed retinotectal pathway and its relation to plasticity studies. *Science* 205: 698–700. [12]

Landis, D. M. D. and T. S. Reese. (1977). Structure of the Purkinje cell membrane in staggerer and weaver mutant mice. *J. Comp. Neurol.* 171: 247–260. [9]

Landis, S. C. (1976). Rat sympathetic neurons and cardiac myocytes developing in microcultures: Correlation of the fine structure of endings with neurotransmitter function in single neurons. *Proc. Natl. Acad. Sci. USA* 73: 4220–4224. [2, 9]

Landis, S. C. (1980). Developmental changes in the neurotransmitter properties of dissociated sympathetic neurons: A cytochemical study of the effects of medium. *Dev. Biol.* 77: 349–361. [2, 9]

Landis, S. C. (1983). Neuronal growth cones. *Annu. Rev. Physiol.* 45: 567–580. [4]

Landis, S. C. and D. Keefe (1983). Evidence for transmitter plasticity *in vivo*: Developmental changes in properties of cholinergic sympathetic neurons. *Dev. Biol.* 98: 349–372. [2]

Landmesser, L. (1971). Contractile and electrical responses of vagus-innervated frog sartorius muscle. *J. Physiol. (Lond.)* 213: 707–725. [9]

Landmesser, L. (1972). Pharmacological properties, cholinesterase activity and anatomy of nerve–muscle junctions in vagus-innervated frog sartorius. *J. Physiol. (Lond.)* 220: 243–256. [9]

Landmesser, L. (1978). The development of motor projection patterns in the chick hind limb. *J. Physiol. (Lond.)* 284: 391–414. [5]

Landmesser, L. (1980). The generation of neuromuscular specificity. *Annu. Rev. Neurosci.* 3: 279–302. [5, 12]

Landmesser, L. and D. G. Morris. (1975). The development of functional innervation in the hind limb of the chick embryo. *J. Physiol. (Lond.)* 249: 301–326. [5, 9]

Landmesser, L. and M. J. O'Donovan. (1984a). Activation patterns of embryonic chick hindlimb muscles recorded *in ovo* and in an isolated spinal cord preparation. *J. Physiol. (Lond.)* 347: 189–204. [14]

Landmesser, L. and M. J. O'Donovan. (1984b). The activation patterns of embryonic chick mononeurones projecting to inappropriate muscles. *J. Physiol. (Lond.)* 347: 205–224. [11]

Landmesser, L. and G. Pilar. (1970). Selective reinnervation of two cell populations in the adult pigeon ciliary ganglion. *J. Physiol. (Lond.)* 211: 203–216. [10]

Landmesser, L. and G. Pilar. (1974a). Synapse formation during embryogenesis on ganglion cells lacking a periphery. *J. Physiol. (Lond.)* 241: 715–736. [6]

Landmesser, L. and G. Pilar. (1974b). Synaptic transmission and cell death during normal ganglionic development. *J. Physiol. (Lond.)* 241: 737–749. [6]

Landmesser, L. and G. Pilar. (1976). Fate of ganglionic synapses and ganglion cell axons during normal and induced cell death. *J. Cell Biol.* 68: 357–374. [6]

Lang, F., C. K. Govind and W. J. Costello. (1978). Experimental transformation of muscle fiber properties in lobster. *Science* 201: 1037–1039. [8]

Langley, J. N. (1892). On the origin from the spinal cord of the cervical and upper thoracic sympathetic fibres, with some observations on white and grey rami communicantes. *Philos. Trans. R. Soc. Lond. [Biol.]* 183: 85–124. [10]

Langley, J. N. (1895). Note on regeneration of pre-ganglionic fibres of the sympathetic. *J. Physiol. (Lond.)* 18: 280–284. [10, 11]

Langley, J. N. (1897). On the regeneration of pre-ganglionic and post-ganglionic visceral nerve fibres. *J. Physiol. (Lond.)* 22: 215–230. [10]

Langley, J. N. (1907). On the contraction of muscle chiefly in relation to the presence of "receptive" substances, Part I. *J. Physiol. (Lond.)* 36: 347–384. [10]

Langley, J. N. (1908a). On the contraction of muscle chiefly in relation to the presence of "receptive" substances, Part II. *J. Physiol. (Lond.)* 37: 165–212. [10]

Langley, J. N. (1908b). On the contraction of muscle chiefly in relation to the presence of "receptive" substances, Part III. *J. Physiol. (Lond.)* 37: 285–300. [10]

Langley, J. N. (1921). *The Autonomic Nervous System*, Part I. Cambridge, England: Heffer and Sons. [10]

Langley, J. N. and H. K. Anderson. (1904). The union of different kinds of nerve fibers. *J. Physiol. (Lond.)* 31: 365–391. [9]

Larrabee, M. G. and D. W. Bronk. (1947). Prolonged facilitation of synaptic excitation in sympathetic ganglia. *J. Neurophysiol.* 10: 139–154. [13]

LaVail, J. H. and M. W. Cowan. (1971). The development of the chick optic tectum. II. Autoradiographic studies. *Brain Res.* 28: 421–441. [4]

LaVail, J. H. and M. M. LaVail. (1972). Retrograde axonal transport in the central nervous system. *Science* 176: 1416–1417. [5]

Law, M. I. and M. Constantine-Paton. (1981). Anatomy and physiology of experimentally produced striped tecta. *J. Neurosci.* 1: 741–759. [12]

Law, M. I. and M. Constantine-Paton. (1982). A banded distribution of retinal afferents within layer 9A of the normal frog optic tectum. *Brain Res.* 247: 201–208. [12]

Lawrence, P. A. (1966). Gradients in the insect segment: The orientation of hairs in the milkweed bug *Oncopeltus fasciatus*. *J. Exp. Biol.* 44: 607–620. [3]

Lawrence, P. A. (1969). Cellular differentiation and pattern formation during metamorphosis of the milkweed bug *Oncopeltus*. *Dev. Biol.* 19: 12–40. [5]

Lawrence, P. A. (1973). A clonal analysis of segment development in *Oncopeltus* (Hemiptera). *J. Embryol. Exp. Morphol.* 30: 681–699. [3]

Lawrence, P. A. (1975). The structure and properties of a compartment border: The intersegmental boundary in *Oncopeltus*. *Ciba Found. Symp.* 29: 3–23. [3]

Lawrence, P. A. (1978). Compartments and the insect nervous system. *Zoon* 6: 157–160. [3]

Lawrence, P. A. (1981). The cellular basis of segmentation in insects. *Cell* 26: 3–10. [3]

Lawrence, P. A. and G. Morata. (1976). Compartments

in the wing of *Drosophila*: A study of the *engrailed* gene. *Dev. Biol. 50*: 321–337. [3]

Lazarides, E. and J. P. Revel. (1979). Molecular basis of cell movement. *Sci. Am. 240(5)*: 100–113. [4]

LeDouarin, N. M. (1980a). The ontogeny of the neural crest in avian embryo chimaeras. *Nature 286*: 663–669. [2, 4]

LeDouarin, N. M. (1980b). Migration and differentiation of neural crest cells. *Curr. Top. Dev. Biol. 16*: 31–85. [4]

LeDouarin, N. M. (1982). *The Neural Crest*. New York: Cambridge University Press. [2, 4]

LeDouarin, N. M. and M.-A. Teillet. (1973). The migration of neural crest cells to the wall of the digestive tract in avian embryo. *J. Embryol. Exp. Morphol. 30*: 31–48. [4]

LeDouarin, N. M. and M.-A. Teillet. (1974). Experimental analysis of the migration and differentiation of neuroblasts of the autonomic nervous system and of the neuroectodermal mesenchymal derivatives, using a biological cell marking technique. *Dev. Biol. 41*: 162–184. [2]

LeDouarin, N. M., M.-A. Teillet and J. Fontaine-Perus. (1984). Chimeras in the study of the peripheral nervous system of birds. In: *Chimeras In Developmental Biology*, N. LeDouarin and A. MacLaren, eds. New York: Academic Press (in press). [4]

Lee, K. S., F. Schottler, M. Oliver and G. Lynch. (1980). Brief bursts of high frequency stimulation produce two types of structural changes in rat hippocampus. *J. Neurophysiol. 44*: 247–258. [13]

Lehmann, F. E. (1938). Regionale Verschiedenheiten des Organisators von Triton, insbesondere in der vorderen und hinteren Kopfregion nachgewiesen durch phasenspezifische Erzeugung von Lithiumbedingten und operative bewirkten Regionaldefekten. *Wilhelm Roux Arch. Entwicklungsmech. Org. 138*: 106–158. [3]

Lemke, G. and J. P. Brockes. (1984). Identification and purification of glial growth factor. *J. Neurosci. 4*: 75–83. [8]

Leonard, R. B., R. E. Coggeshall and W. D. Willis. (1978). A documentation of an age related increase in neuronal and axonal numbers in the stingray *Dasyatis sabina* Leseuer. *J. Comp. Neurol. 179*: 13–22. [6]

Letinsky, M. S. (1974). The development of nerve–muscle junctions in *Rana catesbeiana* tadpoles. *Dev. Biol. 40*: 129–153. [9, 12]

Letinsky, M. S., K. H. Fischbeck and U. J. McMahan. (1976). Precision of reinnervation of original postsynaptic sites in frog muscle after a nerve crush. *J. Neurocytol. 5*: 691–718. [5, 9]

Letinsky, M. S. and K. Morrison-Graham. (1980). Structure of developing frog neuromuscular junctions. *J. Neurocytol. 9*: 321–342. [9]

Letourneau, P. C. (1975a). Possible roles for cell-to-substratum adhesion in neuronal morphogenesis. *Dev. Biol. 44*: 77–91. [5]

Letourneau, P. C. (1975b). Cell-to-substratum adhesion and guidance of axonal elongation. *Dev. Biol. 44*: 92–101. [5]

Letourneau, P. C. (1978). Chemotactic response of nerve fiber elongation to nerve growth factor. *Dev. Biol. 66*: 183–196. [5, 7]

Letourneau, P. C. (1979). Cell–substratum adhesion of neurite growth cones, and its role in neurite elongation. *Exp. Cell Res. 124*: 127–138. [4]

Letourneau, P. C. (1981). Immunocytochemical evidence for colocalization in neurite growth cones of actin and myosin and their relationship to cell–substratum adhesions. *Dev. Biol. 85*: 113–122. [4]

Letourneau, P. C. (1982). Nerve fiber growth and its regulation by extrinsic factors. In: *Neuronal Development*, N. C. Spitzer, ed. New York: Plenum Press. [4]

Letourneau, P. C., P. N. Ray and M. R. Bernfield. (1980). The regulation of cell behavior by cell adhesion. In: *Biological Regulation and Development*, Vol. 2. *Molecular Organization and Cell Function*, R. F. Goldberger, ed. New York: Plenum Press, pp. 339–376. [4]

LeVay, S., M. P. Stryker and C. J. Shatz. (1978). Ocular dominance columns and their development in layer IV of the cat's visual cortex: A quantitative study. *J. Comp. Neurol. 179*: 223–244. [12]

Levi, A., Y. Shechter, E. J. Neufeld and J. Schlessinger. (1980). Mobility, clustering and transport of nerve growth factor in embryonal sensory cells and in a sympathetic neuronal cell line. *Proc. Natl. Acad. Sci. USA 77*: 3469–3473. [7]

Levi-Montalcini, R. (1949). The development of the acoustico-vestibular centers in the chick embryo in the absence of afferent root fiber and of descending fiber tracts. *J. Comp. Neurol. 91*: 209–241. [6, 7, 8]

Levi-Montalcini, R. (1950). The origin and development of the visceral system in the spinal cord of the chick embryo. *J. Morphol. 86*: 253–278. [4, 6]

Levi-Montalcini, R. (1953). Effects of mouse tumor transplantation on the nervous system. *Ann. NY Acad. Sci. 55*: 330–343. [7]

Levi-Montalcini, R. (1964). Events in the developing nervous system. *Prog. Brain Res. 4*: 1–29. [7]

Levi-Montalcini, R. (1972). The morphological effects of immunosympathectomy. In: *Immunosympathectomy*, G. Steiner and E. Schönbaum, eds. Amsterdam: Elsevier, pp. 55–78. [7]

Levi-Montalcini, R. (1975). NGF: an uncharted route. In: *The Neurosciences, Paths of Discovery*. F. G. Worden, J. P. Swazey and G. Adelman, eds. Cambridge: MIT Press, pp. 244–265. [7]

Levi-Montalcini, R. (1976). The nerve growth factor: Its role in growth, differentiation and function of the sympathetic adrenergic neuron. *Prog. Brain Res. 45*: 235–258. [7]

Levi-Montalcini, R. and L. Aloe. (1983). The effect of nerve growth factor on autonomic ganglion cells. In: *Autonomic Ganglia*, L.-G. Elfvin, ed. New York: John Wiley & Sons, pp. 401–426. [7]

Levi-Montalcini, R., L. Aloe, E. Mugnaini, F. Oesch and H. Thoenen. (1975). Nerve growth factor induces volume increase and enhances tyrosine hydroxylase synthesis in chemically axotomized sympathetic ganglia of newborn rats. *Proc. Natl. Acad. Sci. USA* 72: 595–599. [7]

Levi-Montalcini, R. and P. U. Angeletti. (1963). Essential role of the nerve growth factor in the survival and maintenance of dissociated sensory and sympathetic embryonic nerve cells *in vitro. Dev. Biol.* 7: 653–659. [7]

Levi-Montalcini, R. and P. U. Angeletti. (1964). Hormonal control of the NGF content in the submaxillary salivary glands of mouse. In: *Salivary Glands and Their Secretions,* L. M. Srebny and J. Myer, eds. Oxford, England: Pergamon Press, pp. 129–141. [7]

Levi-Montalcini, R. and P. U. Angeletti. (1966). Immunosympathectomy. *Pharmacol. Rev.* 18: 619–628. [7]

Levi-Montalcini, R. and P. U. Angeletti. (1968). Biological aspects of the nerve growth factor. In: *Growth of the Nervous System, Ciba Found. Symp.,* G. E. W. Wolstenholme and M. O'Conner, eds. London: Churchill, pp. 126–147. [7]

Levi-Montalcini, R. and B. Booker. (1960). Destruction of the sympathetic ganglia in mammals by an antiserum to a nerve growth protein. *Proc. Natl. Acad. Sci. USA* 46: 384–391. [7]

Levi-Montalcini, R. and S. Cohen. (1956). *In vitro* and *in vivo* effects of a nerve growth-stimulating agent isolated from snake venom. *Proc. Natl. Acad. Sci. USA* 42: 695–699. [7]

Levi-Montalcini, R. and S. Cohen. (1960). Effects of the extract of the mouse submaxillary salivary glands on the sympathetic system of mammals. *Ann. NY Acad. Sci.* 85: 324–341. [7]

Levi-Montalcini, R. and V. Hamburger. (1951). Selective growth-stimulating effects of mouse sarcoma on the sensory and sympathetic nervous system of the chick embryo. *J. Exp. Zool.* 116: 321–361. [7]

Levi-Montalcini, R. and V. Hamburger. (1953). A diffusible agent of mouse sarcoma, producing hyperplasia of sympathetic ganglia and hyperneurotization of viscera in the chick embryo. *J. Exp. Zool.* 123: 233–287. [7]

Levi-Montalcini, R. and G. Levi. (1942). Les consequences de la destruction d'un territoire d'innervation peripheique sur le développements des centres nerveux correspondents dans l'embryon de poulet. *Arch. Biol. (Liege)* 53: 537–545. [7]

Levi-Montalcini, R. and G. Levi. (1943). Recherches quantitatives sur la marche du processus de differenciation des neurones dans les ganglions spinaux de l'embryon de poulet. *Arch. Biol. (Liege)* 54: 183–206. [7]

Levi-Montalcini, R. and G. Levi. (1944). Correlazioni nell sviluppo tra varie parti del sistema nervoso. *Pontif. Accad. Sci. Commentat.* 8: 529–568. [7]

Levi-Montalcini, R., H. Meyer and V. Hamburger. (1954). *In vitro* experiments on the effects of mouse sarcomas 180 and 37 on the spinal and sympathetic ganglia of the chick embryo. *Cancer Res.* 14: 49–57. [7]

Levine, R. L. and M. Jacobson. (1975). Discontinuous mapping of retina onto tectum innervated by both eyes. *Brain Res.* 98: 172–176. [12]

Levinthal, F., E. Macagno and C. Levinthal. (1975). Anatomy and development of identified cells in isogenic organisms. *Cold Spring Harbor Symp. Quant. Biol.* 40: 321–333. [2]

Levitt, P., M. L. Cooper and P. Rakic. (1981). Coexistence of neuronal and glial precursor cells in the cerebral ventricular zone of the fetal monkey: An ultrastructural immunoperoxidase study. *J. Neurosci.* 1: 27–39. [2]

Levitt, P. and P. Rakic. (1980). Immunoperoxidase localization of glial fibrillary acidic protein in radial glial-cells and astrocytes of the developing rhesus-monkey brain. *J. Comp. Neurol.* 193: 815–840. [2, 4]

Lev-Tov, A. and R. Rahamimoff. (1980). A study of tetanic and post-tetanic potentiation of miniature-endplate potentials at the frog neuromuscular junction. *J. Physiol. (Lond.)* 309: 247–273. [13]

Lewis, E. B. (1978). A gene complex controlling segmentation in *Drosophila. Nature* 276: 565–570. [2, 3]

Lewis, J. (1978). Pathways of axons in the developing chick wing: Evidence against chemo-specific guidance. *Zoon* 6: 175–179. [5]

Lewis, J., A. Chevallier, M. Kieny and L. Wolpert. (1981). Muscle nerve branches do not develop in chick wings devoid of muscle. *J. Embryol. Exp. Morphol.* 64: 211–232. [5]

Lewis, P. D. (1975). Cell death in the germinal layers of the postnatal rat brain. *Neuropathol. Appl. Neurobiol.* 1: 21–29. [6]

Lewis, P. D., A. J. Patel, A. L. Johnson and R. Balazs. (1976). Effect of thyroid deficiency on cell acquisition in the postnatal rat brain: A quantitative histological study. *Brain Res.* 104: 49–62. [6]

Lewis, W. H. (1934). On the locomotion of the polymorphonuclear neutrophils of the rat in autoplasma cultures. *Bull. Johns Hopkins Hosp.* 55: 273–279. [4]

Lichtman, J. W. (1977). The reorganization of synaptic connexions in the rat submandibular ganglion during post-natal development. *J. Physiol. (Lond.)* 273: 155–177. [5, 12]

Lichtman, J. W. (1980). On the predominantly single innervation of submandibular ganglion cells in the rat. *J. Physiol. (Lond.)* 302: 121–130. [12]

Lichtman, J. W. and E. Frank. (1984). Physiological evidence for specificity of synaptic connections between individual sensory and motor neurons in the brachial spinal cord of the bullfrog. *J. Neurosci.* 4: 1745–1753. [10]

Lichtman, J. W. and E. Frank. (1984). On the specificity of sensory-motor and peripheral synaptic connections. In: *Neuronal Growth and Plasticity.* M. Kuno, ed. Tokyo: Japan Scientific Societies Press, pp. 149–164. [12]

Lichtman, J. W., S. Jhaveri and E. Frank. (1984). Anatomical basis of specific connections between sensory axons and motor neurons in the brachial spinal cord of the bullfrog. *J. Neurosci.* 4: 1754–1763. [10]

Lichtman, J. W. and D. Purves. (1980). The elimination of redundant preganglionic innervation to hamster sympathetic ganglion cells in early post-natal life. *J. Physiol. (Lond.)* 301: 213–228. [12]

Lichtman, J. W. and D. Purves. (1981). Regulation of the number of axons that innervate target cells. In: *Development in the Nervous System,* D. R. Garrod and J. D. Feldman, eds. Cambridge. Cambridge University Press, pp. 233–243. [12]

Lichtman, J. W., D. Purves and J. W. Yip. (1979). On the purpose of selective innervation of guinea-pig superior cervical ganglion cells. *J. Physiol. (Lond.)* 292: 69–84 (1979) [10]

Lichtman, J. W., D. Purves and J. W. Yip. (1980). Innervation of neurones in the guinea-pig thoracic chain. *J. Physiol. (Lond.)* 298: 285–299. [10]

Liddell, E. G. T. and C. Sherrington. (1924). Reflexes in response to stretch (myotatic reflexes). *Proc. R. Soc. Lond.* [*Biol.*] 96: 212–242. [10]

Liley, A. W. (1956). An investigation of spontaneous activity at the neuromuscular junction of the rat. *J. Physiol. (Lond.)* 132: 650–656. [13]

Liu, C. N. and W. W. Chambers. (1958). Intraspinal sprouting of dorsal root axons. *Arch. Neurol. Psychiatry* 79: 46–61. [13]

Lloyd, D. P. C. (1943). Reflex action in relation to pattern and peripheral source of afferent stimulation. *J. Neurophysiol.* 6: 111–120. [10]

Lloyd, D. P. C. (1950). Post-tetanic potentiation of response in monosynaptic reflex pathways of the spinal cord. *J. Gen Physiol.* 33: 147–170. [13]

Locke, M. (1959). The cuticular pattern in an insect, *Rhodnius prolixus* Stål. *J. Exp. Biol.* 36: 459-477. [3]

Locke, M. (1967). The development of patterns in the integument of insects. *Adv. Morphog.* 6: 33–87. [3]

Loeb, L. and M. S. Fleisher. (1917). On the factors which determine the movements of tissues in culture media. *J. Med. Res.* 37: 75–99. [4]

Löfberg, J., K. Ahlfors and C. Fällström. (1980). Neural crest cell migration in relation to extracellular matrix organization in the embryonic axolotl trunk. *Dev. Biol.* 75: 148–167. [4]

Lømo, T. (1976). The role of activity in the control of membrane and contractile properties of skeletal muscle. In: *Motor Innervation of Muscle*, S. Thesleff, ed. London: Academic Press, pp. 289–321. [8]

Lømo, T. and J. Rosenthal. (1972). Control of ACh sensitivity by muscle activity in the rat. *J. Physiol. (Lond.)* 221: 493–513. [8]

Lømo, T. and C. R. Slater. (1980). Control of junctional acetylcholinesterase by neural and muscular influences in the rat. *J. Physiol. (Lond.)* 303: 191–202. [9]

Lømo, T. and R. H. Westgaard. (1975). Further studies on the control of ACh sensitivity by muscle activity in the rat. *J. Physiol. (Lond.)* 252: 603–626. [8]

Lømo, T. and R. H. Westgaard. (1976). Control of ACh sensitivity in rat muscle fibers. *Cold Spring Harbor Symp. Quant. Biol.* 40: 263–274. [8]

Lømo, T., R. H. Westgaard and H. A. Dahl. (1974). Contractile properties of muscle: Control by pattern of muscle activity in the rat. *Proc. R. Soc. Lond.* [*Biol.*] 187: 99–103. [8]

Lømo, T., R. H. Westgaard and L. Engebretsen. (1980). Different stimulation patterns affect contractile properties of denervated rat soleus muscles. In: *Plasticity of Muscle*, D. Pette, ed. Berlin: Walter de Gruyter and Co., pp. 297–309. [8]

Lopresti, V., E. R. Macagno and C. Levinthal. (1974). Structure and development of neuronal connections in isogenic organisms—transient gap junctions between growing optic axons and lamina neuroblasts. *Proc. Natl. Acad. Sci. USA* 71: 1098–1102. [5]

Lorch, I. J. and J. F. Danielli. (1950). Transplantation of nuclei from cell to cell. *Nature* 166: 329–330. [1]

Lorenz, K. (1935). Companions as factors in the bird's environment: The conspecific as the eliciting factor for social behaviour patterns. In: K. Lorenz, *Studies in Animal and Human Behaviour*. Translated by R. Martin. Cambridge, MA: Harvard University Press, 1970, pp. 101–254. [14]

Lorenz, K. (1970). *Studies in Animal and Human Behaviour*. Translated by R. Martin. Cambridge, MA.: Harvard University Press. [14]

Luco, J. V. and C. Eyzaguirre. (1955). Fibrillation and hypersensitivity to ACh in denervated muscles: Effect of length of degenerating nerve fibers. *J. Neurophysiol.* 18: 65–73. [8]

Lund, R. D., T. J. Cunningham and J. S. Lund. (1973). Modified optic projections after unilateral eye removal in young rats. *Brain Behav. Evol.* 8: 51–72. [6]

MacIntyre, L. and J. Diamond. (1981). Domains and mechanosensory nerve fields in salamander skin. *Proc. R. Soc. Lond.* [*Biol.*] 211: 471–499. [13]

MacNab, R. M. (1980). Sensing the environment, bacterial chemotaxis. In: *Biological Regulation and Development*, Vol. 2, *Molecular Organization and Cell Function*, R. F. Goldberger, ed. New York: Plenum Press, pp. 377–412. [4]

Maden, M. (1982). Vitamin A and pattern formation in the regenerating limb. *Nature* 295: 672–675. [3]

Maden, M. (1983). The effect of vitamin A on limb regeneration in *Rana temporaria*. *Dev. Biol.* 98: 409–416. [3]

Maehlen, J. and A. Njå. (1981). Selective synapse formation during sprouting and after partial denervation of the guinea-pig superior cervical ganglion. *J. Physiol. (Lond.)* 319: 555–567. [10, 13]

Maehlen, J. and A. Njå. (1982). The effects of electrical stimulation on sprouting after partial denervation of guinea-pig sympathetic ganglion cells. *J. Physiol. (Lond.)* 322: 151–166. [12]

Maehlen, J. and A. Njå. (1984). Rearrangement of synapses on guinea pig sympathetic ganglion cells after partial interruption of the preganglionic nerve. *J. Physiol. (Lond.)* 348: 43–56. [12]

Magleby, K. L. (1973). The effect of tetanic and post-tetanic potentiation on facilitation of transmitter release at the frog neuromuscular junction. *J. Physiol. (Lond.)* 234: 353–371. [13]

Mains, R. E. and P. H. Patterson. (1973). Primary cultures of dissociated sympathetic neurons. I. Establishment of long-term growth in culture and studies of differentiated properties. *J. Cell Biol.* 59: 329–345. [2]

Mallart, A., D. Angaut-Petit, N. F. Zilber-Gachelin, J. Tomás i Ferré and C. Haimann. (1980). Synaptic efficacy and turnover of endings in pauci-innervated muscle fibres of *Xenopus laevis*. In: *Ontogenesis and Functional Mechanisms of Peripheral Synapses, INSERM Symp. 13*, J. Taxi, ed. Amsterdam: Elsevier, pp. 213–223. [13]

Mangold, O. (1929). Experimente zum analyse der Determination und Induktion der Medullarplatte. *Wilhelm Roux Arch. Entwicklungsmech, Org.* 117: 586–696. [3]

Manthorpe, M., S. Skaper, R. Adler, K. Landa and S. Varon. (1980). Cholinergic neuronotrophic factors: Fractionation properties of an extract from selected chick embryonic eye tissues. *J. Neurochem.* 34: 69–75. [7]

Marchase, R. B. (1977). Biochemical investigations of retinotectal adhesive specificity. *J. Cell Biol.* 75: 237–257. [11]

Marchase, R. B., P. Harges and E. R. Jakoi. (1981). Ligatin from embryonic chick neural retina inhibits retinal cell adhesion. *Dev. Biol.* 86: 250–255. [11]

Mariani, J. and J.-P. Changeux. (1980). Multiple innervation of Purkinje cells by climbing fibers in the cerebellum of the adult staggerer mutant mouse. *J. Neurobiol.* 11: 41–50. [12]

Mariani, J. and J.-P. Changeux. (1981). Ontogenesis of olivocerebellar relationships. I. Studies by intracellular recordings of the multiple innervation of Purkinje cells by climbing fibers in the developing rat cerebellum. *J. Neurosci.* 1: 696–702. [12]

Mark, R. F. (1965). Fin movement after regeneration of neuromuscular connections: An investigation of myotypic specificity. *Exp. Neurol.* 12: 292–302. [10]

Mark, R. F. (1974). Selective innervation of muscle. *Br. Med. Bull.* 30: 122–126. [10]

Markelonis, G. J., R. A. Bradshaw, T. H. Oh, J. L. Johnson and J. O. Bates. (1982). Sciatin is a transferrin-like polypeptide. *J. Neurochem.* 39: 315–320. [8]

Markelonis, G. J. and T. H. Oh. (1979). A sciatic nerve protein has a trophic effect on development and maintenance of skeletal muscle cells in culture. *Proc. Natl. Acad. Sci. USA* 76: [8]

Marler, P. (1981). Birdsong: The acquisition of a learned motor skill. *Trends Neurosci.* 4: 88–94. [14]

Marler, P. and S. Peters. (1977). Selective vocal learning in a sparrow. *Science* 198: 519–521. [14]

Marler, P. and M. Tamura. (1964). Culturally transmitted patterns of vocal behavior in sparrows. *Science* 146: 1483–1486. [14]

Marr, D. (1969). A theory of cerebellar cortex. *J. Physiol. (Lond.)* 202: 437–470. [12]

Marshall, L. M., J. R. Sanes and U. J. McMahan. (1977). Reinnervation of original synaptic sites on muscle fiber basement membrane after disruption of the muscle cells. *Proc. Natl. Acad. Sci. USA* 74: 3073–3077. [9]

Marwitt, R., G. Pilar and J. N. Weakly. (1971). Characterization of two ganglion cell populations in avian ciliary ganglia. *Brain Res.* 25: 317–334. [10]

Matsumoto, S. G. and J. G. Hildebrand. (1981). Olfactory mechanisms in the moth *Manduca sexta*: response characteristics and morphology of central neurones in antennal lobes. *Proc. R. Soc. Lond. [Biol.]* 213: 249–277. [14]

Matthews, M. R. and V. H. Nelson. (1975). Detachment of structurally intact nerve endings from chromatolytic neurones of rat superior cervical ganglion during the depression of synaptic transmission induced by postganglionic axotomy. *J. Physiol. (Lond.)* 245: 91–135. [13]

Mathews, M. R. and T. P. S. Powell. (1962). Some observations on transneuronal cell degeneration in the olfactory bulb of the rabbit. *J. Anat. (Lond.)* 96: 89–102. [8]

Matthey, R. (1925). Récupération de la vue après résection des nerfs optiques chez le triton. *C. R. Soc. Biol.* 93: 904–906. [11]

Max, S. R., M. Schwab, M. Dumas and H. Thoenen. (1978). Retrograde axonal transport of nerve growth factor in the ciliary ganglion of the chick and the rat. *Brain Res.* 159: 411–415. [7]

May, R. M. (1925). The relation of nerves to degenerating and regenerating taste buds. *J. Exp. Zool.* 42: 371–410. [8]

McArdle, J. J. (1975). Complex end-plate potentials at the regenerating neuromuscular junction of the rat. *Exp. Neurol.* 49: 629–638. [13]

McGrath, P. A. and M. R. Bennett. (1979). The development of synaptic connections between different segmental motoneurons and striated muscles in an axolotl limb. *Dev. Biol.* 68: 133–145. [5, 6]

McKay, R. D. G., S. Hockfield, J. Johansen, I. Thompson and K. Frederiksen. (1983). Surface molecules identify groups of growing axons. *Science* 222: 788–792. [11]

McLachlan, E. M. (1974). The formation of synapses in mammalian sympathetic ganglia reinnervated with preganglionic or somatic nerves. *J. Physiol. (Lond.)* 237: 217–242. [9]

McLennan, I. S., C. E. Hill and I. A. Hendry. (1980). Glucocorticosteroids modulate transmitter choice in developing superior cervical ganglion. *Nature* 283: 206–207. [2]

McMahan, U. J. and S. W. Kuffler. (1971). Visual identification of synaptic boutons on living ganglion cells and of varicosities in postganglionic axons in the heart of the frog. *Proc. R. Soc. Lond. [Biol.]* 177: 485–508. [8]

McMahan, U. J. and C. R. Slater. (1984). The influence of basal lamina on the accumulation of acetylcholine receptors at synaptic sites in regenerating muscle. *J. Cell Biol.* 98: 1453–1473. [9]

McPherson, A. and J. Tokunaga. (1967). The effects of cross-innervation on the myoglobin concentration of tonic and phasic muscles. *J. Physiol. (Lond.)* 188: 121–129. [8]

Meinertzhagen, I. A. (1973). Development of the compound eye and optic lobe of insects. In: *Developmental Neurobiology of Arthropods*, D. Young, ed. Cambridge: Cambridge University Press, pp. 51–104. [5]

Meinhardt, H. (1978). Space-dependent cell determination under the control of a morphogen gradient. *J. Theoret. Biol.* 74: 307–321. [3]

Meinhardt, H. (1982). *Models of Biological Pattern Formation*. New York: Academic Press. [3]

Mellon, DeF. (1981). Nerves and the transformation of claw type in snapping shrimps. *Trends Neurosci.* 4: 245–248. [8]

Mellon, DeF. and P. J. Stephens. (1978). Limb morphology and function are transformed by contralateral nerve section in snapping shrimps. *Nature* 272: 246–248. [8]

Mendell, L. M. and E. Henneman. (1971). Terminals of single Ia fibers: Location, density, and distribution within a pool of 300 homonymous motoneurons. *J. Neurophysiol.* 34: 171–187. [10]

Mendell, L. M., J. B. Munson and J. G. Scott. (1976). Alterations of synapses on axotomized motoneurones. *J. Physiol. (Lond.)* 255: 67–79. [13]

Menesini-Chen, M. G., J. S. Chen and R. Levi-Montalcini. (1978). Sympathetic nerve fibers ingrowth in the central nervous system of neonatal rodent upon intracerebral NGF injections. *Arch. Ital. Biol.* 116: 53–84. [5,7]

Merrell, R., D. I. Gottlieb and L. Glaser. (1975). Embryonal cell surface recognition: Extraction of an active plasma membrane component. *J. Biol. Chem.* 250: 5655–5659. [11]

Mervis, R. (1978). Structural alterations in neurons of aged canine neocortex: A Golgi study. *Exp. Neurol.* 62: 417–432. [13]

Mesulam, M.-M. (ed.) (1982). *Tracing Neural Connections with Horseradish Peroxidase.* New York: John Wiley & Sons. [5]

Meyer, A. W. (1939). *The Rise of Embryology.* Stanford, CA: Stanford University Press. [1]

Meyer, R. L. (1976). Tests for field regulation in the retinotectal system of goldfish. In: *Developmental Biology, Pattern Formation, Gene Regulation,* D. McMahon and C. F. Fox, eds. Menlo Park, CA: Benjamin, pp. 257–275. [12]

Meyer, R. L. (1978). Evidence from thymidine labeling for continuing growth of retina and tectum in juvenile goldfish. *Exp. Neurol.* 59: 99–111. [11]

Meyer, R. L. (1982). Tetrodotoxin blocks the formation of ocular dominance columns in the goldfish. *Science* 218: 589–591. [12]

Meyer, R. L. and R. W. Sperry. (1976). Retinotectal specificity: Chemoaffinity theory. In: *Neural and Behavioral Specificity. Studies on the Development of Behavior and the Nervous System,* Vol. 3, G. Gottlieb, ed. New York: Academic Press, pp. 111–149. [11,12]

Michler, A. and B. Sakmann. (1980). Receptor stability and channel conversion in the subsynaptic membrane of the developing mammalian neuromuscular junction. *Dev. Biol.* 80: 1–17. [9]

Miledi, R. (1960a). The acetylcholine sensitivity of frog muscle fibres after complete or partial denervation. *J. Physiol. (Lond.)* 151: 1–23. [8]

Miledi, R. (1969b). Junctional and extra-junctional acetylcholine receptors in skeletal muscle fibres. *J. Physiol. (Lond.)* 151: 24–30. [8]

Miledi, R. (1973). Transmitter release induced by injection of calcium ions into nerve terminals. *Proc. R. Soc. Lond. [Biol.]* 183: 421–425. [13]

Miledi, R. and N. C. Spitzer. (1974). Absence of action potentials in frog slow muscle fibres paralysed by botulinum toxin. *J. Physiol. (Lond.)* 241: 183–199. [8]

Miledi, R. and E. Stefani. (1969). Non-selective reinnervation of slow and fast muscle fibres in the rat. *Nature* 222: 569–571. [10]

Miles, F. A. and S. G. Lisberger. (1982). Plasticity in the vestibulo-ocular reflex: A new hypothesis. *Annu. Rev. Neurosci.* 4: 273–299. [13]

Milstein, C. (1980). Monoclonal antibodies. *Sci. Am.* 243 (4): 66–74. [11]

Mintz, B. and K. Illmensee. (1975). Normal genetically mosaic mice produced from malignant teratocarcinoma cells. *Proc. Natl. Acad. Sci. USA* 72: 3585–3589. [2]

Mitchison, G. J., M. Wilcox and R. J. Smith. (1976). Measurement of an inhibitory zone. *Science* 191: 866–868. [3]

Miyata, Y. and K. Yoshioka. (1980). Selective elimination of motor nerve terminals in the rat soleus muscle during development. *J. Physiol. (Lond.)* 309: 631–646. [12]

Mobley, W. C., A. C. Server, D. N. Ishii, R. J. Riopelle and E. M. Shooter. (1977). Nerve growth factor (Parts I, II, and III). *N. Engl. J. Med.* 297: 1096–1104; 1149–1158; 1211–1218. [7]

Molliver, M. E. and H. Van der Loos. (1970). The ontogenesis of cortical circuitry: The spatial distribution of synapses in somesthetic cortex of newborn dog. *Ergeb. Anat. Entwicklungsgesch* 42: 1–54. [9]

Moody-Corbett, F. and M. W. Cohen. (1981). Localization of cholinesterase at sites of high acetylcholine receptor density on embryonic amphibian muscle cells cultured without nerve. *J. Neurosci.* 1: 596–605. [9]

Moody-Corbett, F. and M. W. Cohen. (1982). Influence of nerve on the formation and survival of acetylcholine receptor and cholinesterase patches on embryonic Xenopus muscle cells in culture. *J. Neurosci.* 2: 633-646. [9]

Moody-Corbett, F., P. R. Weldon and M. W. Cohen. (1982). Cholinesterase localization at sites of nerve contact on embryonic amphibian muscle cells in culture. *J. Neurocytol.* 11: 381–394. [9]

Morata, G. and P. A. Lawrence. (1975). Control of compartment development by the *engrailed* gene in Drosophila. *Nature* 255: 614–617. [3]

Morata, G. and P. A. Lawrence. (1977). Homeotic genes, compartments and cell determination in Drosophila. *Nature* 265: 211–216. [3]

Morgan, T. H. (1927). *Experimental Embryology.* New York: Columbia University Press. [1]

Moscona, A. A. (1962). Analysis of cell recombinations in experimental synthesis of tissues *in vitro. J. Cell. Comp. Physiol.* 60(Suppl): 65–79. [4]

Moscona, A. A. (1963). Studies on cell aggregation: Demonstration of materials with selective cell-binding activity. *Proc. Natl. Acad. Sci. USA* 49: 742–747. [4]

Moscona, A. A. and H. Moscona. (1952). The disassociation and aggregation of cells from organ rudiments of the early chick embryo. *J. Anat.* 86: 287–301. [4]

Motorina, M. V., Z. A. Tamarova, A. I. Shapovalov and B. I. Shiryaev. (1982). Investigation of synaptic connections between primary efferents and motoneurons in the frog spinal cord by intracellular injection of horseradish peroxidase. *Neurophysiology (Transl. of Neirofiziologiya)* 14: 48–560. [12]

Mountcastle, V. B. (1957). Modality and topographic properties of single neurons of cat's somatic sensory cortex. *J. Neurophysiol.* 20: 408–434. [12, 14]

Muller, K. J. (1979). Synapses between neurones in the central nervous system of the leech. *Biol. Rev.* 54: 99–134. [10]

Muller, K. J., J. G. Nicholls and G. S. Stent (1981). *Neurobiology of the Leech.* Cold Spring Harbor, NY: Cold Spring Harbor Laboratory. [10]

Murphy, R. A., J. D. Saide, M. H. Blanchard and M. Young. (1977). Nerve growth factor in mouse serum and saliva: Role of the submandibular gland. *Proc. Natl. Acad. Sci. USA* 74: 2330–2333. [7]

Murphy, R. A., R. H. Singer, J. D. Saide, N. J. Pantazis, M. H. Blanchard, K. S. Byron and B. G. W. Arnason. (1977). Synthesis and secretion of a high-molecular-weight form of nerve growth factor by skeletal muscle cells in culture. *Proc. Natl. Acad. Sci USA* 74: 4496–4500. [7]

Murray, J. G. and J. W. Thompson. (1957). The occurrence and function of collateral sprouting in the sympathetic nervous system of the cat. *J. Physiol. (Lond.)* 135: 133–162. [13]

Naef, A. (1926). Über die Urformen der Anthropomorphen und die Stammesgaschichte des Menschenschädels. *Naturwiss.* 14: 445–452. [1]

Nakamura, O. S. Toivonen. (1978). *Organizer. A Milestone of a Half-Century from Spemann.* Amsterdam: Elsevier. [3]

Narayanan, C. H. and V. Hamburger. (1971). Motility in chick embryos with substitution of lumbrosacral by brachial and brachial by lumbrosacral spinal cord segments. *J. Exp. Zool.* 178: 415–432. [14]

Narayanan, Y. and C. H. Narayanan. (1981). Ultrastructural and histochemical observations in the developing iris musculature in the chick. *J. Embryol. Exp. Morphol.* 62: 117–127. [6]

Nardi, J. B. (1983). Neuronal pathfinding in developing wings of the moth *Manduca sexta. Dev. Biol.* 95: 163–174. [5]

Nardi, J. B. and F. C. Kafatos. (1976). Polarity and gradients in lepidopteran wing epidermis. II. The differential adhesiveness model: Gradient of a nondiffusible cell surface parameter. *J. Embryol. Exp. Morphol.* 36: 489–512. [5]

Needham, A. E. (1952). *Regeneration and Wound-healing.* New York: John Wiley & Sons. [8]

Needham, J. (1959). *A History of Embryology.* 2nd Ed. Cambridge: Cambridge University Press. [1]

Needham, J., C. H. Waddington and D. M. Needham. (1934). Physico-chemical experiments on the amphibian organizer. *Proc. R. Soc. Lond. (Biol.)* 114: 393–422. [3]

Nelson, S. G. and L. M. Mendell. (1978). Projection of single knee flexor Ia fibers to homonymous and heteronymous motoneurons. *J. Neurophysiol.* 41: 778–787. [10]

Nestler, E. J. and P. Greengard. (1983). Protein phosphorylation in the brain. *Nature* 305: 583–589. [13]

Newgreen, D. F., I. L. Gibbins, J. Sauter, B. Wallenfels and R. Wütz. (1982). Ultrastructural and tissue-culture studies on the role of fibronectin, collagen, and glycos-

aminoglycans in the migration of neural crest cells in the fowl embryo. *Cell Tissue Res.* 221: 521–549. [4]

Newgreen, D. F. and J.-P. Thiery. (1980). Fibronectin in early avian embryos: Synthesis and distribution along the migration pathways of neural crest cells. *Cell Tissue Res.* 211: 269–291. [4]

Nijhout, H. F. (1978). Wing pattern formation in Lepidoptera: A Model. *J. Exp. Zool.* 206: 119–136. [3]

Nijhout, H. F. (1980a). Ontogeny of the color pattern on the wings of *Precis coenia* (Lepidoptera: Nymphalidae). *Dev. Biol.* 80: 275-288. [3]

Nijhout, H. F. (1980b). Pattern formation on lepidopteran wings: Determination of an eyespot. *Dev. Biol.* 80: 267–274. [3]

Nijhout, H. F. (1981). The color patterns of butterflies and moths. *Sci. Am.* 245(5): 140–151. [3]

Nisbett, A. (1976). *Konrad Lorenz.* London: J. M. Dent and Sons, Ltd. [14]

Nishi, R. and D. K. Berg. (1977). Dissociated ciliary ganglion neurons *in vitro*: Survival and synapse formation. *Proc. Natl. Acad. Sci. USA* 74: 5171–5175. [7]

Nishi, R. and D. K. Berg. (1979). Survival and development of ciliary ganglion neurones grown alone in cell culture. *Nature* 277: 232–234. [7]

Nishi, R. and D. K. Berg. (1981). Two components from eye tissue that differentially stimulate the growth and development of ciliary ganglion neurons in cell culture. *J. Neurosci.* 1: 505–513. [7]

Nishi, S., H. Soeda and K. Koketsu. (1965). Studies on sympathetic B and C neurons and patterns of preganglionic innervation. *J. Cell. Comp. Physiol.* 66: 19–32. [10]

Niu, M. C. (1958). The role of ribonucleic acid in embryonic differentiation. *Anat. Rec.* 131: 43. [3]

Njå, A. and D. Purves. (1977a). Specific innervation of guinea-pig superior cervical ganglion cells by preganglionic fibres arising from different levels of the spinal cord. *J. Physiol. (Lond.)* 264: 565–583. [10, 12]

Njå, A. and D. Purves. (1977b). Re-innervation of guinea-pig superior cervical ganglion cells by preganglionic fibres arising from different levels of the spinal cord. *J. Physiol. (Lond.)* 272: 633-651. [10]

Njå, A. and D. Purves. (1978a). The effects of nerve growth factor and its antiserum on synapses in the superior cervical ganglion of the guinea-pig. *J. Physiol. (Lond.)* 277: 53–75. [13]

Njå, A. and D. Purves. (1978b). Specificity of initial synaptic contacts made on guinea-pig superior cervical ganglion cells during regeneration of the cervical sympathetic trunk. *J. Physiol. (Lond.)* 281: 45–62. [10]

Noden, D. M. (1975). Analysis of migratory behavior of avian cephalic neural crest cells. *Dev. Biol.* 42: 106–130. [4]

Nornes, H. O. and G. D. Das. (1974). Temporal pattern of neurogenesis in spinal cord of rat. I. An autoradiographic study—time and sites of origin and migration and settling patterns of neuroblasts. *Brain Res.* 73: 121–138. [1]

Nottebohm, F. (1970). Ontogeny of birdsong. *Science* 167: 950–956. [14]

Nottebohm, F. (1971). Neural lateralization of vocal control in a passerine bird. I. Song. *J. Exp. Zool.* 177: 229–261. [14]

Nottebohm, F. (1977). Asymmetries in neural control of vocalization in the canary. In: *Lateralization in the Nervous System*, S. R. Harnad et al., eds. New York: Academic Press, pp. 23–44. [14]

Nottebohm, F. (1980a). Brain pathways for vocal learning in birds: A review of the first 10 years. In: *Progress in Psychobiology and Physiological Psychology*, Vol. 9, J. M. S. Sprague and A. N. E. Epstein, eds. New York: Academic Press, pp. 85–124. [14]

Nottebohm, F. (1980b). Testosterone triggers growth of brain vocal control nuclei in adult female canaries. *Brain Res.* 189: 429–436. [14]

Nottebohm, F. (1981). A brain for all seasons: Cyclical anatomical changes in song control nuclei of the canary brain. *Science* 214: 1368–1370. [14]

Nottebohm, F. and A. P. Arnold. (1976). Sexual dimorphism in vocal control areas of the songbird brain. *Science* 194: 211–213. [14]

Nottebohm, F., S. Kasparian and C. Pandazis. (1981). Brain space for a learned task. *Brain Res.* 213: 99–109. [14]

Nottebohm, F., E. Manning and M. Nottebohm. (1979). Reversal of hypoglossal dominance in canaries following unilateral syringeal denervation. *J. Comp. Physiol.* 134: 227–240. [14]

Nottebohm, F. and M. E. Nottebohm. (1978). Relationship between song repertoire and age in the canary, *Serinus canarius*. *Z. Tierpsychol.* 46: 298–305. [14]

Nottebohm, F., T. M. Stokes and C. M. Leonard. (1976). Central control of song in the canary, *Serinus canarius*. *J. Comp. Neurol.* 165: 457–486. [14]

Nudell, B. M. and A. D. Grinnell. (1982). Inverse relationship between transmitter release and terminal length in synapses on frog muscle fibers of uniform input resistance. *J. Neurosci.* 2: 216–224.

Nudell, B. M. and A. D. Grinnell. (1983). Regulation of synaptic position, size, and strength in anuran skeletal muscle. *J. Neurosci.* 3: 161–176. [12]

Nurcombe, V. and M. R. Bennett. (1981). Embryonic chick retinal ganglion cells identified *in vitro*. Their survival is dependent on a factor from the optic tectum. *Exp. Brain Res.* 44: 249–254. [7]

Nurcombe, V., P. A. McGrath and M. R. Bennett. (1981). Postnatal death of motor neurons during the development of the brachial spinal cord of the rat. *Neurosci. Lett.* 27: 249–254. [12]

Nusslein-Volhard, C. and E. Wieschaus. (1980). Mutations affecting segment number and polarity in *Drosophila*. *Nature* 287: 795–801. [3]

Nyström, B. (1968a). Histochemical studies of endplate bound esterases in "slow- red" and "fast-white" cat muscles during postnatal development. *Acta Neurol. Scand.* 44: 295–318. [9]

Nyström, B. (1968b). Postnatal development of motor nerve terminals in "slow-red" and "fast-white" cat muscles. *Acta Neurol. Scand.* 44: 363-383. [12]

Oakley, B. (1974). On the specification of taste neurons in the rat tongue. *Brain Res.* 75: 85–96. [8]

O'Brien, R. A. D., A. J. C. Ostberg and G. Vrbová. (1978). Observations on the elimination of polyneuronal innervation in developing mammalian skeletal muscle. *J. Physiol. (Lond.)* 282: 571–582. [12]

Oger, J., B. G. W. Arnason, N. Pantazis, J. Lehrich and M. Young. (1974). Synthesis of nerve growth factor by L and 3T3 cells in culture. *Proc. Natl. Acad. Sci. USA* 71: 1554–1558. [7]

Oh, T. H. and G. J. Markelonis. (1978). Neurotrophic protein regulates muscle acetylcholinesterase in culture. *Science* 200: 337–339. [8]

Oh, T. H. and G. J. Markelonis. (1980). Dependence of *in vitro* myogenesis on a trophic protein present in chick embryo extract. *Proc. Natl. Acad. Sci. USA* 77: 6922–6955. [8]

Oh, T. H. and G. J. Markelonis. (1982). Chicken serum transferrin duplicates the myotrophic effects of sciatin on cultured muscle cells. *J. Neurosci. Res.* 8: 535–545. [8]

Oh, T. H., C. A. Sofia, Y. C. Kim, C. Carroll, H. H. Kim, G. J. Markelonis and P. J. Reier. (1981). Sciatin. Immunocytochemical localization of a myotrophic protein in chicken neural tissues. *J. Histochem. Cytochem.* 29: 1205–1212. [8]

Okado, N. and R. W. Oppenheim. (1984). Cell death of motoneurons in the chick embryo spinal cord. IX. The loss of motoneurons following removal of afferent inputs. *J. Neurosci.* 4: 1639–1652. [6]

O'Lague, P. H., K. Obata, P. Claude, E. J. Furshpan and D. D. Potter. (1974). Evidence for cholinergic synapses between dissociated rat sympathetic neurons in cell culture. *Proc. Natl. Acad. Sci. USA* 71: 3602–3606. [9]

O'Leary, D. D. M. and W. M. Cowan. (1982). Further studies on the development of the isthmo-optic nucleus with special reference to the occurrence and fate of ectopic and ipsilaterally projecting neurons. *J. Comp. Neurol.* 212: 399–416. [6]

O'Leary, D. D. M. and W. M. Cowan. (1984). Survival of isthmo-optic neurons after early removal of one eye. *Dev. Brain Res.* 12: 293–310. [6]

O'Leary, D. D. M., J. W. Fawcett and W. M. Cowan. (1983). The early postnatal restriction of the ipsilateral retino-collicular projection is due to cell death rather than collateral elimination. *Soc. Neurosci. Abs. 9: 856.* [12]

O'Leary, D. D. M., C. R. Gerfen and W. M. Cowan. (1983). The development and restriction of the ipsilateral retinofugal projection in the chick. *Dev. Brain Res.* 10: 93–109. [12]

O'Leary, D. D. M., B. B. Stanfield and W. M. Cowan. (1981). Evidence that the early postnatal restriction of the cells or origin of the callosal projection is due to the elimination of axonal collaterals rather than to the death of neurons. *Dev. Brain Res.* 1: 607–617. [12]

Olek, A. J. (1980). Effects of α- and β-bungarotoxin on motor neuron loss in *Xenopus* larvae. *Neuroscience* 5: 1557–1563. [6]

Olmsted, J. M. D. (1920a). The nerve as a formative influence in the development of taste-buds. *J. Comp. Neurol.* 31: 465–468. [8]

Olmsted, J. M. D. (1920b). The results of cutting the seventh cranial nerve in *Amiurus nebulosus* (Lesueur). *J. Exp. Zool. 31*: 369–402. [8]

Olson, L. and T. Malmfors. (1970). Growth characteristics of adrenergic nerves in the adult rat. Fluorescence, histochemical, and ³H-noradrenaline uptake studies using tissue transplanted to the anterior chamber of the eye. *Acta Physiol. Scand. 348(Suppl.)*: 1–111. [7, 13]

Oppenheimer, J. M. (1967). *Essays in the History of Embryology.* Cambridge, MA: MIT Press. [1]

Oppenheim, R. W. (1981a). Neuronal cell death and some related regressive phenomena during neurogenesis: A selective historical review and a progress report. In: *Studies in Developmental Neurobiology. Essays in Honor of Viktor Hamburger,* W. M. Cowan, ed. New York: Oxford University Press, pp. 74–133. [6]

Oppenheim, R. W. (1981b). Cell death of motoneurons in the chick embryo spinal cord. V. Evidence on the role of cell death and neuromuscular function in the formation of specific peripheral connections. *J. Neurosci. 1*: 141–151. [6]

Oppenheim, R. W. (1982). The neuroembryological study of behavior: Progress, problems, perspectives. *Curr. Top. Dev. Biol. 17*: 257–309. [14]

Oppenheim, R. W. (1984). Cell death of motoneurons in the chick embryo spinal cord. VIII. Motoneurons prevented from dying in the embryo persist after hatching. *Dev. Biol. 101*: 35–39. [5]

Oppenheim, R. W. and I.-W. Chu-Wang. (1983). Aspects of naturally-occurring motoneuron death in the chick spinal cord during embryonic development. In: *Somatic and Autonomic Nerve–Muscle Interactions,* G. Burnstock and G. Vrbová eds. Amsterdam: Elsevier, pp. 57–107. [9]

Oppenheim, R. W., I.-W. Chu-Wang and J. L. Maderdrut. (1978). Cell death of motoneurons in the chick embryo spinal cord. III. The differentiation of motoneurons prior to their induced degeneration following limb-bud removal. *J. Comp. Neurol. 177*: 87–111. [6]

Oppenheim, R. W., J. L. Maderdrut and D. J. Wells. (1982). Cell death of motoneurons in the chick embryo spinal cord. VI. Reduction of naturally occurring cell death in the thoracolumbar column of Terni by nerve growth factor. *J. Comp. Neurol. 210*: 174–189. [6]

Oppenheim, R. W. and C. Majors-Willard. (1978). Neuronal cell death in the brachial spinal cord of the chick is unrelated to the loss of polyneuronal innervation in wing muscle. *Brain Res. 154*: 148–152. [12]

Oppenheim, R. W. and R. Núñez. (1982). Electrical stimulation of hindlimb increases neuronal cell death in chick embryo. *Nature 295*: 57–59. [6]

Oppenheimer, J. M. (1967). *Essays in the History of Embryology.* Cambridge, MA: MIT Press. [1]

Ostberg, A.-J. C., G. Raisman, P. M. Field, L. L. Iversen and R. E. Zigmond. (1976). A quantitative comparison of the formation of synapses in the rat superior cervical sympathetic ganglion by its own and by foreign nerve fibres. *Brain Res. 107*: 445–470. [9]

Otten, U., M. Schwab, C. Gagnon and H. Thoenen. (1977). Selective induction of tyrosine hydroxylase and dopamine β-hydroxylase by nerve growth factor: Comparison between adrenal medulla and sympathetic ganglia of adult and newborn rats. *Brain Res. 133*: 291–303. [7]

Owman, C. (1981). Pregnancy induces degenerative and regenerative changes in the autonomic innervation of the female reproductive tract. In: *Development of the Autonomic Nervous System, CIBA Found. Symp. 83,* K. Elliott and G. Lawrenson, eds. London: Pittman Books Ltd., pp. 252-279. [13]

Packman, S., H. Avin, J. Ross and P. Leder. (1972). Comparison of globin genes in duck reticulocytes and liver cells. *Biochem. Biophys. Res. Commun. 49*: 813–819. [2]

Palay, S. L. and V. Chan-Palay. (1975). A guide to the synaptic analysis of the neuropil. *Cold Spring Harbor Symp. Quant. Biol. 40*: 1–16. [9]

Palka, J. (1982). Genetic manipulation of sensory pathways in *Drosophila.* In: *Neuronal Development,* N. C. Spitzer, ed. New York: Plenum Press, pp. 121–170. [3]

Palka, J., M. Schubiger and R. L. Ellison. (1983). The polarity of axon growth in the wings of *Drosophila melanogaster. Dev. Bio. 98*: 481–492. [3]

Palmatier, M. A., B. K. Hartman and E. M. Johnson. (1984). Demonstration of retrogradely transported endogenous nerve growth factor in axons of sympathetic neurons. *J. Neurosci. 4*: 751–756. [7]

Parker, G. H. (1932). On the trophic impulse so-called, its rate and nature. *Am. Nat. 66*: 147–158. [8]

Parks, T. N. (1979). Afferent influences on the development of the brainstem auditory nuclei of the chicken: Otocyst ablation. *J. Comp. Neurol. 183*: 665–678. [6]

Patel, N. B. and M.-M. Poo. (1982). Orientation of neurite growth by extracellular electric fields. *J. Neurosci. 2*: 483–496. [5]

Patel, N. B. and M.-M. Poo. Perturbation of the direction of neurite growth by pulsed and focal electric fields. *J. Neurosci.* (in press). [5]

Patterson, P. H. (1978). Environmental determination of autonomic neurotransmitter functions. *Annu. Rev. Neurosci. 1*: 1–17. [2]

Patterson, P. H. and L. L. Y. Chun. (1974). The influence of non-neuronal cells on catecholamine and acetylcholine synthesis and accumulation in cultures of dissociated sympathetic neurons. *Proc. Natl. Acad. Sci. USA 71*: 3607–3610. [2]

Patterson, P. H. and L. L. Y. Chun. (1977). The induction of acetylcholine synthesis in primary cultures of dissociated rat sympathetic neurons. I. Effects of conditioned medium. *Dev. Biol. 56*: 263–280. [2]

Pearlman, A. L. (1985). The visual cortex of the normal mouse and the reeler mutant. In: *The Cerebral Cortex,* E. G. Jones and A. A. Peters, eds. New York: Plenum Press (in press). [6]

Pearson, J. (1979). Familial dysautonomia (a brief review). *J. Auton. Nerv. Syst. 1*: 119–126. [7]

Pearson, J., E. M. Johnson and L. Brandeis. (1983). Effects of antibodies to nerve growth factor on intrauterine development of derivatives of cranial neural crest and placode in the guinea pig. *Dev. Biol. 96*: 32–36. [7]

Pearson, K. G. and A. B. Bradley. (1972). Specific regeneration of excitatory motoneurons in two leg muscles in the cockroach. *Brain Res. 47*: 492–496. [10]

Peng, H. B. and P.-C. Cheng. (1982). Formation of postsynaptic specializations induced by latex beads in cultured muscle cells. *J. Neurosci. 2*: 1760–1774. [9]

Pestronk, A., D. B. Drachman and J. W. Griffin. (1980). Effects of aging on nerve sprouting and regeneration. *Exp. Neurol. 70*: 65–82. [13]

Peters, A. and D. W. Vaughan. (1981). Central nervous system. In: *Aging and Cell Structure*, Vol. 1, J. E. Johnson, ed. New York: Plenum Press, pp. 1–34. [13]

Pette, D., W. Müller, E. Leisner and G. Vrbová. (1976). Time dependent effects on contractile properties, fibre population, myosin light chains and enzymes of energy metabolism in intermittently and continuously stimulated fast-twitch muscles of the rabbit. *Pflügers Arch. 364*: 103–112. [8]

Pettigrew, A. G., B. Lindeman and M. R. Bennett. (1979). Development of the segmental innervation of the chick forelimb. *J. Embryol. Exp. Morphol. 49*: 115–137. [5, 6]

Pettigrew, J. D. and R. D. Freeman. (1973). Visual experience without lines: Effect on developing cortical neurons. *Science 182*: 599–601. [14]

Pettigrew, J. D. and L. J. Garey. (1974). Selective modification of single neuron properties in the visual cortex of kittens. *Brain Res. 66*: 160–164. [14]

Pfenninger, K. H. and R. P. Rees. (1976). From the growth cone to the synapse. Properties of membranes involved in synapse formation. In: *Neuronal Recognition*, S. H. Barondes, ed. New York: Plenum Press, pp. 131–178. [9]

Piatt, J. (1942). Transplantation of aneurogenic forelimbs in *Amblystoma punctatum*. *J. Exp. Zool. 91*: 79–101. [8]

Piatt, J. (1946). The influence of the peripheral field on the development of the mesencephalic V nucleus in *Amblystoma*. *J. Exp. Zool. 102*: 109–141. [6]

Piatt, J. (1956). Studies on the problem of nerve pattern. I. Transplantation of the forelimb primordium to ectopic sites in *Amblystoma*. *J. Exp. Zool. 131*: 173–202. [5]

Pilar, G. and L. Landmesser. (1972). Axotomy mimicked by localized colchicine application. *Science 177*: 1116–1118. [13]

Pilar, G. and L. Landmesser. (1976). Ultrastructural differences during embryonic cell death in normal and peripherally deprived ciliary ganglia. *J. Cell Biol. 68*: 339–356. [6]

Pilar, G., L. Landmesser and L. Burstein. (1980). Competition for survival among developing ciliary ganglion cells. *J. Neurophysiol. 43*: 233–254. [6]

Pinsker, H., I. Kupfermann, V. Castellucci and E. R. Kandel. (1970). Habituation and dishabituation of the gill-withdrawal reflex in *Aplysia*. *Science 167*: 1740–1742. [13]

Pintar, J. E. (1978). Distribution and synthesis of glycosaminoglycans during quail neural crest morphogenesis. *Dev. Biol. 67*: 444-464. [4]

Pittman, R. and R. W. Oppenheim. (1979). Cell death of motoneurons in the chick embryo spinal cord. IV. Evidence that a functional neuromuscular interaction is involved in the regulation of naturally occurring cell death and the stabilization of synapses. *J. Comp. Neurol. 187*: 425–446. [6]

Pockett, S. (1981). Elimination of polyneuronal innervation in proximal and distal leg muscles of chick embryos. *Dev. Brain Res. 1*: 299–302. [12]

Podleski, T. R., D. Axelrod, P. Ravdin, I. Greenberg, M. M. Johnson and M. M. Saltpeter. (1979). Nerve extract induces increase and redistribution of acetylcholine receptors on cloned muscle cells. *Proc. Natl. Acad. Sci. USA 75*: 2035–2039. [9]

Poo, M.-M. (1981). *In situ* electrophoresis of membrane components. *Annu. Rev. Biophys. Bioeng. 10*: 245–276. [5]

Poole, T. J. and M. S. Steinberg. (1982). Evidence for the guidance of pronephric duct migration by a craniocaudally traveling adhesion gradient. *Dev. Biol. 92*: 144–158. [4]

Postlethwait, J. H. and H. A. Schneiderman. (1971). Pattern formation and determination in the antenna of the homoeotic mutant *Antennapedia* of *Drosophila melanogaster*. *Dev. Biol. 25*: 606–640. [3]

Potter, D. D., S. C. Landis and E. J. Furshpan. (1980). Dual function during development of rat sympathetic neurones in culture. *J. Exp. Biol. 89*: 57–71. [2]

Potter, D. D., S. C. Landis and E. J. Furshpan. (1981). Adrenergic–cholinergic dual function in cultured sympathetic neurones of the rat. In: *Development of the Autonomic Nervous System, Ciba Found. Symp. 83*, K. Elliott and G. Lawrenson, eds. London: Pitman Books, pp. 123–138. [2]

Powell, T. P. S. and S. D. Erulkar. (1962). Transneuronal cell degeneration in the auditory relay nuclei of the cat. *J. Anat. 91*: 249–268. [8]

Pratt, R. M., M. A. Larsen and M. C. Johnston. (1975). Migration of cranial neural crest cells in a cell-free hyaluronate-rich matrix. *Dev. Biol. 44*: 298–305. [4]

Prestige, M. C. (1967a). The control of cell number in the lumbar ventral horns during the development of *Xenopus laevis* tadpoles. *J. Embryol. Exp. Morphol. 18*: 359–387. [6]

Prestige, M. C. (1967b). The control of cell number in the lumbar spinal ganglia during the development of *Xenopus laevis* tadpoles. *J. Embryol. Exp. Morphol. 17*: 453–471. [6]

Prestige, M. C. and M. A. Wilson. (1974). A quantitative study of the growth and development of the ventral root in normal and experimental conditions. *J. Embryol. Exp. Morphol. 32*: 819–833. [6]

Preyer, W. (1885). *Die Specielle Physiologie des Embryo*. Leipzig: Grieben's Verlag. [14]

Proctor, W., S. Roper and B. Taylor. (1982). Somatic motor axons can innervate autonomic neurones in the frog heart. *J. Physiol. (Lond.) 326*: 173–188. [9]

Provine, R. R. (1973). Neurophysiological aspects of behavior development in the chick embryo. In: *Studies on the Development of Behavior and the Nervous System*, Vol. I,

G. Gottlieb, ed. New York: Academic Press, pp. 77–102. [14]

Pumplin, D. W. (1983). Normal variations in presynaptic active zones of frog neuromuscular junctions. *J. Neurocytol.* 12: 317–323. [13]

Purves, D. (1975). Functional and structural changes in mammalian neurones following interruption of their axons. *J. Physiol. (Lond.)* 252: 429–463. [12, 13]

Purves, D. (1976a). Competitive and non-competitive reinnervation of mammalian sympathetic neurones by native and foreign fibers. *J. Physiol. (Lond.)* 261: 453–475. [9]

Purves, D. (1976b). Functional and structural changes in mammalian sympathetic neurones following colchicine application to post-ganglionic nerves. *J. Physiol. (Lond.)* 259: 159–175. [13]

Purves, D. (1976c). Long-term regulation in the vertebrate peripheral nervous system. In: *International Review of Physiology, Nerophysiology II*, Vol. 10, R. Porter, ed. Baltimore: University Park Press, pp. 125–177. [8]

Purves, D. (1977). The formation and maintenance of synaptic connections. In: *Function and Formation of Neural Systems*, G. S. Stent, ed. Berlin: Dahlem Konferenzen, pp. 21–49. [12, 13]

Purves, D. (1980). Neuronal competition. *Nature* 287: 585-586. [6]

Purves, D. (1983). Modulation of neuronal competition by postsynaptic geometry in autonomic ganglia. *Trends Neurosci.* 6: 10–16. [12]

Purves, D. and R. I. Hume. (1981). The relation of postsynaptic geometry to the number of presynaptic axons that innervate autonomic ganglion cells. *J. Neurosci.* 1: 441–452. [5, 12]

Purves, D. and J. W. Lichtman. (1978). The formation and maintenance of synaptic connections in autonomic ganglia. *Physiol. Rev.* 58: 821–862. [12]

Purves, D. and J. W. Lichtman. (1980). Elimination of synapses in the developing nervous system. *Science* 210: 153–157. [12]

Purves, D. and J. W. Lichtman. (1983). The relationship of convergence and postsynaptic geometry in mammalian sympathetic ganglia. *Soc. Neurosci. Abst.:* 320. [12]

Purves, D. and A. Njå. (1978). Trophic maintenance of synaptic connections in autonomic ganglia. In: *Neuronal Plasticity*, C. W. Cotman, ed. New York: Raven Press, pp. 27-47. [12, 13]

Purves, D. and B. Sakmann. (1974). The effect of contractile activity on fibrillation and extrajunctional acetylcholine-sensitivity in rat muscle maintained in organ culture. *J. Physiol. (Lond.)* 237: 157–182. [8]

Purves, D. and W. Thompson. (1979). The effects of post-ganglionic axotomy on selective synaptic connexions in the superior cervical ganglion of the guinea-pig. *J. Physiol. (Lond.)* 297: 95–110. [10]

Purves, D., W. Thompson and J. W. Yip. (1981). Reinnervation of ganglia transplanted to the neck from different levels of the guinea-pig sympathetic chain. *J. Physiol. (Lond.)* 313: 49–63. [10]

Purves, D. and D. J. Wigston. (1983). Neural units in the superior cervical ganglion of the guinea-pig. *J. Physiol. (Lond.)* 334: 169–178. [10]

Radice, G. P. (1980). The spreading of epithelial cells during wound closure in *Xenopus* larvae. *Dev. Biol.* 76: 26–46. [4]

Raff, M. C., R. H. Miller and M. Noble. (1983). A glial progenitor that develops *in vitro* into an astrocyte or an oligodendrocyte depending on culture medium. *Nature* 303: 390–396. [2]

Raff, M. C., R. Mirsky, K. L. Fields, R. P. Lisak, S. H. Dorfman, D. H. Silberberg, N. A. Gregson, S. Leibowitz and M. C. Kennedy. (1978). Galactocerebroside is a specific cell-surface antigenic marker for oligodendrocytes in culture. *Nature* 274: 813–816. [2]

Rager, G. (1980). Development of the retino-tectal projection in the chicken. *Adv. Anat. Embryol. Cell Biol.* 63: 1–92. [6]

Rahamimoff, R., A. Lev-Tov and H. Meiri. (1980). Primary and secondary regulation of quantal transmitter release: Calcium and sodium. *J. Exp. Biol.* 89: 5–18. [13]

Raisman, G. (1969). Neuronal plasticity in the septal nuclei of the adult rat. *Brain Res.* 14: 25–48. [13]

Raisman, G. and P. M. Field. (1973). A quantitative investigation of the development of collateral reinnervation after partial deafferentiation of the septal nuclei. *Brain Res.* 50: 241–264. [13]

Raisman, G., P. M. Field, A. J. C. Ostberg, L. L. Iverson and R. E. Zigmond. (1974). A quantitative ultrastructural and biochemical analysis of the process of reinnervation of the superior cervical ganglion in the adult rat. *Brain Res.* 71: 1–16. [9]

Rakic, P. (1971a). Guidance of neurons migrating to the fetal monkey neocortex. *Brain Res.* 33: 471–476. [4]

Rakic, P. (1971b). Neuron–glia relationship during granule cell migration in developing cerebellar cortex. A Golgi and electromicroscopic study in *Macacus rhesus*. *J. Comp. Neurol.* 141: 283–312. [4]

Rakic, P. (1972). Mode of cell migration to the superficial layers of fetal monkey neocortex. *J. Comp. Neurol.* 145: 61–84. [4]

Rakic, P. (1974). Neurons in rhesus monkey visual cortex: Systematic relation between time of origin and eventual disposition. *Science* 183: 425–427. [1, 4]

Rakic, P. (1975). Synaptic specificity in the cerebellar cortex: Study of anomalous circuits induced by single gene mutations in mice. *Cold Spring Harbor Symp. Quant. Biol.* 40: 333–346. [9]

Rakic, P. (1976). Prenatal genesis of connections subserving ocular dominance in the rhesus monkey. *Nature* 261 : 467–471. [12]

Rakic, P. (1977). Prenatal development of the visual system in rhesus monkey. *Philos. Trans. R. Soc. Lond. [Biol.]* 278: 245–260. [12,14]

Rakic, P. (1978). Neuronal migration and contact guidance in the primate telencephalon. *Postgrad. Med. J.* 54: 25–37. [4]

Rakic, P. (1981a). Development of visual centers in the primate brain depends on binocular competition before birth. *Science* 214: 928–931. [12, 14]

Rakic, P. (1981b). Neuronal–glial interaction during brain development. *Trends Neurosci.* 4: 184–187. [2]

Rakic, P. and K. P. Riley. (1983). Overproduction and elimination of retinal axons in fetal rhesus monkey. *Science* 219: 1441–1444. [6]

Rakic, P. and R. L. Sidman. (1973a). Weaver mutant mouse cerebellum: Defective neuronal migration secondary to specific abnormality of Bergmann glia. *Proc. Natl. Acad. Sci. USA* 70: 240–244. [4]

Rakic, P. and R. L. Sidman. (1973b). Sequence of developmental abnormalities leading to granule cell deficit in cerebellar cortex of weaver mutant mice. *J. Comp. Neurol.* 152: 103–132. [4]

Rakic, P., L. J. Stensaas, E. P. Sayre and R. L. Sidman. (1974). Computer-aided three-dimensional reconstruction and quantitative analysis of cells from serial electron microscopic montages of foetal monkey brain. *Nature* 250: 31–34. [4]

Ramirez, B. and J. V. Luco. (1973). Some physiological and biochemical features of striated muscles reinnervated by preganglionic sympathetic fibers. *J. Neurobiol.* 4: 525–533. [9]

Ramón y Cajal, S. (1890). Sur l'origine et les ramifications des fibres nerveuses de la moelle embryonaire. *Anat. Ang.* 5: 609–613. [4]

Ramón y Cajal, S. (1892). *The Structure of the Retina.* Transl. 1972. Springfield, IL: Charles Thomas. [11]

Ramón y Cajal, S. (1911). *Histologie du Système Nerveux de l'homme et des Vertébrés.* Vol. 1. A. Maloine, Paris. Reprinted by Consejo Superior de Investigaciónes Científicas, Inst. Ramón y Cajal, Madrid, 1955. [4, 9]

Ramón y Cajal, S. (1928). *Degeneration and Regeneration of the Nervous System.* (Facsimile of 1928 edition in two volumes, translated by R. M. May.) New York: Hafner Press. [9]

Ramón y Cajal, S. (1929). *Studies on Vertebrate Neurogenesis.* (Translation of the 1929 edition by L. Guth.) Springfield, IL: Charles Thomas. [4, 5, 6, 7, 9]

Ramón y Cajal, S. (1937). *Recollections of My Life.* (Translated by H. Craigie.) Philadelphia: American Philosophical Society. [9]

Raper, J. A., M. Bastiani and C. S. Goodman. (1983a). Pathfinding by neuronal growth cones in grasshopper embryos. I. Divergent choices made by the growth cones of sibling neurons. *J. Neurosci.* 3: 20–30. [5]

Raper, J. A., M. Bastiani and C. S. Goodman. (1983b). Pathfinding by neuronal growth cones in grasshopper embryos. II. Selective fasciculation onto specific axonal pathways. *J. Neurosci.* 3: 31–41. [5]

Rawles, M. E. (1948). Origin of melanophores and their role in development of color patterns in vertebrates. *Physiol. Rev.* 28: 383–408. [4]

Raymond, P. A. and S. S. Easter. (1983). Post-embryonic growth of the optic tectum in goldfish. I. Location of

germinal cells and numbers of neurons produced. *J. Neurosci.* 3: 1077–1091. [11]

Ready, D. F. and J. G. Nicholls. (1979). Identified neurones isolated from leech CNS make selective connections in culture. *Nature* 281: 67–69. [10]

Redfern, P. A. (1970). Neuromuscular transmission in new-born rats. *J. Physiol. (Lond.)* 209: 701–709. [12]

Redman, S. and B. Walmsley. (1981). The synaptic basis of the monosynaptic stretch reflex. *Trends Neurosci.* 4: 248–251. [10]

Rees, R. P., M. B. Bunge and R. P. Bunge. (1976). Morphological changes in the neuritic growth cone and target neuron during synaptic junction development in culture. *J. Cell Biol.* 68: 240–263. [9]

Reh, T. A. and M. Constantine-Paton. (1984a). Retinal ganglion cell terminals change their projection sites during larval development of *Rana pipiens. J. Neurosci.* 4: 442–457. [11]

Reh, T. A. and M. Constantine-Paton. (1984b). Eye-specific segregation requires neural activity in three-eyed *Rana pipiens. J. Neurosci.* (in press). [12]

Reichardt, L. F. and P. H. Patterson. (1977). Neurotransmitter synthesis and uptake by isolated sympathetic neurones in microcultures. *Nature* 270: 147–151. [2]

Reiness, C. G. and C. B. Weinberg. (1981). Metabolic stabilization of acetylcholine receptors at newly formed neuromuscular junctions in rat. *Dev. Biol.* 84: 247–254. [9]

Riesen, A. H. (1961). Stimulation as a requirement for growth and function in behavioral development. In: *Functions of Varied Experience,* D. W. Fiske and S. R. Maddi, ed. Homewood, IL: Dorsey Press, pp. 57–105. [14]

Riley, C. M., R. L. Day, D. M. Greeley and W. S. Langford. (1949). Central autonomic dysfunction with defective lacrimation. I. Report of five cases. *Pediatrics* 3: 468–478. [7]

Riley, D. A. (1976). Multiple axon branches innervating single endplates of kitten soleus myofibers. *Brain Res.* 110: 158–161. [12]

Riley, D. A. (1977a). Spontaneous elimination of nerve terminals from the endplates of developing skeletal myofibers. *Brain Res.* 134: 279–285. [12]

Riley, D. A. (1977b). Multiple innervation of fiber types in the soleus muscles of postnatal rats. *Exp. Neurol.* 56: 400–409. [12]

Riley, D. A. (1978). Tenotomy delays the postnatal development of the motor innervation of the rat soleus. *Brain Res.* 143: 162–167. [12]

Riley, D. A. (1981). Ultrastructural evidence for axon retraction during the spontaneous elimination of polyneural innervation of the rat soleus muscle. *J. Neurocytol.* 10: 425–440. [12]

Ripley, K. L. and R. R. Provine. (1972). Neural correlates of embryonic motility in the chick. *Brain Res.* 45: 127–134. [14]

Robbins, N. (1967). The role of the nerve in maintenance of frog taste buds. *Exp. Neurol.* 17: 364–380. [8]

Rogers, L. A. and W. M. Cowan. (1973). The development of the mesencephalic nucleus of the trigeminal nerve in the chick. *J. Comp. Neurol. 147*: 291–320. [6]

Rohrer, H., T. Schäfer, S. Korsching and H. Thoenen. (1982). Internalization of nerve growth factor by pheochromocytoma PC12 cells: Absence of transfer to the nucleus. *J. Neurosci. 2*: 687–697. [7]

Romanes, G. J. (1901). *Darwin and After Darwin*. London: Open Court Publishing Co. [1]

Romanul, F. C. A. and E. L. Hogan. (1965). Enzymatic changes in denervated muscle. I. Histochemical studies. *Arch. Neurol. 13*: 263–273. [8]

Romanul, F. C. A. and J. P. van der Meulen. (1967). Slow and fast muscles after cross innervation: Enzymatic and physiological changes. *Arch. Neurol. 17*: 387–402. [8]

Rootman, D. S., W. G. Tatton and M. Hay. (1981). Postnatal histogenetic death of rat forelimb motoneurons. *J. Comp. Neurol. 199*: 17–27. [6]

Roper, S. (1976a). Sprouting and regeneration of synaptic terminals in the frog cardiac ganglion. *Nature 261*: 148–149. [13]

Roper, S. (1976b). The acetylcholine sensitivity of the surface membrane of multiply-innervated parasympathetic ganglion cells in the mudpuppy before and after partial denervation. *J. Physiol. (Lond.) 254*: 455–473. [8]

Roper, S. and C.-P. Ko. (1978). Synaptic remodeling in the partially denervated parasympathetic ganglion in the heart of the frog. In: *Neuronal Plasticity*, C. W. Cotman, ed. New York: Raven Press, pp. 1–25. [13]

Roseman, S. (1970). The synthesis of complex carbohydrates by multiglycosyltransferase systems and their potential function in intercellular adhesion. *Chem. Phys. Lipids 5*: 270–297. [11]

Rosenthal, J. (1969). Post-tetanic potentiation at the neuromuscular junction of the frog. *J. Physiol. (Lond.) 203*: 121–133. [13]

Rosenthal, J. L. and P. S. Taraskevich. (1977). Reduction of multiaxonal innervation at the neuromuscular junction of the rat during development. *J. Physiol. (Lond.) 270*: 299–310. [12]

Rosenthal, L. J., M. A. Reiner and M. A. Bleicher. (1979). Nonoperative management of distal fingertip amputations in children. *Pediatrics 64*: 1–3. [3]

Roth, S. (1968). Studies on intercellular adhesive selectivity. *Dev. Biol. 18*: 602–631. [11]

Roth, S. and R. B. Marchase. (1976). An *in vitro* assay for retino-tectal specificity. In: *Neuronal Recognition*, S. H. Barondes, ed. New York: Plenum Press, pp. 227–248. [11]

Roth, S., E. J. MacGuire and S. Roseman. (1971). Evidence for cell-surface glycosyltransferases. Their potential role in cellular recognition. *J. Cell Biol. 51*: 536–547. [11]

Rothbard, J. B., R. Brackenbury, B. A. Cunningham and G. M. Edelman. (1982). Differences in the carbohydrate structures of neural cell–adhesion molecules from adult and embryonic chicken brains. *J. Biol. Chem. 257*: 11064–11069. [11]

Roux, W. (1888). Beiträge zur Entwicklungsmechanik des Embryo. *Virchows Arch. path. Anat. u. Physiol. u. kl. Med. 114*: 113–153. Tafel II und III. Translated by H. Laufer. In: *Foundations of Experimental Embryology*, 2nd Ed., 1974, B. H. Willier and J. M. Oppenheimer, eds. New York: Hafner Press, pp. 2–37. [1]

Rovasio, R. A., A. Delouvée, K. M. Yamada, R. Timpl and J.-P. Thiery. (1983). Neural crest cell migration: Requirements for exogenous fibronectin and high cell density. *J. Cell Biol. 96*: 462–473. [4]

Rovensky, Y. A. and I. L. Slavnaya. (1974). Spreading of fibroblast-like cells on grooved surfaces. A study by scanning electron microscopy. *Exp. Cell Res. 84*: 199–206. [4]

Rovensky, Y. A., I. L. Slavnaya, and J. M. Vasiliev. (1971). Behaviour of fibroblast-like cells on grooved surfaces. *Exp. Cell Res. 65*: 193–201. [4]

Rubin, E. (1985a). Development of the rat superior cervical ganglion: Ganglion cell maturation. *J. Neurosci.* (in press). [9, 10, 12]

Rubin, E. (1985b). Development of the rat superior cervical ganglion: Ingrowth of preganglionic axons. *J. Neurosci.* (in press). [5, 9, 10, 12]

Rubin, E. (1985c). Development of the rat superior cervical ganglion: Initial stages of synapse formation. *J. Neurosci.* (in press). [10, 12]

Rubin, E. and D. Purves. (1980). Segmental organization of sympathetic preganglionic neurons in the mammalian spinal cord. *J. Comp. Neurol. 192*: 163–174. [10]

Rubin, L. L., S. M. Schuetze, C. L. Weill and G. D. Fischbach. (1980). Regulation of acetylcholinesterase appearance at neuromuscular junctions *in vitro*. *Nature 283*: 264–267. [9]

Ruppenthal, G. C., G. L. Arling, H. F. Harlow, G. P. Sackett and S. J. Suomi. (1976). A 10-year perspective of motherless-mother monkey behavior. *J. Abnorm. Psychol. 85*: 341–349. [14]

Rutishauser, U., W. E. Gall and G. M. Edelman. (1978). Adhesion among neural cells of the chick embryo. IV. Role of the cell surface molecule CAM in the formation of neurite bundles in cultures of spinal ganglia. *J. Cell Biol. 79*: 382–393. [11]

Saito, A. and S. I. Zacks. (1969). Fine structure of neuromuscular junctions after nerve section and implantation of nerve in denervated muscle. *Exp. Mol. Pathol. 10*: 256–273. [9]

Sakmann, B. (1975). Reappearance of extrajunctional acetylcholine sensitivity in denervated rat muscle after blockage with α-bungarotoxin. *Nature 255*: 415–416. [8]

Sakmann, B. and H. R. Brenner. (1978). Change in synaptic channel gating during neuromuscular development. *Nature 276*: 401–402. [9]

Salmons, S. and F. A. Sréter. (1976). Significance of impulse activity in the transformation of skeletal muscle type. *Nature 263*: 30–34. [8]

Salmons, S. and G. Vrbová. (1969). The influence of activity on some contractile characteristics of mammalian fast and slow muscles. *J. Physiol. (Lond.) 201*: 535–549. [8]

Salpeter, M. M., S. Spanton, K. Holley and T. R. Pod-leski. (1982). Brain extract causes acetylcholine receptor redistribution which mimics some early events at developing neuromuscular junctions. *J. Cell Biol. 93*: 417–425. [9]

Salzer, J. L. and R. P. Bunge. (1980). Studies of Schwann cell proliferation. I. An analysis in tissue culture of proliferation during development, Wallerian degeneration, and direct injury. *J. Cell Biol. 84*: 739–752. [8]

Salzer, J. L., R. P. Bunge and L. Glaser. (1980b). Studies of Schwann cell proliferation. III. Evidence for the surface localization of the neurite mitogen. *J. Cell Biol. 84*: 767–778. [8]

Salzer, J. L., A. K. Williams, L. Glaser and R. P. Bunge. (1980a). Studies of Schwann cell proliferation. II. Characterization of the stimulation and specificity of the response to a neurite membrane fraction. *J. Cell Biol. 84*: 753–766. [8]

Sanes, D. H. and M. Constantine-Paton. (1983). Altered activity patterns during development reduce neural tuning. *Science 221*: 1183–1185. [12]

Sanes, J. R. (1983). Roles of extracellular matrix in neural development. *Annu. Rev. Physiol. 45*: 581–600. [4, 9]

Sanes, J. R., D. H. Feldman, J. M. Cheney and J. G. Lawrence. (1984). Brain extract induces synaptic characteristics in the basal lamina of cultured myotubes. *J. Neurosci. 4*: 464–473. [9]

Sanes, J. R. and Z. W. Hall. (1979). Antibodies that bind specifically to synaptic sites on muscle fiber basal lamina. *J. Cell Biol. 83*: 357–370. [9]

Sanes, J. R. and J. G. Hildebrand. (1975). Nerves in the antennae of pupal *Manduca sexta Johanssen* (Lepidoptera: Sphingidae). *Wilhelm Roux Arch. Entwicklungsmech. Org. 178*: 71–78. [5]

Sanes, J. R. and J. G. Hildebrand. (1976). Origin and morphogenesis of sensory neurons is an insect antenna. *Dev. Biol. 51*: 300–319. [5]

Sanes, J. R., J. G. Hildebrand and D. J. Prescott. (1976). Differentiation of insect sensory neurons in the absence of their normal synaptic targets. *Dev. Biol. 52*: 121–127. [6]

Sanes, J. R., L. M. Marshall and U. J. McMahan. (1978). Reinnervation of muscle fiber basal lamina after removal of myofibers. *J. Cell Biol. 78*: 176–198. [9]

Sanes, J. R., L. M. Marshall and U. J. McMahan. (1980). Reinnervation of skeletal muscle: Restoration of the normal synaptic pattern. In: *Nerve Repair and Regeneration: Its Clinical and Experimental Basis*, D. L. Jewett and H. R. McCarroll, eds. St. Louis: Mosby, pp. 130–138. [5, 9]

Sargent, P. B. and M. J. Dennis. (1977). Formation of synapses between parasympathetic neurones deprived of preganglionic innervation. *Nature 268*: 456–458. [13]

Sargent, P. B. and M. J. Dennis. (1981). The influence of normal innervation upon abnormal synaptic connections between frog parasympathetic neurons. *Dev. Biol. 81*: 65–73. [13]

Sauer, F. C. (1935). Mitosis in the neural tube. *J. Comp. Neurol. 62*: 377–405. [1,2]

Saunders, J. W. (1948). The proximo-distal sequence of origin of the parts of the chick wing and the role of the ectoderm. *J. Exp. Zool. 108*: 363–403. [3]

Saunders, J. W. (1970). *Patterns and Principles of Animal Development*. New York: Macmillan. [1, 2]

Saunders, J. W. and J. F. Fallon. (1966). Cell death in morphogenesis. In: *Major Problems in Developmental Biology*, M. Locke, ed. New York: Academic Press, pp. 289–314. [6]

Saunders, J. W. and M. T. Gasseling. (1968). Ectodermal–mesenchymal interactions in the origin of limb symmetry. In: *Epithelial–Mesenchymal Interactions*, R. Fleischmajer and R. E. Billingham, eds. Baltimore: Williams and Wilkins, pp. 78–97. [3]

Saunders, J. W. and M. T. Gasseling. (1983). New insights into the problem of pattern regulation in the limb bud of the chick embryo. In: *Limb Development and Regeneration, Part A*, J. F. Fallon and A. I. Caplan, eds. New York: Alan R. Liss, pp. 67–76. [3]

Saxen, L. and S. Toivonen. (1962). *Primary Embryonic Induction*. London: Logos Press. [3]

Saxod, R. (1972). Rôle du nerf et du territoire cutané dans le développement des corpuscules de Herbst et de Grandry. *J. Embryol. Exp. Morphol. 27*: 277–300. [8]

Saxod, R. (1978). Development of cutaneous sensory receptors in birds. In: *Handbook of Sensory Physiology*, Vol. IX: *Development of Sensory Systems*, M. Jacobson, ed. New York: Springer-Verlag, pp. 337–417. [8]

Saxod, R. and P. Sengel. (1968). Sur les conditions de la différenciation des corpuscules sensoriels cutanés chez le Poulet et le Canard. *C. R. Hebd. Séances Acad. Sci. (Paris) Series D. 267*: 1149–1152. [8]

Sayers, H. and D. A. Tonge. (1982). Differences between foreign and original innervation of skeletal muscle in the frog. *J. Physiol. (Lond.) 330*: 57–68. [10]

Schafer, T., M. E. Schwab, and H. Thoenen. (1983). Increased formation of preganglionic synapses and axons due to a retrograde trans-synaptic action of nerve growth factor in the rat sympathetic nervous system. *J. Neurosci. 3*: 1501–1510. [13]

Schaller, H. C. (1975). A neurohormone from hydra is also present in the rat brain. *J. Neurochem. 25*: 187–188. [3]

Schaller, H. C. and H. Bodenmüller. (1981). Isolation and amino acid sequence of a morphogenetic peptide from hydra. *Proc. Natl. Acad. Sci. USA 78*: 7000–7004. [3]

Schaller, H. C., T. Schmidt and C. J. P. Grimmelikhuijzen. (1979). Separation and specificity of action of four morphogens from hydra. *W. Roux. Arch. Dev. Biol. 186*: 139–149. [3]

Scheibel, A. B. (1982). Age-related changes in the human forebrain. *Neurosci. Res. Program Bull. 20*: 577–583. [13]

Scheibel, M. E., R. D. Lindsay, U. Tomiyasu and A. B. Scheibel. (1975). Progressive dendritic changes in aging human cortex. *Exp. Neurol. 47*: 392–403. [13]

Scheibel, M. E., R. D. Lindsay, U. Tomiyasu and A. B. Scheibel. (1976). Progressive dendritic changes in the aging human limbic system. *Exp. Neurol. 53*: 420–430. [13]

Scheibel, M. E., U. Tomiyasu and A. B. Scheibel. (1977). The aging human Betz cell. *Exp. Neurol. 56*: 598–609. [13]

Schiffmann, E. (1982). Leukocyte chemotaxis. *Annu. Rev. Physio. 44*: 553–568. [4]

Schmidt, H. and E. Stefani. (1976). Re-innervation of twitch and slow muscle fibres of the frog after crushing the motor nerves. *J. Physiol. (Lond.) 258*: 99–123. [10]

Schmidt, H. and E. Stefani. (1977). Action potentials in slow muscle fibres of the frog during regeneration of motor nerves. *J. Physiol. (Lond.) 270*: 507–517. [10]

Schmidt, J. T. (1978). Retinal fibers alter tectal positional markers during the expansion of the half-retinal projection in goldfish. *J. Comp. Neurol. 177*: 279–300. [11, 12]

Schmidt, J. T., C. M. Cicerone and S. S. Easter. (1978). Expansion of the half retinal projection to the tectum in goldfish: An electrophysiological and anatomical study. *J. Comp. Neurol. 177*: 257–278. [11]

Schmidt, J. T. and D. L. Edwards. (1983). Activity sharpens the map during the regeneration of the retinotectal projection in goldfish. *Brain Res. 269*: 29–39. [12]

Schneider, G. E. (1973). Early lesions of the superior colliculus: Factors affecting the formation of abnormal retinal projections. *Brain Behav. Evol. 8*: 73–109. [13]

Schneiderman, H. A. and L. I. Gilbert. (1964). Control of growth and development in insects. *Science 143*: 325–333. [1]

Scholes, J. H. (1979). Nerve fibre topography in the retinal projection to the tectum. *Nature 278*: 620–624. [11]

Scholes, J. H. (1982). Ribbon optic nerves and axonal growth patterns in the retinal projection to the tectum. In: *Development in the Nervous System*, D. R. Garrod and J. D. Feldman, eds. Cambridge: Cambridge University Press, pp. 181–214. [11]

Schotté, O. E. and E. G. Butler. (1941). Morphological effects of denervation and amputation of urodele larvae. *J. Exp. Zool. 87*: 279–322. [8]

Schwab, M. E., R. Heumann and H. Thoenen. (1982). Communication between target organs and nerve cells: Retrograde axonal transport and site of action of nerve growth factor. *Cold Spring Harbor Symp. Quart. Biol. 46*: 125–134. [7]

Schwab, M. E., K. Stöckel and H. Thoenen. (1976). Immunocytochemical localization of nerve growth factor (NGF) in the submandibular gland of adult mice by light and electron microscopy. *Cell Tissue Res. 169*: 289–299. [7]

Schwab, M. E. and H. Thoenen. (1983). Retrograde axonal transport. In: *Handbook of Neurochemistry*, Vol. 5, A. Lajtha, ed. New York: Plenum, pp. 381–404. [7]

Schwanwitsch, B. N. (1924). On the ground plan of wing pattern in nymphalids and certain other families of Rhopalocerous Lepidoptera. *Proc. Zool. Soc. London 34*: 509–525. [3]

Schwartz, J. P. and X. P. Breakefield. (1980). Altered nerve growth factor in fibroblasts from patients with familial dysautonomia. *Proc. Natl. Acad. Sci. USA 77*: 1154–1158. [7]

Schwob, J. and J. Price. (1984). The development of axonal connections in the central olfactory system of rats. *J. Comp. Neurol. 223*: 177–202. [12]

Scott, B. E., V. E. Engelbert and K. C. Fisher. (1969). Morphological and electrophysiological characteristics of dissociated chick embryonic spinal ganglion cells in culture. *Exp. Neurol. 23*: 230–248. [2]

Scott, J. G. and L. M. Mendell. (1976). Individual EPSPs produced by single triceps surae Ia afferent fibers in homonymous and heteronymous motoneurons. *J. Neurophysiol. 39*: 679–692. [10]

Scott, J., M. Selby, M. Urdes, M. Quiroga, G. I. Bell and W. J. Rutter. (1983). Isolation and nucleotide sequence of a cDNA encoding the precursor of mouse nerve growth factor. *Nature 302*: 538–539. [7]

Scott, S. A. (1982). The development of the segmental pattern of skin sensory innervation in the embryonic chick hindlimb. *J. Physiol. (Lond.) 303*: 203–220. [5]

Seeley, J. P., K. H. Charles, M. L. Shelanski and L. A. Greene. (1983). Pressure microinjection of nerve growth factor and anti-nerve growth factor into the nucleus and cytoplasm: Lack of effects on neurite outgrowth from pheochromcytoma cells. *J. Neurosci. 3*: 1488–1494. [7]

Sengel, P. (1975). Feather pattern development. In: *Cell Patterning, Ciba Found. Symp. 29* (new series), R. Porter and J. Rivers eds. Amsterdam: Elsevier, pp. 51–70. [2]

Sengelaub, D. R. and B. L. Finlay. (1981). Early removal of one eye reduces normally occurring cell death in the remaining eye. *Science 213*: 573–574. [6]

Server, A. C. and E. M. Shooter. (1977). Nerve growth factor. *Adv. Protein Chem. 31*: 339–409. [7]

Shankland, M. (1984). Positional determination of supernumerary blast cell death in the leech embryo. *Nature 307*: 541–543. [5]

Shatz, C. J. (1983). Prenatal development of the cat's retinogeniculate pathway. *J. Neurosci. 3*: 482–499. [12]

Shatz, C. J. and M. P. Stryker. (1978). Ocular dominance in layer IV of the cat's visual cortex and the effects of monocular deprivation. *J. Physiol. (Lond.) 281*: 267–283. [12]

Shaw, G. and D. Bray. (1977). Movement and extension of isolated growth cones. *Exp. Cell Res. 104*: 55–62. [4]

Shellswell, G. B. and L. Wolpert. (1977). The pattern of muscle and tendon development in the chick wing. In *Vertebrate Limb and Somite Morphogenesis*, D. A. Ede, J. R. Hinchliffe and M. Balls, eds. Cambridge: Cambridge University Press, pp. 71–87. [3]

Shelton, D. L. and L. F. Reichert. (1984). Expression of the β-nerve growth factor gene correlates with the density of sympathetic innervation in effector organs. *Proc. Natl. Acad. USA.* (in press). [7]

Shorey, M. L. (1909). The effect of the destruction of peripheral areas on the differentiation of the neuroblasts. *J. Exp. Zool. 7*: 25–63. [6]

Shy, G. M. and G. A. Drager. (1960). A neurological syndrome associated with orthostatic hypotension: A clinical pathologic study. *AMA Arch. Neurol. 2*: 511–527. [7]

Siggers, D. C., J. G. Rogers, S. H. Boyer, L. Margolet, H. Dorkin, S. P. Banerjee and E. M. Shooter. (1976). Increased nerve growth factor β-chain cross-reacting material in familial dysautonomia. *N. Engl. J. Med. 295*: 629–634. (See also editorial comments by R. Levi-Montalcini following this article, pp. 671–673.) [7]

Silver, J. and R. M. Robb. (1979). Studies on the development of the eye cup and optic nerve in normal mice and in mutants with congenital optic nerve aplasia. *Dev. Biol. 68*: 175–190. [5]

Silver, J. and R. S. Sidman. (1980). A mechanism for the guidance and topographic patterning of retinal ganglion cell axons. *J. Comp. Neurol. 189*: 101–111. [5]

Singer, M. (1952). Induction of regeneration of the forelimb of the postmetamorphic frog by augmentation of the nerve supply. *J. Exp. Zool. 126*: 419–471. [8]

Singer, M. (1965). A theory of the trophic nervous control of amphibian limb regeneration, including a re-evaluation of quantitative nerve requirement. In: *Regeneration in Animals and Related Problems*, V. Kiortsis and H. A. L. Trampush, eds. Amsterdam: Elsevier, pp. 20–32. [8]

Singer, M. (1973). *Limb Regeneration in the Vertebrates*, Module in Biology, No. 6. Reading, MA: Addison-Wesley, pp. 1–27. [8]

Singer, M. (1978). On the nature of the neurotrophic phenomenon in urodele limb regeneration. *Am. Zool. 18*: 829–841. [8]

Singer, M., R. H. Nordlander and M. Egar. (1979). Axonal guidance during embryogenesis and regeneration in the spinal cord of the newt. "The blueprint hypothesis" of neuronal pathway patterning. *J. Comp. Neurol. 185*: 1–22. [5]

Sisto-Daneo, L. and G. Filogamo. (1974). Ultrastructure of developing myoneural junctions. Evidence for two patterns of synaptic area differentiation. *J. Submicrosc. Cytol. 6*: 219–228. [9]

Sisto-Daneo, L. and G. Filogamo. (1975). Differentiation of synaptic area in "slow" and "fast" muscle fibers. *J. Submicrosc. Cytol. 7*: 121–131. [9]

Skene, J. H. P. (1983). An oncogene abounds in brains. *Trends Neurosci. 6*: 353–354. [7]

Slack, J. M. W. (1983). *From Egg to Embryo: Determinative Events in Early Development*. Cambridge: Cambridge University Press. [1]

Sloan, H. E., S. E. Hughes and B. Oakley. (1983). Chronic impairment of axonal transport eliminates taste responses and taste buds. *J. Neurosci. 3*: 112–128. [8]

Smith, C. G. and M. Hollyday. (1984). The development of postnatal organization of motor nuclei in the rat spinal cord. *J. Comp. Neurol.* (in press). [5]

Smith, D. O. (1979). Reduced capabilities of synaptic transmission in aged rats. *Exp. Neurol. 66*: 650–666. [13]

Smith, D. O. and J. L. Rosenheimer. (1982). Decreased sprouting and degeneration of nerve terminals of active muscles in aged rats. *J. Neurophysiol. 48*: 100–109. [13]

Smith, J. C. and J. M. W. Slack. (1983). Dorsalization and neural induction: Properties of organizer in *Xenopus laevis. J. Embryol. Exp. Morphol. 78*: 299–317. [3]

Smith, J. C., C. Tickle and L. Wolpert. (1978). Attenuation of positional signalling in the chick limb by high doses of γ-radiation. *Nature 272*: 612–613. [3]

Smolen, A. (1981). Postnatal development of ganglionic neurons in the absence of preganglionic input: Morphological synapse formation. *Dev. Brain Res. 1*: 49–58. [9]

Smolen, A. J. and G. Raisman. (1979). Synapse formation in the superior cervical sympathetic ganglion of the rat during normal development and after neonatal deafferentation. *Anat. Rec. 193*: 688. [12]

Sohal, G. S. (1976a). An experimental study of cell death in the developing trochlear nucleus. *Exp. Neurol. 51*: 684–698. [6]

Sohal, G. S. (1976b). Effects of deafferentiation on the development of the isthmo- optic nucleus in the duck (*Anas platyrhynchos*). *Exp. Neurol. 50*: 161–173. [6]

Sohal, G. S., T. L. Creazzo and T. G. Oblak. (1979). Effects of chronic paralysis with α-bungarotoxin on development of innervation. *Exp. Neurol. 66*: 619–628. [6]

Sohal, G. S. and C. H. Narayanan. (1974). The development of the isthmo-optic nucleus in the duck (*Anas platyrhynchos*). I. Changes in cell number and cell size during normal development. *Brain Res. 77*: 243–255. [6]

Sohal, G. S. and T. A. Weidman. (1978). Ultrastructural sequence of embryonic cell death in normal and peripherally deprived trochlear nucleus. *Exp. Neurol. 61*: 53–64. [6]

Solomon, F. (1979). Detailed neurite morphologies of sister neuroblastoma cells are related. *Cell 16*: 165–169. [4]

Sondhi, K. C. (1963). The biological foundations of animal patterns. *Q. Rev. Biol. 38*: 289–327. [3]

Sotelo, C. and S. L. Palay. (1971). Altered axons and axon terminals in the lateral vestibular nucleus of the rat. Possible example of axonal remodeling. *Lab. Invest. 25*: 653–671. [13]

Sotelo, C. and J. P. Rio. (1980). Cerebellar malformation obtained in rats by early postnatal treatment with 6-aminonicotinamide. Role of neuron–glia interactions in cerebellar development. *Neuroscience 5*: 1737–1759. [4]

Speidel, C. C. (1933). Studies of living nerves. II. Activities of ameboid growth cones, sheath cells, and myelin segments, as revealed by prolonged observation of individual nerve fibers in frog tadpoles. *Am. J. Anat. 52*: 1–75. [5]

Speidel, C. C. (1941). Adjustments of nerve endings. *Harvey Lect. 36*: 126–158. [5]

Speidel, C. C. (1947). Correlated studies of sense organs and nerves of the lateral-line in living frog tadpoles. *J. Comp. Neurol. 87*: 29–55. [8]

Speidel, C. C. (1948). Correlated studies of sense organ and nerves of the lateral line in living frog tadpoles. II. The trophic influence of specific nerve of denervated and reinnervated organs. *Am. J. Anat. 82*: 277–320. [8]

Spemann, H. (1938). *Embryonic Development and Induction*. New Haven: Yale University Press. [1, 2, 3]

Spemann, H. and H. Mangold. (1924). Induction von embryonolanlagen durch implantation artfremder organisatoren. *Arch. Mikrosk. Anat. Entwicklungsmech. 100*: 599–638. English translation by V. Hamburger reprinted in *Foundations of Experimental Embryology*, B. H. Willier and J. Oppenheimer, eds., 2nd Ed., 1974. New York: Hafner Press, pp. 144–184. [3]

Sperry, R. W. (1941). The effect of crossing nerves to antagonistic muscles in the hind-limb of the rat. *J. Comp. Neurol.* 75: 1–19. [11]

Sperry, R. W. (1943a). Effect of 180° rotation of the retinal field on visuomotor coordination. *J. Exp. Zool.* 92: 263–279. [11]

Sperry, R. W. (1943b). Visuomotor coordination in the newt *(Triturus viridescens)* after regeneration of the optic nerve. *J. Comp. Neurol.* 79: 33–35. [11]

Sperry, R. W. (1944). Optic nerve regeneration with return of vision in anurans. *J. Neurophysiol.* 7: 57–69. [11]

Sperry, R. W. (1956). The eye and the brain. *Sci. Am.* 194(5): 48–52. [11]

Sperry, R. W. (1963). Chemoaffinity in the orderly growth of nerve fiber patterns and connections. *Proc. Natl. Acad. Sci. USA* 50: 703–710. [11]

Sperry, R. W. (1965). Embryogenesis of behavioral nerve nets. In: *Organogenesis*, R. L. DeHaan and H. Ursprung, eds. New York: Holt, Rinehart and Winston, pp.161–171. [11]

Sperry, R. W. (1968). Mental unity following surgical disconnection of the cerebral hemispheres. *Harvey Lect.* 62: 293–323. [11]

Sperry, R. W. (1982). Some effects of disconnecting the cerebral hemispheres. *Science* 217: 1223–1226. [11]

Sperry, R. W. and H. L. Arora. (1965). Selectivity in regeneration of the oculomotor nerve in the cichlid fish, *Astronatus ocellatus. J. Embryol. Exp. Morphol.* 14: 307–317. [5, 10]

Spitzer, N. C. (1979). Ion channels in development. *Annu. Rev. Neurosci.* 2: 363–397. [2]

Spitzer, N. C. (1981). Development of membrane properties in vertebrates. *Trends Neurosci.* 4: 169–172. [2]

Spitzer, N. C. (1982). The development of electrical excitability. In: *Neuronal and Glial Interrelationships*, T. A. Sears, ed. Berlin: Springer Verlag. [2]

Spitzer, N. C. and J. E. Lamborghini. (1976). The development of the action potential mechanism of amphibian neurons isolated in culture. *Proc. Natl. Acad. Sci. USA* 73: 1641–1645. [2]

Srihari, T. and G. Vrbová. (1978). The role of muscle activity in the differentiation of neuromuscular junctions in slow and fast chick muscles. *J. Neurocytol.* 7: 529–540. [12]

Stanfield, B. B., D. D. M. O'Leary and C. Fricks. (1982). Selective collateral elimination in early postnatal development restricts cortical distribution of rat pyramidal tract neurones. *Nature* 298: 371–373. [12]

Stefanelli, A. (1950). Studies on the development of Mauthner's cell. In: *Genetic Neurology*, P. Weiss, ed. Chicago: University of Chicago Press, pp. 161–165. [6]

Stefanelli, A. (1951). The Mauthnerian apparatus in the ichthyopsida; its nature and function and correlated problems of neurohistogenesis. *Q. Rev. Biol.* 26: 17–34. [5]

Steinbach, J. H. (1981). Developmental changes in acetylcholine receptor aggregates at rat skeletal neuromuscular junctions. *Dev. Biol.* 84: 267–276. [9]

Steinberg, M. S. (1978). Cell-cell recognition in multicellular assembly: Levels of specificity. In: *Cell-Cell Recognition*, A. S. G. Curtis, ed. Cambridge: Cambridge University Press, pp. 25–49. [4]

Stent, G. S. (1973). A physiological mechanism for Hebb's postulate of learning. *Proc. Natl. Acad. Sci. USA* 70: 997–1001. [12]

Stent, G. S. (1977). Explicit and implicit semantic content of the genetic information. In: *Foundational Problems in the Special Sciences*, R. E. Butts and J. Hintikka, eds. Dordrecht, Holland: D. Reidel Publishing Company, pp. 131–149. [2]

Stent, G. S. (1981). Strength and weakness of the genetic approach to the development of the nervous system. *Annu. Rev. Neurosci.* 4: 163–194. [2]

Stent, G. S., D. A. Weisblat, S. S. Blair and S. L. Zackson. (1982). Cell lineage in the development of the leech nervous system. In: *Neural Development*, N. C. Spitzer, ed. New York: Plenum Press, pp. 1–44. [2, 3]

Stephenson, R. S. (1979). Axon reflexes in axolotl limbs: Evidence that branched motor axons reinnervate muscles selectively. *Exp. Neurol.* 64: 174–189. [10]

Stirling, R. V. and D. Summerbell. (1983). Familiarity breeds contempt: The behavior of axons in foreign and familiar environments. In: *Limb Development and Regeneration, Part A.* J. F. Fallon and A. I. Caplan, eds. New York: Alan R. Liss, pp. 217–226. [5]

Stirling, R. V. and D. C. Summerbell. (1979). The segmentation of axons from the segmental nerve roots to the chick wing. *Nature* 278: 640–642. [5]

Stöckel, K., G. Guroff, M. Schwab and H. Thoenen. (1976). The significance of retrograde axonal transport for the accumulation of systemically administered nerve growth factor (NGF) in the rat superior cervical ganglion. *Brain Res.* 109: 271–284. [7]

Stöckel, K., U. Paravicini and H. Thoenen. (1974). Specificity of the retrograde axonal transport of nerve growth factor. *Brain Res.* 76: 413–421. [7]

Stöckel, K., M. Schwab and H. Thoenen. (1975). Specificity of retrograde transport of nerve growth factor (NGF) in sensory neurons: A biochemical and morphological study. *Brain Res.* 89: 1–14. [7]

Stöckel, K. and H. Thoenen. (1975). Retrograde axonal transport of nerve growth factor: Specificity and biological importance. *Brain Res.* 85: 337–341. [7]

Stone, L. S. (1941). Transplantation of the vertebrate eye and return of vision. *Trans. NY Acad. Sci.* 3: 208–212. [11]

Stone, L. S. (1944). Functional polarization in the retinal development and its reestablishment in regenerating retinae of rotated grafted eyes. *Proc. Soc. Exp. Biol. Med.* 57: 13–14. [11]

Stone, L. S. and L. S. Farthing. (1942). Return of vision four times in the same adult salamander eye *(Triturus viridescens)* repeatedly transplanted. *J. Exp. Zool.* 91: 265–285. [11]

Stone, L. S. and I. S. Zaur. (1940). Reimplantation and transplantation of adult eyes in the salamander *(Triturus viridescens)* with return of vision. *J. Exp. Zool. 85:* 243–269. [11]

Stout, J. F. and F. Huber. (1972). Responses of central auditory neurons of female crickets *(Gryllis campestris L.)* to the calling song of the male. *Z. Vgl. Physiol. 76:* 302–313. [14]

Stratton, G. M. (1896–1897). Vision without inversion of the retinal image. (In 3 parts). *Psychol. Rev. 3:* 611–617; *4:* 341–360, 463–481. [13]

Strausfeld, N. J. (1980). Male and female visual neurones in dipterous insects. *Nature 283:* 381–383. [14]

Straznicky, C., R. M. Gaze and M. J. Keating. (1981). The development of the retinotectal projections from compound eyes in *Xenopus. J. Embryol. Exp. Morphol. 62:* 13–35. [11]

Stretton, A. O. W. and E. A. Kravitz. (1968). Neuronal geometry determination with a technique of intracellular dye injection. *Science 162:* 132–134. [5]

Struhl, G. (1981). A gene product required for the correct initiation of segmental determination in *Drosophila. Nature 293:* 36–41. [3]

Stryker, M. (1981). Late segmentation of geniculate afferents to the cat's visual cortex after recovery from binocular impulse blockade. *Soc. Neurosci. Abs. 7:* 842. [12]

Stryker, M. P., H. Sherk, A. G. Leventhal and H. V. B. Hirsch. (1978). Physiological consequences for the cat's visual cortex of effectively restricting early visual experience with oriented contours. *J. Neurophysiol. 41:* 896–909. [14]

Stuermer, C. A. O. and S. S. Easter. (1984). Rules of order in the retinotectal fascicles of goldfish. *J. Neurosci. 4:* 1045–1051. [11]

Sulston, J. E. and H. R. Horvitz. (1977). Post-embryonic cell lineages of the nematode *Caenorhabditis elegans. Dev. Biol. 56:* 110–156. [2, 6]

Sulston, J. E. and H. R. Horvitz. (1981). Abnormal cell lineages in mutants of the nematode *Caenorhabditis elegans. Dev. Biol. 82:* 41–55. [2]

Sulston, J. E., E. Schierenberg, J. G. White and J. N. Thomson. (1983). The embryonic cell lineage of the nematode *Caenorhabditis elegans. Dev. Biol. 100:* 64–119. [2]

Sulston, J. E. and J. G. White. (1980). Regulation and cell autonomy during postembryonic development of *Caenorhabditis elegans. Dev. Biol. 78:* 577–597. [2]

Summerbell, D. (1979). The zone of polarizing activity: Evidence for a role in normal chick limb morphogenesis. *J. Embryol. Exp. Morphol. 50:* 217–233. [3]

Summerbell, D. (1981). Evidence for regulation of growth, size and pattern in the developing chick limb. *J. Embryol. Exp. Morphol. 65:* 129–150. [3]

Summerbell, D., J. H. Lewis and L. Wolpert. (1973). Positional information in chick limb morphogenesis. *Nature 244:* 492–496. [3]

Summerbell, D. and R. V. Stirling. (1981). The innervation of dorsoventrally reversed chick wings: Evidence that motor axons do not actively seek out their appropriate targets. *J. Embryol. Exp. Morphol. 61:* 233–247. [5]

Sumner, B. E. H. (1975). A quantitative analysis of boutons with different types of synapse in normal and injured hypoglossal nuclei. *Exp. Neurol. 49:* 406–417. [13]

Sumner, B. E. H. (1976). Quantitative ultrastructural observations on the inhibited recovery of the hypoglossal nucleus from the axotomy response when regeneration of the hypoglossal nerve is prevented. *Exp. Brain Res. 26:* 141–150. [13]

Sumner, B. E. H. and F. I. Sutherland. (1973). Quantitative electron microscopy on the injured hypoglossal nucleus in the rat. *J. Neurocytol. 2:* 315–328. [13]

Swanson, L. W., T. J. Teyler and R. F. Thompson (eds.). (1982). Hippocampal long-term potentiation: Mechanisms and implications for memory. *Neurosci. Res. Program Bull. 20:* 613–769. [13]

Sytkowski, A. J., Z. Vogel and M. W. Nirenberg. (1973). Development of acetylcholine receptor clusters on cultured muscle cells. *Proc. Natl. Acad. Sci. USA 70:* 270–274. [9]

Taghert, P. H., M. J. Bastiani, R. K. Ho and C. S. Goodman. (1982). Guidance of pioneer growth cones: Filopodial contacts and coupling revealed with an antibody to Lucifer Yellow. *Dev. Biol. 94:* 391–399. [5]

Taghert, P. H., C. Q. Doe and C. S. Goodman. (1984). Cell determination and regulation during development of neuroblasts and neurones in the grasshopper embryo. *Nature 307:* 163–166. [5]

Tassava, R. A. and W. D. McCullough. (1978). Neural control of cell cycle events in regenerating salamander limbs. *Am. Zool. 18:* 843–854. [8]

Taylor, D. L. and J. S. Condeelis. (1979). Cytoplasmic structure and contractility in amoeboid cells. *Int. Rev. Cytol. 56:* 57–144. [4]

Tello, J. F. (1917). Genesis de las terminaciones nerviosas motrices y sensitivas. *Trab. Lab. Invest. Biol. Univ. Madr. 15:* 101–199. [12]

Teräväinen, H. (1968). Development of the myoneural junction in the rat. *Z. Zellforsch. Mikrosk. Anat. 90:* 372–388. [9]

Thanos, S., F. Bonhoeffer, and U. Rutishauser (1984). Fiber-fiber interaction and tectal cues influence the development of the chicken retinotectal projection. *Proc. Natl. Acad. Sci. USA 81:* 1906–1910. [11]

Thiery, J. P., R. Brackenbury, U. Rutishauser and G. M. Edelman. (1977). Adhesion among neural cells of the chick embryo. II. Purification and characterization of a cell adhesion molecule from neural retina. *J. Biol. Chem. 252:* 6841–6845. [11]

Thoenen, H. and Y.-A. Barde. (1980). Physiology of nerve growth factor. *Physiol. Rev. 60:* 1284–1335. [7]

Thoenen, H., Y.-A. Barde and D. Edgar. (1981). Physiology of nerve growth factor (NGF) and related factors for the survival of peripheral neurons. *Adv. Biochem. Psychopharmacol. 28:* 263–273. [7]

Thoenen, H., U. Otten and M. Schwab. (1979). Orthograde and retrograde signals for the regulation of neuronal gene expression: The peripheral sympathetic nervous system as a model. In: *The Neurosciences, 4th Study*

Program, F. O. Schmitt and F. G. Worden, eds. Cambridge, MA: MIT Press, pp. 911–928. [7]

Thompson, W. (1983a). Lack of segmental selectivity in elimination of synapses from soleus muscle of newborn rats. *J. Physiol. (Lond.) 335*: 343–352. [12]

Thompson, W. (1983b). Synapse elimination in neonatal rat muscle is sensitive to pattern of muscle use. *Nature 302*: 614–616. [12]

Thompson, W. and J. K. S. Jansen. (1977). The extent of sprouting of remaining motor units in partly denervated immature and adult rat soleus muscle. *Neuroscience 2*: 523–535. [8,12]

Thompson, W., D. P. Kuffler and J. K. S. Jansen. (1979). The effect of prolonged, reversible block of nerve impulses on the elimination of polyneuronal innervation of new-born rat skeletal muscle fibers. *Neuroscience 2*: 271–281. [12]

Thorpe, W. H. (1958). The learning of song patterns by birds, with especial reference to the song of the chaffinch *(Fringiella coelebs). Ibis 100*: 535–570. [14]

Thorpe, W. H. (1961). *Bird Song: The Biology of Vocal Communication and Expression in Birds.* Cambridge: Cambridge University Press. [14]

Thorpe, W. H. (1963). *Learning and Instinct in Animals*, 2nd Ed. Cambridge, MA: Harvard University Press. [14]

Thulin, C. A. (1960). Electrophysiological studies of peripheral nerve regeneration with special reference to the small diameter (γ) fibres. *Exp. Neurol. 2*: 598–612. [5]

Tickle, C., B. Alberts, L. Wolpert and J. Lee. (1982). Local application of retinoic acid to the limb bud mimics the action of the polarizing region. *Nature 296*: 564–566. [3]

Tickle, C., D. Summerbell and L. Wolpert. (1975). Positional signalling and specification of digits in chick limb morphogenesis. *Nature 254*: 199–202. [3]

Tiedemann, H. (1968). Factors determining embryonic differentiation. *J. Cell Physiol. 72(Suppl. I)*: 129–144. [3]

Tinbergen, N. (1953). *The Herring Gull's World.* New York: Harper & Row. [14]

Tinbergen, N. (1969). *Curious Naturalists.* Garden City, NY: Doubleday. [14]

Todd, T. J. (1823). On the process of reproduction of the members of the aquatic salamander. *Q. J. Sci., Lit. Arts. 16*: 84–96. [8]

Toole, B. P. (1976). Morphogenetic role of glycosaminoglycans (acid micropolysaccharides) in brain and other tissues. In: *Neuronal Recognition*, S. H. Barondes, ed. New York: Plenum Press, pp. 275–329. [4]

Torrey, T. W. (1934). The relation of taste buds to their nerve fibers. *J. Comp. Neurol. 59*: 203–220. [8]

Torvik, A. (1956). Transneuronal changes in the inferior olive and pontine nuclei in kittens. *J. Neuropathol. Exp. Neurol. 15*: 119–145. [8]

Tower, S. S. (1939). The reaction of muscle to denervation. *Physiol. Rev. 19*: 1–48. [8]

Townes, P. L. and J. Holtfreter. (1955). Directed movements and selective adhesion of embryonic amphibian cells. *J. Exp. Zool. 128*: 53–118. [4]

Townes-Anderson, E. and G. Raviola. (1978). Degeneration and regeneration of autonomic nerve endings in the anterior part of rhesus monkey ciliary muscle. *J. Neurocytol. 7*: 583–600. [13]

Trinkaus, J. P. (1969). *Cells into Organs: The Forces That Shape the Embryo.* Englewood Cliffs, NJ: Prentice-Hall. [1]

Trisler, C. D., M. D. Schneider and M. Nirenberg. (1981). A topographic gradient of molecules in retina can be used to identify neuron position. *Proc. Natl. Acad. Sci. USA 78*: 2145–2149. [11]

Truman, J. W. (1983). Programmed cell death in the nervous system of an adult insect. *J. Comp. Neurol. 216*: 445–452. [6]

Truman, J. W. and L. M. Schwartz. (1982). Insect systems for the study of programmed neuronal death. *Neurosci. Comment. 1*: 66–72. [6]

Tsukahara, N. (1978). Synaptic plasticity in the red nucleus. In: *Neuronal Plasticity*, Carl. W. Cotman, ed. New York: Raven Press, pp. 113–130. [13]

Tsukahara, N. (1981). Synaptic plasticity in the mammalian central nervous system. *Annu. Rev. Neurosci. 4*: 351–379. [13]

Tuffery, A. R. (1971). Growth and degeneration of motor end-plates in normal cat hind limb muscles. *J. Anat. 110*: 221–247. [13]

Turner, C. D. and J. T. Bagnara. (1971). *General Endocrinology*, 5th Ed. Philadelphia: Saunders. [1]

Turner, N. E., J.-A. Barde, M. E. Schwab and H. Thoenen. (1983). Extract from brain stimulates neurite outgrowth from fetal rat retinal explants. *Dev. Brain Res. 6*: 77–83. [7]

Ullrich, A., A. Gray, C. Berman, and T. J. Dull. (1983). Human β-nerve growth factor gene sequence highly homologous to that of mouse. *Nature 303*: 821–825. [7]

Unsicker, K. and J. H. Chamley. (1977). Growth characteristics of postnatal rat adrenal medulla in culture. *Cell Tissue Res. 177*: 247–268. [7]

Unsicker, K., B. Krisch, U. Otten and H. Thoenen. (1978). Nerve growth factor-induced fiber outgrowth from isolated rat adrenal chromaffin cells: Impairment by glucocorticoids. *Proc. Natl. Acad. Sci. USA 75*: 3498–3502. [7]

Usherwood, P. N. R. (1969). Glutamate sensitivity of denervated insect muscle fibres. *Nature 233*: 411–413. [8]

Van der Loos, H. (1965). The "improperly" oriented pyramidal cell in the cerebral cortex and its possible bearing on problems of neuronal growth and cell orientation. *Bull. Johns Hopkins Hosp. 117*: 228–250. [5]

Van der Loos, H. and J. Dörfl. (1978). Does the skin tell the somatosensory cortex how to construct a map of the periphery? *Neurosci. Lett. 7*: 23–30. [8]

Van der Loos, H. and T. A. Woolsey. (1973). Somatosensory cortex: Structural alterations following early injury to sense organs. *Science 179*: 395–398. [8]

Van Essen, D. C. (1982). Neuromuscular synapse elimination: Structural, functional and mechanistic aspects. In: *Neuronal Development*, N. C. Spitzer, ed. New York: Plenum Press, pp. 333–371. [12]

Van Essen, D. C. and J. K. S. Jansen. (1977). The specificity of re-innervation by identified sensory and motor neurons in the leech. *J. Comp. Neurol.* 171: 433–454. [10]

Van Sluyters, R. C. and C. Blakemore. (1973). Experimental creation of unusual neuronal properties in visual cortex of kitten. *Nature* 246: 506–508. [14]

Varon, S., J. Nomura and E. M. Shooter. (1967a). The isolation of the mouse nerve growth factor protein in a high molecular weight form. *Biochemistry* 6: 2202–2209. [7]

Varon, S., J. Nomura and E. M. Shooter. (1967b). Subunit structure of a high molecular weight form of the nerve growth factor from mouse submaxillary gland. *Proc. Natl. Acad. Sci. USA* 57: 1782–1789. [7]

Varon, S., J. Nomura and E. M. Shooter. (1968). Reversible dissociation of mouse nerve growth factor protein into different subunits. *Biochemistry* 7: 1296–1303. [7]

Varon, S., C. Raiborn and E. Tyszka. (1973). In vitro studies of dissociated cells from newborn mouse dorsal root ganglia. *Brain Res.* 54: 51–63. [7]

Vaughan, D. W. (1977). Age-related deterioration of pyramidal cell basal dendrites in rat auditory cortex. *J. Comp. Neurol.* 171: 501–516. [13]

Vaughan, R. B. and J. P. Trinkaus. (1966). Movements of epithelial cell sheets *in vitro*. *J. Cell Sci.* 1: 407–413. [4]

Vijayashankar, N. and H. Brody. (1979). A quantitative study of the pigmented neurons in the nuclei locus coeruleus and subcoeruleus in man as related to aging. *J. Neuropathol. Exp. Neurol.* 38: 490–497. [13]

Vogt, M. (1925). Gestaltungsanalyse am Amphibienkeim mit örtlacher vitalfärbung. 1. *Wilhelm Roux Arch. Entwicklungsmech. Org.* 106: 542–610. [2]

Vogt, M. (1929). Gestaltungsanalyse am Amphibienkeim mit örtlacher Vitalfärbung. 2. *Wilhelm Roux Arch. Entwicklungsmech. Org.* 120: 384–706. [2]

von Baer, K. E. (1828). *Entwicklungsgeschichte de Thiere: Beobachtung und Reflexion.* Königsberg: Bornträger. [1]

von der Marlsburg, C. and D. J. Willshaw. (1977). How to label nerve cells so that they can interconnect in an ordered fashion. *Proc. Natl. Acad. Sci. USA* 74: 5176–5178. [11]

von Schilcher, F. and J. C. Hall. (1979). Neural topography of courtship song in sex mosaics of *Drosophila melanogaster*. *J. Comp. Physiol.* 129: 85–95. [14]

von Senden, M. (1932). Raum–und Gestaltauffassung bei operierten Blindgeborenen vor und nach der Operation. Leipzig: Barth. (English translation, 1960. *Space and Sight: The Perception of Space and Shape in the Congenitally Blind Before and After Operation.* Glencoe, IL: The Free Press.) [4]

von Vintschgau, M. (1880). Beobachtungen über die veränderungen der Schmeckbecher nach Durchschneidung des n. Glossopharyngeus. *Arch. Gen. Physiol.* 23: 1–13. [8]

Vrensen, G., D. De Groot and J. Nuñes-Cardozo. (1977). Postnatal development of neurons and synapses in the visual and motor cortex of rabbits: A quantitative light and electron microscopic study. *Brain Res. Bull.* 2: 405–416. [9]

Waddington, C. H. (1936). *How Animals Develop.* New York: W. W. Norton. [1]

Waddington, C. H. (1952). *The Epigenetics of Birds.* Cambridge: Cambridge University Press. [1]

Walicke, P. A., R. B. Campenot and P. H. Patterson. (1977). Determination of transmitter function by neuronal activity. *Proc. Natl. Acad. Sci. USA* 74: 5767–5771. [2]

Walker, B. E. (1960). Renewal of cell populations in the female mouse. *Am. J. Anat.* 107: 95–105. [8]

Wallace, B. (1984). Selective loss of neurites during differentiation of cells in the leech central nervous system. *J. Comp. Neurol.* 228: 149–153. [12]

Wallace, B. G., M. N. Adal and J. G. Nicholls. (1977). Regeneration of synaptic connexions by sensory neurones in leech ganglia maintained in culture. *Proc. R. Soc. Lond. (Biol.)* 199: 567–585. [10]

Wallace, H. (1981). *Vertebrate Limb Regeneration.* New York: John Wiley & Sons. [3]

Wallace, L. J. and L. M. Partlow. (1976). α-Adrenergic regulation of secretion of mouse saliva rich in nerve growth factor. *Proc. Natl. Acad. Sci. USA* 73: 4210–4214. [7]

Watson, W. E. (1974). Cellular responses to axotomy and to related procedures. *Br. Med. Bull.* 30: 112–115. [13]

Weber, M. (1981). A diffusible factor responsible for the determination of cholinergic functions in cultured sympathetic neurons. Partial purification and characterization. *J. Biol. Chem.* 256: 3447–3453. [2]

Weber, M. and A. Le Van Thai. (1982). Progress in the purification of a factor involved in the neurotransmitter choice made by cultured sympathetic neurons. In: *Embryonic Development. Part B: Cellular Aspects*, M. M. Burger and R. Weber, eds. New York: Alan R. Liss, pp. 473–483. [2]

Weber, R. (1962). Induced metamorphosis in isolated tails of *Xenopus* larvae. *Experientia* 18: 84–85. [6]

Weinberg, C. B., J. R. Sanes and Z. W. Hall. (1981). Formation of neuromuscular junctions in adult rats: Accumulation of acetylcholine receptors, acetylcholinesterase, and components of synaptic basal lamina. *Dev. Biol.* 84: 255–266. [9]

Weinreich, D. (1971). Ionic mechanism of post-tetanic potentiation at the neuromuscular junction of the frog. *J. Physiol. (Lond.)* 212: 431–446. [13]

Weisblat, D. A. (1981). Development of the nervous system. In: *The Neurobiology of the Leech.* K. Muller, J. G. Nicholls and G. S. Stent, eds. Cold Spring Harbor, NY: Cold Spring Harbor Laboratory, pp. 173–195. [1, 2, 3]

Weisblat, D. A., G. Harper, G. S. Stent and R. T. Sawyer. (1980). Embryonic cell lineages in the nervous system of the glossiphoniid leech, *Helobdella triserialis*. *Dev. Biol.* 76: 58–78. [1, 2]

Weisblat, D. A., R. T. Sawyer and G. S. Stent. (1978). Cell lineage analysis by intracellular injection of a tracer enzyme. *Science* 202: 1295–1298. [2,3]

Weiss, G. M. and J. J. Pysh. (1978). Evidence for loss of Purkinje cell dendrites during late development: A morphometric Golgi analysis in the mouse. *Brain Res. 154*: 219–230. [13]

Weiss, P. (1924). Die funktion transplantierter amphibienextremitaten. Aufstellung einer resonanztheorie der motorischen nerventatigkeit auf grund abgestimmter endorgane. *Arch. Mikrosk. Anat. Entwicklungsmech. 102*: 635–672. [11]

Weiss, P. (1928). Erregungspecifität and Erregungsresonanz. *Ergeb. Biol. 3*: 1–115. [11]

Weiss, P. (1934). *In vitro* experiments on the factors determining the course of the outgrowing nerve fiber. *J. Exp. Zool. 68*: 393–448. [5, 11]

Weiss, P. A. (1936). Selectivity controlling the central-peripheral relations in the nervous system. *Biol. Rev. 11*: 494–531. [11]

Weiss, P. (1939). *Principles of Development*. New York: Henry Holt and Company. [3, 4, 11]

Weiss, P. (1941a). Self differentiation of the basic patterns of coordination. *Comp. Psychol. Monogr. 17*: 1–96. [11]

Weiss, P. (1941b). Nerve patterns: Mechanics of nerve growth. *Growth (Suppl. 5)*: 163–203. [4, 5, 11]

Weiss, P. (1945). Experiments on cell and axon orientation *in vitro*: The role of colloidal exudates in tissue organisation. *J. Exp. Zool. 100*: 353–386. [11]

Weiss, P. (1955). Nervous system (neurogenesis). In: *The Analysis of Development*, B. H. Willier, P. Weiss and V. Hamburger, eds. Philadelphia: Saunders, pp. 346–401. [14]

Weiss, P. (1961). Guiding principles in cell locomotion and cell aggregation. *Exp. Cell Res. (Suppl. 8)*: 260–281. [4]

Weiss, P. (1965). Specificity in the neurosciences. *Neurosci. Res. Program Bull. 3*: 5–36. [11]

Weiss, P. (1968). Research in retrospect. Reprinted from G. Gabbiani, *Reflections on Biologic Research*. St. Louis, MO: Warren H. Green, Inc., pp. 237–244. [11]

Weiss, P. and H. B. Hiscoe. (1948). Experiments on the mechanism of nerve growth. *J. Exp. Zool. 107*: 315–396. [5, 11]

Weiss, P. and A. Hoag. (1946). Competitive reinnervation of rat muscles by their own and foreign nerves. *J. Neurophysiol. 9*: 413–418. [10]

Weiss, P. and F. Rossetti. (1951). Growth responses of opposite sign among different neuron types exposed to thyroid hormone. *Proc. Natl. Acad. Sci. USA 37*: 540–556. [6]

Welker, C. (1976). Receptive fields of barrels in the somatosensory neocortex of the rat. *J. Comp. Neurol. 166*: 173–190. [8]

Weller, W. L. and J. I. Johnson. (1975). Barrels in cerebral cortex altered by receptor disruption in newborn but not five-day-old mice (*Cricetidae and Muridae*). *Brain Res. 83*: 504–508. [8]

Werner, J. K. (1974). Trophic influence of nerves on the development and maintenance of sensory receptors. *Am. J. Phys. Med. 53*: 127–142. [8]

Wernig, A., A. P. Anzil and A. Bieser. (1981). Light and electron microscopic identification of a nerve sprout in muscle of normal adult frog. *Neurosci. Lett. 21*: 261–266. [13]

Wernig, A., J. J. Carmody, A. P. Anzil, E. Hansert, M. Marciniak and H. Zucker. (1984). Persistence of nerve sprouting with features of synapse remodelling in soleus muscles of adult mice. *Neuroscience 11*: 241–253. [13]

Wernig, A., M. Pećot-Dechavassine and H. Stöver. (1980a). Sprouting and regression of the nerve at the frog neuromuscular junction in normal conditions and after prolonged paralysis with curare. *J. Neurocytol. 9*: 277–303. [13]

Wernig, A., M. Pećot-Dechavassine and H. Stöver. (1980b). Signs of nerve regression and sprouting in the frog neuromuscular synapse. In: *Ontogenesis and Functional Mechanisms of Peripheral Synapses, INSERM Symp. 13*, J. Taxi, ed. Amsterdam: Elsevier, pp. 225–238. [13]

Wessells, N. K., S. R. Johnson and R. P. Nuttall. (1978). Axon initiation and growth cone regeneration in cultured motor neurons. *Exp. Cell Res. 117*: 335–345. [4]

Wessells, N. K., M. A. Ludueña, P. C. Letourneau, J. T. Wrenn and B. S. Spooner. (1974). Thorotrast uptake and transit in embryonic glia, heart, fibroblasts, and neurons *in vitro*. *Tissue Cell 6*: 757–776. [4]

Wessels, N. K. and R. P. Nuttall. (1978). Normal branching, induced branching, and steering of cultured parasympathetic motor neurons. *Exp. Cell Res. 114*: 111–122. [5]

Weston, J. A. (1963). A radioautographic analysis of the migration and localization of trunk neural crest cells in the chick. *Dev. Biol. 6*: 279–310. [4]

Weston, J. A. (1982). Motile and social behavior of neural crest cells. In: *Cell Behavior*, R. Bellairs, A. Curtis and G. Dunn, eds. New York: Cambridge University Press, pp. 429–470. [4]

White, J. G., R. H. Horvitz and J. E. Sulston. (1982). Neurone differentiation in cell lineage mutants of *Caenorhabditis elegans*. *Nature 297*: 584–587. [2]

White, J. G., E. Southgate, J. N. Thomson and S. Brenner. (1976). The structure of the ventral nerve cord of *Caenorhabditis elegans*. *Philos. Trans. R. Soc. Lond. (Biol.) 275*: 327–348. [2]

Whitelaw, V. and M. Hollyday. (1983a). Thigh and calf discrimination in the motor innervation of the chick hindlimb following deletions of limb segments. *J. Neurosci. 3*: 1199–1215. [5]

Whitelaw, V. and M. Hollyday. (1983b). Position-dependent motor innervation of the chick hindlimb following serial and parallel duplications of limb segments. *J. Neurosci. 3*: 1216–1225. [5]

Whitelaw, V. and M. Hollyday. (1983c). Neural pathway constraints in the motor innervation of the chick hindlimb following dorsoventral rotations of distal limb segments. *J. Neurosci. 3*: 1226–1233. [5]

Whitington, P. M. (1979). The specificity of innervation of regenerating motor neurons in the cockroach. *J. Comp. Neurol. 186*: 465–472. [10]

Whitington, P. M., M. Bate, E. Seifert, K. Ridge and C. S. Goodman. (1982). Survival and differentiation of identified embryonic neurons in the absence of their target muscles. *Science* 215: 973–975. [6]

Whitington, P. M. and E. Seifert. (1982). Axon growth from limb motoneurons in the locust embryo: The effect of target limb removal on the path taken out of the central nervous system. *Dev. Biol.* 93: 206–215. [6]

Wiersma, C. A. G. (1931). An experiment on the "resonance theory" of muscular activity. *Arch. Neerl. Physiol.* 16: 337–345. [11]

Wiesel, T. N. (1982). Postnatal development of the visual cortex and the influence of environment. *Nature* 299: 583–591. [14]

Wiesel, T. N. and D. H. Hubel. (1963a). Effects of visual deprivation on morphology and physiology of cells in the cat's lateral geniculate body. *J. Neurophysiol.* 26: 978–993. [8]

Wiesel, T. N. and D. H. Hubel. (1963b). Single cell responses in striate cortex of kittens deprived of vision in one eye. *J. Neurophysiol.* 26: 1003–1017. [12, 14]

Wiesel, T. N. and D. H. Hubel. (1965). Comparison of the effects of unilateral and bilateral eye closure on cortical unit responses in kittens. *J. Neurophysiol.* 28: 1029–1040. [8,12,14]

Wigglesworth, V. B. (1940). Local and general factors in the development of "pattern" in *Rhodnius prolixus* (Hemiptera). *J. Exp. Biol.* 17: 180–200. [3]

Wigglesworth, V. B. (1953). The origin of sensory neurones in an insect *Rhodnius prolixus* (Hemiptera). *Q. J. Microsc. Sci.* 94: 93–112. [3, 5]

Wigglesworth, V. B. (1959). *The Control of Growth and Form: A Study of the Epidermal Cell in an Insect.* Ithaca, NY: Cornell University Press. [5]

Wigston, D. J. (1980). Suppression of sprouted synapses in axolotl muscle by transplanted foreign nerves. *J. Physiol. (Lond.)* 307: 355–366. [10]

Wigston, D. J. (1983). Innervation of individual guinea-pig superior cervical ganglion cells by axons with similar conduction velocities. *J. Physiol. (Lond.)* 334: 179–187. [10]

Wigston, D. J. and J. R. Sanes. (1982). Selective reinnervation of adult mammalian muscle by axons from different segmental levels. *Nature* 299: 464–467. [10]

Wigston, D. J. and J. R. Sanes. (1985). Axons from different segmental levels selectively reinnervate rat intercostal muscles. *J. Neurosci.* (in press). [10]

Wilcox, M., G. J. Mitchison and R. J. Smith. (1973). Pattern formation in the blue-green alga, *Anabaena*. I. Basic mechanisms. *J. Cell Sci.* 12: 707–723. [3]

Willard, A. L. (1980). Electrical excitability of outgrowing neurites of embryonic neurones in cultures of dissociated neural plate of *Xenopus laevis. J. Physiol. (Lond.)* 301: 115–128. [2]

Williams, P. E. and G. Goldspink. (1971). The effect of immobilization on the longitudinal growth of striated muscle fibres. *J. Anat.* 116: 45–55. [9]

muscle fibres. *J. Anat.* 116: 45–55. [9]

Williams, R. W. and P. Rakic. (1984). Form, ultrastructure, and selectivity of growth cones in the developing primate optic nerve: 3-dimensional reconstructions from serial electron micrographs. *Soc. Neurosci. Abs.* [11]

Willier, B. H. and J. M. Oppenheimer. (1974). *Foundations of Experimental Embryology,* 2nd Ed. New York: Hafner Press. [3]

Willier, B. H. and M. E. Rawles. (1935). Organ forming areas in the early chick blastoderm. *Proc. Soc. Exp. Biol.* 32: 1293–1296. [3]

Wilson, E. B. (1903). Notes on the reversal of asymmetry in the regeneration of the chelae in *Alpheus heterochelis. Biol. Bull.* 4: 197–210. [8]

Wilson, E. B. (1911). *The Cell in Development and Inheritance,* 2nd Ed. New York: Macmillan. [1]

Wilson, H. V. (1907). On some phenomena of coalescence and regeneration in sponges. *J. Exp. Zool.* 5: 245–258. [4]

Wilson, H. V. and J. T. Penney. (1930). The regeneration of sponges *(Microciana)* from dissociated cells. *J. Exp. Zool.* 56: 73–147. [4]

Wolpert, L. (1969). Positional information and the spatial pattern of cellular differentiation. *J. Theor. Biol.* 25: 1–47. [3]

Wolpert, L. (1978). Pattern formation in biological development. *Sci. Am.* 239(4): 154–164. [3]

Wolpert, L., J. H. Lewis and D. Summerbell. (1975). Morphogenesis of the vertebrate limb in cell patterning. *Ciba Found. Symp.* 29: 95–130. [3]

Wong, R., R. D. Hadley, S. B. Kater and G. C. Hauser. (1981). Neurite outgrowth in molluscan organ and cell cultures: The role of conditioning factor(s). *J. Neurosci.* 1: 1008–1021. [10]

Woolsey, T. A. (1978). Some anatomical bases of cortical somatotopic organization. *Brain Behav. Evol.* 15: 325–371. [8]

Woolsey, T. A., D. Durham, R. M. Harris, D. J. Simons and K. L. Valentino. (1981). Somatosensory development. In: *Development of Perception,* Vol. 1. New York: Academic Press, pp. 259–292. [8]

Woolsey, T. A. and H. Van der Loos. (1970). The structural organization of layer IV in the somatosensory region (SI) of mouse cerebral cortex. The description of a cortical field composed of discrete cytoarchitectonic units. *Brain Res.* 17: 205–242. [8]

Woolsey, T. A. and J. R. Wann. (1976). Areal changes in mouse cortical barrels following vibrissal damage at different postnatal ages. *J. Comp. Neurol.* 170: 53–66. [8]

Wright, D. A. and P. A. Lawrence. (1981a). Regeneration of the segment boundary in *Oncopeltus. Dev. Biol.* 85: 317–327. [3]

Wright, D. A. and P. A. Lawrence. (1981b). Regeneration of the segment boundaries in *Oncopeltus:* Cell lineage. *Dev. Biol.* 85: 328–333. [3]

Wright, L. L., T. J. Cunningham and A. J. Smolen. (1983). Developmental neuron death in the rat superior cervical sympathetic ganglion: Cell counts and ultrastructure. *J. Neurocytol.* 12: 727–738. [6]

Wright, M. R. (1947). Regeneration and degeneration experiments on lateral line nerves and sense organs in anurans. *J. Exp. Zool. 105*: 221–257. [8]

Yamada, K. M., B. S. Spooner and N. K. Wessells. (1971). Ultrastructure and function of growth cones and axons of cultured nerve cells. *J. Cell Biol. 49*: 614–635. [4]

Yankner, B. A. and E. M. Shooter. (1979). Nerve growth factor in the nucleus: Interaction with receptors on the nuclear membrane. *Proc. Natl. Acad. Sci. USA 76*: 1269–1273. [7]

Yankner, B. A. and E. M. Shooter. (1982). The biology and mechanism of action of nerve growth factor. *Annu. Rev. Biochem 51*: 845–868. [7]

Yellin, H. (1967a). Muscle fiber plasticity and the creation of localized motor units. *Anat. Rec. 157*: 345. [8]

Yellin, H. (1967b). Neural regulation of enzymes in muscle fibers of red and white muscle. *Exp. Neurol. 19*: 92–103. [8]

Yip, H. K. and B. Grafstein. (1982). Effect of nerve growth factor on regeneration of goldfish optic axons. *Brain Res. 238*: 329–339. [7]

Yip, H. K. and E. M. Johnson. (1983). Retrograde transport of nerve growth factor in lesioned goldfish retinal ganglion cells. *J. Neurosci. 3*: 2172–2182. [7]

Yoon, M. G. (1971). Reorganization of retinotectal projection following surgical operations on the optic tectum in goldfish. *Exp. Neurol. 33*: 395–411. [11]

Yoon, M. G. (1972). Transposition of the visual projection from the nasal hemiretina onto the foreign rostral zone of the optic tectum in goldfish. *Exp. Neurol. 37*: 451–462. [11]

Yoon, M. G. (1976). Progress of topographic regulation of the visual projection in the halved optic tectum of adult goldfish. *J. Physiol. (Lond.) 257*: 621–643. [11]

Young, M., J. Oger, M. H. Blanchard, H. Asdourian, H. Amos and B. J. W. Arnason. (1975). Secretion of a nerve growth factor by primary chick fibroblast cultures. *Science 187*: 361–362. [7]

Young, P. T. (1928). Auditory localization with acoustical transposition of the ears. *J. Exp. Psychol. 11*: 399–429. [13]

Zacks, S. I. (1974). *The Motor Endplate*. Huntington, NY: R. E. Krieger Publishing Co. [9,10]

Zackson, S. L. (1982). Cell clones and segmentation in leech development. *Cell 31*: 761–770. [3]

Zalewski, A. A. (1969a). Combined effects of testosterone and motor, sensory or gustatory nerve reinnervation on the regeneration of taste buds. *Exp. Neurol. 24*: 285–297. [8]

Zalewski, A. A. (1969b). Regeneration of taste buds after reinnervation by peripheral or central sensory fibers of vagal ganglia. *Exp. Neurol. 25*: 429–437. [8]

Zalewski, A. A. (1972). Regeneration of taste buds after transplantation of tongue and ganglia grafts to the anterior chamber of the eye. *Exp. Neurol. 35*: 519–528. [8]

Zalewski, A. A. (1974). Neuronal and tissue specifications involved in taste bud formation. *Ann. NY Acad. Sci. 228*: 344–349. [8]

Zalewski, A. A. (1981). Regeneration of taste buds after reinnervation of a denervated tongue papilla by a normally non-gustatory nerve. *J. Comp. Neurol. 200*: 309–314. [8]

Zigmond, S. H. (1978). Chemotaxis by polymorphonuclear leukocytes. *J. Cell Biol. 77*: 269–287. [4]

Zipser, B. and R. McKay. (1981). Monoclonal antibodies distinguish identifiable neurones in the leech. *Nature 289*: 549–554. [11]

Ziskind, L. and M. J. Dennis. (1978). Depolarising effect of curare on embryonic rat muscles. *Nature 276*: 622–623. [9]

Zucker, R. S. (1972). Crayfish escape behavior and central synapses. I. Neural circuit exciting lateral giant fiber. II. Physiological mechanisms underlying behavioral habituation. *J. Neurophysiol. 35*: 621–637. [13]

Zucker, R. S. (1982). Processes underlying one form of synaptic plasticity: Facilitation. In: *Conditioning*, C. D. Woody, ed. New York: Plenum Press, pp. 249–264. [13]

Index